TREATMENT PLANS AND INTERVENTIONS IN COUPLE THERAPY

TREATMENT PLANS AND INTERVENTIONS FOR EVIDENCE-BASED PSYCHOTHERAPY

Robert L. Leahy, Series Editor

Each volume in this practical series synthesizes current information on a particular disorder or clinical population; shows practitioners how to develop specific, tailored treatment plans; and describes interventions proven to promote behavior change, reduce distress, and alleviate symptoms. Step-by-step guidelines for planning and implementing treatment are illustrated with rich case examples. User-friendly features include reproducible self-report forms, handouts, and symptom checklists, all in a convenient large-size format. Specific strategies for handling treatment roadblocks are also detailed. Emphasizing a collaborative approach to treatment, books in this series enable practitioners to offer their clients the very best in evidence-based practice.

TREATMENT PLANS AND INTERVENTIONS
FOR DEPRESSION AND ANXIETY DISORDERS, SECOND EDITION
Robert L. Leahy, Stephen J. F. Holland, and Lata K. McGinn

TREATMENT PLANS AND INTERVENTIONS
FOR BULIMIA AND BINGE-EATING DISORDER
Rene D. Zweig and Robert L. Leahy

TREATMENT PLANS AND INTERVENTIONS FOR INSOMNIA:
A CASE FORMULATION APPROACH
Rachel Manber and Colleen E. Carney

TREATMENT PLANS AND INTERVENTIONS
FOR OBSESSIVE–COMPULSIVE DISORDER
Simon A. Rego

CBT WITH JUSTICE-INVOLVED CLIENTS:
INTERVENTIONS FOR ANTISOCIAL AND SELF-DESTRUCTIVE BEHAVIORS
Raymond Chip Tafrate, Damon Mitchell, and David J. Simourd

CBT TREATMENT PLANS AND INTERVENTIONS
FOR DEPRESSION AND ANXIETY DISORDERS IN YOUTH
Brian C. Chu and Sandra S. Pimentel

TREATMENT PLANS AND INTERVENTIONS IN COUPLE THERAPY:
A COGNITIVE-BEHAVIORAL APPROACH
Norman B. Epstein and Mariana K. Falconier

Treatment Plans and Interventions in Couple Therapy

A Cognitive-Behavioral Approach

Norman B. Epstein

Mariana K. Falconier

Series Editor's Note by Robert L. Leahy

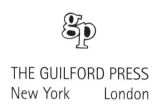

THE GUILFORD PRESS

New York   London

Library of Congress Cataloging-in-Publication Data

Names: Epstein, Norman, 1947– author. | Falconier, Mariana K., author.
Title: Treatment plans and interventions in couple therapy : a
   cognitive-behavioral approach / Norman B. Epstein, Mariana K. Falconier.
Description: New York, NY : The Guilford Press, [2024] | Series: Treatment
   plans and interventions for evidence-based psychotherapy | Includes
   bibliographical references and index.
Identifiers: LCCN 2023054961 | ISBN 9781462554195 (paperback : acid-free
   paper) | ISBN 9781462554201 (hardcover : acid-free paper)
Subjects: LCSH: Couples therapy. | Marital psychotherapy. | Cognitive
   therapy. | BISAC: PSYCHOLOGY / Psychotherapy / Couples & Family |
   PSYCHOLOGY / Movements / Cognitive Behavioral Therapy (CBT)
Classification: LCC RC488.5 .E67 2024 | DDC 616.89/15—dc23/eng/20231212
LC record available at *https://lccn.loc.gov/2023054961*

About the Authors

Norman B. Epstein, PhD, is Professor Emeritus in the Department of Family Science in the School of Public Health at the University of Maryland, College Park, and a licensed clinical psychologist. He is a Fellow of the American Psychological Association, Fellow of the Association for Behavioral and Cognitive Therapies, Professional Member of the American Association for Marriage and Family Therapy, Founding Fellow of the Academy of Cognitive Therapy, and Diplomate of the American Board of Assessment Psychology. Dr. Epstein is a pioneer in the development of cognitive-behavioral therapy with couples and families. His research, teaching, and training of clinicians have focused on cognitive, emotional, and behavioral processes in relationship adjustment and dysfunction; couple and family coping with stress; treatments for distressed couples and families; and culturally sensitive adaptations of Western-derived models of therapy. Dr. Epstein is author or editor of five previous books, has published over 150 journal articles and book chapters, and has presented numerous research papers and training workshops nationally and internationally. He has served on editorial boards of leading journals and has maintained a clinical practice throughout his career.

Mariana K. Falconier, PhD, is Professor and Director of the Couple and Family Therapy Master's Program at the University of Maryland, College Park. Previously, she was Associate Professor, Director of the Center for Family Services, and Director of the Master's Program in Marriage and Family Therapy at Virginia Polytechnic and State University. Dr. Falconier is a licensed marriage and family therapist in both Maryland and Virginia, a licensed psychologist in Argentina, and an approved supervisor and clinical fellow of the American Association for Marriage and Family Therapy. Her research focuses on how couples cope with stress, primarily economic stress among low-income couples and immigration stress in Latine couples. She developed TOGETHER, an evidence-based, interdisciplinary group program designed to help couples improve their communication, coping, and financial management skills; adapted the program to serve Latine couples and LGBTQ couples; and has received federal funding to offer TOGETHER to various underserved communities, for which she received an Excellence in Professional/Clinical Practice Award from the National Council on Family Relations. Dr. Falconier has published and widely presented nationally and internationally. She has served on editorial boards of leading journals, directed mental health clinics, and maintained a clinical practice.

Series Editor Note

It is hard to imagine any therapist who works effectively with individual clients who will not confront relationship issues as a significant part of their clinical picture. Even if you are working with children and adolescents, it is very likely at some point that the parents' relationship will become a target for therapy. Parental conflicts—especially about how to parent—can affect the child, and parental depression can create significant distress for children and adolescents. If you are dealing with a depressed client, the depression may be partly a result of relationship conflict, or the depression may impact the relationship, or, even more likely, these factors will work in both directions. We live in an interpersonal world, and this book is an absolutely essential resource for any clinician.

Norman Epstein and Mariana Falconier build a foundation by providing an excellent summary of some of the basic concepts in cognitive-behavioral therapy and how they can be utilized in couple therapy. This basic foundation is a common thread throughout each chapter. This volume is not simply a cookbook of techniques, but rather it provides the right balance of academic and practical knowledge so that the clinician will understand why the interventions make sense. There are chapters on dealing with aggression, infidelity, financial problems, co-parenting, and individual psychopathology, such as depression, anxiety, and substance abuse. What is especially helpful for the clinician is that the authors are not overly committed to one specific approach, but rather incorporate ideas and techniques and interventions from a wide range of approaches. I think this integrative approach is a much more realistic model for clinical practice since clients do not come in to see us because we belong to a particular school of therapy, but rather because we have helpful approaches that can be adapted to the individual. The goal is to fit the therapy to the client, rather than fit the client to the therapy. Flexibility and openness are key features in this thoughtful, insightful, and helpful book.

There are extensive handouts for clients, guides to interventions, assessment instruments, and specific plans for treatment. Illustrative case examples bring important ideas to life and give you a sense that you are in the "room" with experienced clinicians. The style of writing is quite accessible, which makes this book even more user-friendly. We don't have to slog through difficult jargon. Rather, each chapter is written in a clear and pragmatic style. Readers will be very fortunate to be able to turn to almost any chapter of this book and find pearls of wisdom. I know I was enriched by reading this excellent book. In fact, I believe many readers will find that these ideas are useful not only in helping clients, but also in helping ourselves.

ROBERT L. LEAHY, PhD
Director, American Institute for Cognitive Therapy;
Clinical Professor of Psychology, Department of Psychiatry,
Weill Cornell Medical College, New York, New York

Preface

Both of us have devoted a major portion of our professional lives to understanding the complexities of intimate relationships and developing and implementing effective clinical interventions to assist distressed couples and families. Based on our educational and clinical training backgrounds, we both also have strong foundations in understanding individual psychological functioning (intrapsychic cognitive and emotional processes), including personal historical influences on development. Furthermore, we share an emphasis on understanding the strong bidirectional link between the quality of relationship functioning and the well-being of its members, underscoring the crucial role that interventions at the relationship level have in the mental health field.

We both have practiced and taught a variety of couple and family therapy (CFT) models (e.g., emotion focused, solution focused, narrative, psychodynamic, collaborative, structural, strategic, experiential, multigenerational) for many years, as well as ways of integrating models based on common factors they possess that can be highly complementary. In addition, both of us have directed graduate CFT training programs that provide therapists with a strong foundation in diverse models and an ability to select interventions based on careful case conceptualization. We are highly experienced clinical researchers and clinicians who bring our first-hand knowledge of the therapy process to our teaching and clinical supervision, guided by systemic conceptualization and intervention with relationship problems, qualities that we have attempted to convey throughout this text. Our approach to understanding and treating couples and families also includes a focus on the multiple contextual factors, within an ecological framework, that influence people's lives and their intimate relationships, such as extended family relations, community institutions such as schools and health care systems, work environments, and the socioeconomic, legal, and political environment responsible for discrimination, inequities, structural racism, lack of opportunities, and community violence, among others. NBE is a pioneer in the development of cognitive-behavioral approaches to couple and family therapy. He has published extensively on cognitive-behavioral models, and yet he integrates components of other models in all of his work. MKF's clinical, teaching, and research careers, heavily influenced by social constructionism and postmodern models, have focused on marginalized couples, including immigrant, financially distressed, Latine, African American, and LGBTQ+ couples. Her work has emphasized sociocultural humility and attunement, with a strong commitment to affirmative practices that protect and foster diversity, inclusion, and equity.

Given the breadth of the theoretical concepts we bring to all of our work, the reader may wonder why we decided to focus on cognitive-behavioral couple therapy (CBCT) and its detailed application to a variety of very common presenting problems in couple therapy. Prior books on couple therapy have tended to have one of two foci. Many focus on a detailed presentation of one particular model for use in reducing couples' overall conflict and distress, without attending to specific aspects of presenting concerns and diverse client populations. They may include brief chapters on how to adapt that therapy model to treating a particular problem such as partner aggression or infidelity, but their overall approach is fairly generic. Those books are important contributions to the therapy literature, as they help readers develop a deep understanding of core aspects of relationship functioning that are strengths or risk factors, and they provide extensive knowledge of assessment and intervention methods consistent with the model. In contrast, the focus of other couple therapy books has been on providing easily accessible resources for students and practicing clinicians who are searching for effective treatments of the diverse problems they encounter in their clinical practices. Those handbooks attend to specific problem areas (e.g., parenting, sexual problems, partner aggression, infidelity) or specific populations (e.g., therapy with African American couples, Latine couples, sexual-minority couples), with each chapter focused on one problem or population, written by proponents of a particular theoretical model and varying in detail about the model concepts and methods. Those books are convenient references for clinicians who often need to switch gears from one couple's issues to another's.

Even though both types of books are valuable, our goal in the present book was to bridge the two types by presenting concepts and methods of a particular model in depth and then demonstrating how clinicians can apply it widely across various presenting concerns that couples commonly bring to their offices. Thus, the therapist can have the experience of shifting from understanding the most relevant factors influencing one presenting problem to focusing on the factors relevant to a different presenting problem while maintaining a consistent theoretical model and set of interventions that can be adapted as needed for each issue. This book is unique in that regard. We chose CBCT as the organizing model for this book because (1) it is a top model in terms of established empirical support for treating both relational problems and problems in partners' individual functioning; (2) it has very strong foci on all three realms of individual and relational functioning of cognition, emotion (and associated physiological responses), and behavior, and how they can be understood; and (3) it allows for consideration of contextual dimensions (e.g., sociocultural, economic, policy, and legal) that shape individuals' experiences and create constraints and opportunities for clients and therapists depending on their social location. A CBCT model also bridges the personal histories of the partners and their shared relationship history with their current experiences (not just focused on the here and now). This model selection obviously was especially not a stretch for NBE, but we believe a similar approach could be used in future books on other major CFT models. It also is important to state that even though we present CBCT as an evidence-based, comprehensive theoretical approach, by no means are we advocating that all therapists should practice primarily from a CBCT framework. Other major models of couple therapy also address the three realms of behavior, cognition, and emotion to varying degrees and attend to contextual factors. We believe that therapists who practice those models also will be able to find much in the present book that they can identify with and implement in their work.

In this book, we bring together CBCT concepts and empirical knowledge that we and our colleagues have developed in the field over several decades and our own experience with clinical practice and training, to present the nuanced CBCT model that has evolved and its application to contemporary clinical issues. The book provides an in-depth description of core CBCT concepts and methods for assessing couple problems experienced by diverse clients, planning appropriate treatment tailored to the characteristics and needs of each couple, and selecting and implementing interventions within a strong therapeutic alliance with each couple. We include detailed descriptions of applications to the treatment of the most common presenting concerns that couple therapists encounter in their practices, drawing on those core CBCT concepts and methods but applying them in ways that address the characteristics of each type of presenting problem. Of course, it is not possible to cover in one book all possible couple presenting issues in sufficient detail to convey nuanced clinical decision making to readers. We have chosen to concentrate on a set of common problems based on both our own experiences as clinicians and research surveys of the top problems. Nonetheless, in the final chapter we list other presenting problems and relevant clinical literature on each issue as a resource for therapists.

Throughout the writing of this book, we consistently aimed for it to be scholarly and based on research evidence, while at the same time highly accessible as a guide to everyday clinical practice. We want to share how we think about our client couples and the challenges they experience in their relationships, how we collaborate with them in improving their lives together, and how we are mindful of self-of-the-therapist factors that may influence our clinical work (e.g., different cultural backgrounds and social location of therapists and their clients, presenting problems that "hit close to home" for the therapist). Throughout the book, our goal is to achieve clinical work with diverse clients (in terms of race, ethnicity, religion, sexual orientation, gender identity, social position, etc.) that is attuned to their lived experiences and applies our interventions in a nuanced, flexible manner relevant to conditions they face in daily life. The chapters that focus on particular presenting problems all address diversity, issues in establishing a strong therapeutic alliance (including self-of-the-therapist issues), and ways to adapt one's theoretical model to be relevant and palatable to the clients. In trying to be inclusive of all gender identities, we have referred to partners in general as "they," but we have also provided examples in which partners were identified as male, female, queer, or nonbinary, with appropriate corresponding pronouns. For the sake of inclusivity, we have also avoided the gendered nouns and adjectives "Latina" or "Latino" unless we are describing a specific cisgender example. Instead we have referred to "Latine" individuals and "Latines" as the plural form, consistent with the inclusive ending "-e" used in the Spanish language in Latin American Spanish-speaking countries.

We believe this book can be used in clinically oriented programs that include education and training in couple therapy. It can help students learn about couple therapy in general and the CBCT model and its application to concrete problem areas in particular. The book also can be a great resource for experienced practicing couple therapists who want to enhance their familiarity with CBCT and ways that it can contribute to their work with couples with a variety of concerns. It also can help clinicians who have been practicing cognitive-behavioral therapy with individuals but want to learn ways of extending their expertise to treatment of their clients' relationship problems and ways of using couple interventions to supplement individual therapy for treating problems involving individual psychological functioning (e.g., depression, anxiety).

We hope after reading this book beginning therapists and experienced therapists who have used other approaches to couple therapy can feel comfortable with the CBCT model, see the degree to which it is conceptually integrative and relevant to working with their clients, and see that it can address various couples' presenting problems. We also hope the reader can expand their view of CBCT beyond old stereotypes of it being mechanistic and focused only on communication skills, contracts to change behaviors, and challenging irrational beliefs, and can incorporate it to understand the complex interplay among cognitions, behaviors, emotions, and contextual factors when assessing and treating couples. We also wish that the reader agrees with us that CBCT offers a clear, solid conceptual framework to identify the individual, relational, and contextual factors in the past and in the present that affect couple relationships, and allows the therapist to develop a deep understanding of their clients' internal and external experiences. Finally, we hope that experienced individual cognitive-behavioral therapists can make use of this model with its systemic and relational perspectives.

Acknowledgments

Norman B. Epstein: At this point in my long career, I have much to reflect on to identify the people who influenced the development of the work represented in this book. Before I turn to those reflections, I want to acknowledge my coauthor, Mariana Falconier, whose contributions played a major role in shaping the book from its inception. Her in-depth knowledge of the range of models in the couple and family therapy (CFT) field, substantial cultural sensitivity and attunement, and breadth of clinical experience have enriched this book immensely.

My early clinical psychology education and training at the University of California, Los Angeles was a complex mix of psychodynamic approaches, cognitive models such as George Kelly's role construct approach, early versions of behavioral couple and family therapy, and family systems theory. My research mentors Albert Mehrabian and Seymour Feshbach got me excited about conducting empirical studies, especially regarding socially important topics such as empathy, altruism, and aggression. The early groundbreaking work on family communication patterns and psychopathology (and family interventions to treat severe disorders) by clinical psychology professors Eliot Rodnick and Mike Goldstein also contributed to my focus on bidirectional influences between intrapsychic and interpersonal processes.

My empirical research focused on cognition in couple relationships began with my collaboration with Roy Eidelson at the University of Pennsylvania on the development of the Relationship Belief Inventory, a measure of unrealistic relationship beliefs. I subsequently had the great fortune to work with Aaron (Tim) Beck at his Center for Cognitive Therapy at the University of Pennsylvania in the early 1980s, a period of great growth for the "cognitive revolution" in psychology and excitement at the Center as scholars from around the world came to visit. I deeply appreciated Tim's support for my work at the Center on applying a cognitive-behavioral model to couple and family relationships. I collaborated with Jim Pretzer and Barbara Fleming on the development of the Marital Attitude Scale (assessing attributions) and with Art Freeman and Karen Simon to produce the edited book *Depression in the Family* in 1986. Also, Windy Dryden was a visiting scholar from England at the Center during that period, and our rich discussions eventually led to our collaboration (along with Steve Schlesinger) on the edited book *Cognitive-Behavioral Therapy with Families* in 1988. My experiences at the Center led to significant enduring professional relationships and personal friendships, such as Bob Leahy, Frank Dattilio, and John Riskind. My close collaboration over the years with Frank Dattilio, a leader in the application of CBT with couples and families, has included numerous coauthored publications, as well as our joint training workshops for clinicians.

The next major development in my career occurred when Don Baucom (University of North Carolina, Chapel Hill) and I discovered each other's work. Don's strong background in behavioral couple therapy and mine in the interface between intrapsychic processes and intimate interactions were a perfect fit that launched a long-term program of collaboration on research and therapy model development, with our first book on cognitive-behavioral couple therapy published in 1990. Several of Don's grad students (Charles Burnett, Rob Carels, Anthony Daiuto, Lynn Rankin-Esquer, Kristina Coop Gordon, Steve Sayers, Tamara Goldman Sher) made valuable contributions to this work over the years and became professional colleagues. In addition, many graduate students in our CFT program at the University of Maryland (in alphabetical order)—Janey Cunningham, Taryn Dezfulian, John Evans, Linda Evans, Mariana Falconier, Nicole Finkbeiner, John Hart, Heather Helms-Erikson, Katie Hrapczynski, Kirsten Jimerson, Leanne Juzaitis, April McDowell, Justin Neylon, Katelyn Opel, Elise Resnick, Ashley Southard, and Sherylls Valladares—collaborated on research papers and presentations. Don and I also benefited tremendously from consultation with anxiety experts Dianne Chambless and Alan Goldstein.

In addition to my focus on interventions for distressed couples, I developed a psychoeducation program for families with a member diagnosed with a major mental disorder (e.g., schizoaffective disorder, bipolar disorder), in collaboration with a local Maryland provider of mental health services for individuals with those disorders (Vesta, Inc.). Experts on family psychoeducation and behavioral family therapy for major disorders, Kim Mueser and David Miklowitz, were invaluable consultants in the design of the program and training of the therapists for its implementation. My department colleague Roger Rubin was my close collaborator on all stages of this project, as the cotherapist teams that met with families each consisted of a clinician from Vesta and a graduate student from our CFT program.

In 1995, Fuguo Chen from Shanghai Second Medical University became a visiting scholar in my department to learn about cognitive-behavioral therapy with couples and families, an enriching year that led to an enduring friendship and professional collaboration. Dr. Chen subsequently invited me to present training workshops in Shanghai on a number of occasions, which also led to Chinese students applying to the Family Science PhD program at the University of Maryland. In addition, this led to a major collaboration with Xiaoyi Fang of the Developmental Psychology program at Beijing Normal University (BNU), a pioneer in research and clinical training in couple and family therapy in China. I visited BNU several times to provide training, and in 2008 a dozen of my CFT program students traveled with me to Beijing to participate with Dr. Fang and many of his graduate students in a joint seminar on family therapy. This collaboration led to journal publications on cultural factors influencing families and ways of adapting Western-derived therapy models for application in China. My grad students Le Zheng and Jennifer Young played significant roles in this work. Furthermore, my former doctoral students Woochul Park (now a faculty member at Duksung Women's University in Seoul) and Haedong Kim (now a faculty member at Towson University in Maryland) and former University of Maryland visiting scholar Jung Eun Kim (a faculty member at Suwon University in Hwaseong, Gyeonggi Province, South Korea) have continued to collaborate with me on research and presentations regarding family processes in diverse cultures and adaptations of Western-derived therapy models to meet the needs of culturally diverse families.

Another application of cognitive-behavioral couple therapy to a common presenting problem involved a long-term professional collaboration and friendship with Michael Metz, an expert on sex therapy, whom I originally met at the University of Pennsylvania. Mike had a longstanding collaboration with Barry McCarthy, another major figure in the field. Mike and I planned and began writing a professional guide to cognitive-behavioral sex therapy for couples, which tragically was derailed by Mike's premature death. Barry offered to work with me on completing this testament to Mike's significant contributions to the field, which we did.

I also want to acknowledge the roles that my CFT program colleagues Carol Werlinich and Jaslean LaTaillade had in developing with me a cognitive-behavioral couple intervention to treat psychological and mild to moderate physical partner aggression. Christopher Murphy of the University of Maryland Baltimore County provided invaluable help in our designing an intervention that would address empirically identified risk factors for partner aggression and conceptualizing ways to intervene safely at a couple level. This work was inspired by Dan O'Leary's pioneering research demonstrating that with careful screening, conjoint treatment of milder forms of partner aggression can be safe and effective. My colleagues and I also are indebted to several cohorts of students in our CFT training program who served as therapists in the initial clinical trial of the program, which was conducted in our department's Center for Healthy Families outpatient clinic. CFT students (in alphabetical order) Rachel Alexander, Irina Beyder-Kamjou, Holly Bramble, Morgan Childers, David Curtis, Andrew Dauler, BreAnna Davis, Taryn Dezfulian, Laura Evans, Serena Galloway, John Hart, Lindsey Hoskins, Katie Hrapczynski, M. Sarah Kursch, Lynda Lee, Paige Murtagh, Elizabeth Ott, Ken Parnell, Deanna Pruitt, Ashley Southard, Mark Treimel, Sherylls Valladares, Anna White, and Katy Wilder also participated in research on outcomes of the program and clinical presentations at national professional meetings.

I especially want to thank Jim Nageotte and Jane Keislar at The Guilford Press for their wise feedback as the drafts of the chapters of this book took shape, and for their warm encouragement and support throughout the course of the project. It's been a pleasure working with them.

I have been so fortunate to have all of these wonderful mentors, colleagues, and students over the years whose expertise, enthusiasm, creativity and support have shaped my work. I can clearly see threads of their influence throughout this book.

Last, but most special to me, I want to acknowledge my family—my wife, Carolyn, and daughters, Meredith and Christine, and their families—whose love and support have made the completion of a challenging project such as this book possible. They mean the world to me.

Mariana K. Falconier: I feel fortunate to have had incredible training instructors, supervisors, therapists, and colleagues and rich clinical experiences both in my home country, Argentina, and in the United States. I have to first thank my own first therapist, Perla Brodsky, who introduced me to systems-oriented therapy (*terapia sistémica,* as it was called in Argentina) when I was only 17 years old and inspired me to become a systems thinker and pursue training in CFT first in Argentina and later on in the United States. As well, I was fortunate to be trained and to work with the leading figures in systemic and cognitive-behavioral therapy in Argentina in the 1990s, such as Hugo Hirsch, Martin Wainstein, Hector Fernandez Alvarez, and Dora Schnitman. Dr. Wainstein gave me the unique opportunity to teach one of the sections of the elective course Theory and Techniques in Systemic Therapy (CFT) at the University of Buenos Aires, which allowed me to study CFT models in more detail. Dr. Alvarez introduced me to cognitive-behavioral therapy at his institute, the AIGLE Foundation, and his dedication to and belief in the need for rigorous research taught me about its importance. I want to reserve a special thanks to Dr. Schnitman, whose 2-year postgraduate training in postmodern epistemology and systemic therapy models transformed my personal views on therapy and science and eventually solidified my decision to continue my studies in the United States. Dr. Schnitman built the best postgraduate program in systemic therapies ever offered until that time in Argentina by bringing together national and international leading figures whose work emphasized language and discourse analysis as critical in therapy to open or constrain change. Dr. Gergen's conceptualization of the relational self and Sheila McNamee's writings on social constructivism and therapy as social construction in the 1990s taught me to continuously see all human behaviors, beliefs, and scientific ideas in context and in relation to sociocultural political forces, which prepared me to understand and integrate issues of power, gender, racism, heterosexism, ableism, and other -isms in my clinical work and in my personal life.

I am equally thankful for all the training experiences in couple and family therapy in Argentina in clinics and psychiatric hospitals such as Hospital Torcuato de Alvear, Hospital Borda, and Hospital Cuenca Alta. I am especially thankful to the Centro Privado de Psicoterapias (Private Center of Psychotherapies), where I learned the most enduring lessons as a therapist in my home country. Its founder and director, Lic. Hugo Hirsch, offered not only a job to the therapists but also a rich learning experience. In this clinic intakes were conducted by the most experienced therapists, who recorded that initial intake session and provided the recorded tape and an intake summary to the therapist assigned to the case. This process allowed all beginning therapists, like me at the time, to listen and learn from hundreds of outstanding first intake sessions. In addition, and even more remarkable, was the opportunity to learn from Hugo himself on Monday evenings during live sessions dedicated to the most challenging cases. Four or 5 hours of challenging cases, sometimes my own, every Monday for 3 years taught me how to be an effective therapist and embrace clinical challenges.

My training, clinical, and teaching experiences in Argentina in the first decade of my professional career were undoubtedly foundational, but I am forever thankful for my decision to come to the United States to continue my training and clinical work and add research as a critical component of my work. The lead author of this book has been my lifelong professional mentor and one of my godparents in this country. Thanks to his love for research, his generosity, and his inexhaustible patience for teaching, I embraced research and decided to follow his steps in academia. But, most importantly for writing this book, it has been Norman Epstein who introduced me to cognitive-behavioral couple therapy (CBCT) in 2000 and who has since then continued to strengthen my CBCT knowledge and skills through our ongoing collaborations. I am also indebted to Dr. Epstein for the tremendous number of doors that he has opened in my academic and clinical career, for his solid, wise guidance in these last 24 years, and for being such an extraordinary role model as a leader, a therapist, an instructor, a trainer, an author, and a researcher.

Carol Werlinich, Director of the Training Clinic at University of Maryland at the time and recipient of the first license as a marriage and family therapist in the state of Maryland, supervised most of my clinical work and played a key role in strengthening my clinical skills and helping me integrate my knowledge and experience as a therapist. I am also grateful for Leigh Leslie's course on Gender and Ethnicity, which introduced me 24 years ago to the key concepts of diversity, inclusion, social justice, intersectionality, power, privilege, and cultural competence and sensitivity, which helped me not only understand, honor, and affirm my clients' identities but also make sense of my own experiences as an immigrant Latina in the United States and the role of my social identities in my clinical, teaching, and research work. Her early teachings and her mentorship, together with my postmodern, social constructionist views, were critical in working with marginalized, minority identities in my research and clinical practice and are present in every chapter of this book.

I would also like to thank Guy Bodenmann, whose concept of dyadic coping transformed my research and clinical work and whose generosity and mentorship allowed me to develop and provide programmatic interventions for couples dealing with a variety of stressors related to immigration, finances, and discrimination. The psychoeducational program TOGETHER/JUNTOS en PAREJA, which has served low-income African American, Latine immigrant, and LGBTQ+ couples since 2011, was inspired by Dr. Bodenmann's Couples Coping Enhancement Training and was developed around the central idea that by strengthening dyadic coping skills couples can better manage all stressors, including financial ones. Thanks to his work, dyadic coping skills are viewed today as essential to couples' healthy functioning in the same way that communication and problem-solving skills are. I am very thankful to my colleagues Celia Hayhoe and Jinhee Kim, cocreators with me of the TOGETHER program, for believing in the idea of integrating relationship and financial education and bringing this interdisciplinary program to life.

I also have immense gratitude for all the leading figures in the CFT field from whom I had the privilege to learn directly or indirectly, particularly to those devoted to couple therapy, such as Andrew Christensen, Neil Jacobson, Sue Johnson, and John and Julie Gottman. I am equally thankful to the many students and supervisees whose questions have helped me advance my knowledge and understanding of couple relationships, especially to those who, with their challenging questions, made me revisit concepts and established practices. I have enormous gratitude to the many clients whom I have seen over the years who allowed me to share part of their journeys, taught me about resilience, and helped me become a better therapist. Finally, my deepest gratitude is to my husband, Cesar Costantino, and my children, Milena and Lucca, for the numerous ways in which they have helped me grow as a person and as a therapist, and for all the strength, support, and space that they have given me to devote myself to this wonderful profession and to coauthor this book.

Contents

PART II. TREATMENT PLANNER

List of Reproducible Handouts (Online)

TREATMENT PLANS AND INTERVENTIONS IN COUPLE THERAPY

PART I

INTRODUCTION AND OVERVIEW

CHAPTER 1

Introduction to Cognitive–Behavioral Couple Therapy Concepts and Methods

Cognitive-behavioral concepts and methods for understanding and treating problems in couple relationships constitute a major theoretical model that has developed since the 1960s and is well supported by research (for reviews, see Baucom, Epstein, Fischer, Kirby, & LaTaillade, 2023; Baucom, Shoham, Mueser, Daiuto, & Stickle, 1998; Fischer, Baucom, & Cohen, 2016; Lebow & Snyder, 2022). Consequently, cognitive-behavioral couple therapy (CBCT) is routinely included in couple and family therapy textbooks (e.g., Lebow & Snyder, 2023; Nichols & Davis, 2016). CBCT methods are widely used by clinicians, including many who adhere primarily to other theoretical models but integrate cognitive-behavioral interventions in their treatment plans (Northey, 2002). The conceptual model of CBCT and the range of assessment methods and interventions have expanded substantially over the years to complex influences among partners' cognitions, emotional responses, and behavioral interactions. An increased focus on multiple layers of contextual factors that influence a couple and its members (ranging from personal histories, needs and personality characteristics to broader ecological influences such as extended family, jobs, culture, and societal conditions) has resulted in a much more comprehensive systemic model for assessment and treatment. Thus, CBCT can help therapists understand opportunities and challenges that contexts create for couples, making it an excellent model for treating couples whose lives are affected by discrimination, social inequities, climate disasters, disease pandemics, and the like.

The popularity and wide applicability of CBCT as a treatment framework have been due to its comprehensiveness in addressing the major realms of intimate relationships: individuals' internal *cognitions* and *emotions* regarding their experiences with significant others and the overt *behavioral interactions* between partners. In addition, CBCT procedures for assessment and intervention (e.g., identifying thoughts that elicit partners' aggressive actions; teaching communication and problem-solving skills) are straightforward and easy to explain to clients. CBCT developed as an integrative framework representing the merging of several components that capture individual partners' intrapsychic processes, intergenerational influences from partners' families of origin, a couple's current behavioral interactions (e.g., the common circular demand–withdraw pattern), and ecological contextual influences. Furthermore, the attention in CBCT to each couple's contextual stressors broadens assessment and treatment planning to address conditions that influence a relationship as it develops over time. The conceptual richness and clinical sophistication of CBCT allow therapists to apply it to complex relationship issues such as infidelity, partner aggression, and sexual problems, a member's physical or mental health problem, and couples coping with external stressors such as discrimination and limited material resources.

This chapter presents an overview of (1) the theoretical roots of CBCT, (2) core behavioral, cognitive, and emotional domains that are addressed, (3) the range of interventions used to modify problematic behavioral patterns, cognitions, and emotional responses (described in detail in Chapter 4), and (4) how CBCT is applied to relational problems and problems involving individuals' physical or mental health issues. It also touches on (5) how CBCT practitioners attend to "common factors" (e.g., the therapeutic alliance, therapist cultural sensitivity) that have been found to influence the effectiveness of various therapy models. Finally, we describe examples of how CBCT can be integrated with other theoretical orientations, and we provide a summary of existing research support.

This book emphasizes treatment of couples that are in relationships involving some degree of commitment, not those who are casually dating. However, the interventions are relevant for relationships at all stages of development. Some of the concepts and methods can be applied in premarital counseling in a preventive way, as they often are used in relationship education and enhancement programs (e.g., Carlson, Rhoades, Johnson, Stanley, & Markman, 2023; Halford, 2011; Halford & Moore, 2002; Markman & Rhoades, 2012; Markman, Stanley, & Blumberg, 2010). CBCT can be applied with couples who are diverse in age, race, ethnicity, gender identity, sexual orientation, and socioeconomic status, although therapists must be culturally attuned to understanding the concerns couples bring to therapy based on their backgrounds.

THEORETICAL ROOTS OF CBCT

The core theoretical concepts of CBCT have been derived from a few major sources: (1) learning theory, (2) family systems theory, (3) basic research findings in cognitive psychology regarding human information processing, (4) the theoretical base underlying cognitive therapy, and (5) models of emotional experience and expression. The following are brief summaries of these roots that are integrated into CBCT.

Learning Theory Combined with Social Exchange Concepts

The earliest forms of CBCT focused on behavioral interactions between partners that contribute to individuals' levels of satisfaction with their relationship, as well as principles regarding learning from one's experiences. Behaviorally oriented couple therapists (Jacobson & Margolin, 1979; Stuart, 1980; Weiss, Hops, & Patterson, 1973) applied social exchange theory (Thibaut & Kelley, 1959), which proposes that an individual's level of satisfaction with a relationship depends on the ratio of benefits to costs experienced in the relationship. An individual will be relatively dissatisfied with a relationship that is perceived as providing a poor benefit-to-cost ratio, especially when comparing the existing ratio to a more favorable ratio that one predicts would occur in an alternative relationship. This model of relationship satisfaction is consistent with Western cultures within which CBCT was developed (Epstein, Falconier, & Dattilio, 2020).

A related premise of the behavioral model is that members of a relationship continually provide consequences for each other's actions that influence the likelihood that each person will exhibit those actions. Learning theory concepts focus on processes through which both constructive and problematic behaviors are acquired and controlled through interactions with one's environment, especially with other people. Even though learned patterns may become fairly persistent, learning theory proposes that they can be modified through similar types of experiences with one's environment.

Concepts that have been applied to understanding and treating couple relationship problems derive from B. F. Skinner's (1953, 1971) model of *operant conditioning*, which involves increasing or decreasing an individual's specific action by controlling consequences of the action. Behaviors that lead to rewards tend to increase (positive reinforcement), as will those behaviors that lead to removal of an aversive condition; for example, an individual nags until the partner complies with the request, leading the partner to become more compliant with the person's requests (negative reinforcement). In contrast to reinforcement processes, a person's behavior can be decreased when it is followed by a consequence assumed to be aversive (punishment), or by discontinuing the reinforcement (extinction) (Weiss, 1978). Thus, when members of a couple provide each other with reinforcing and punishing consequences, they shape each other's behaviors. The partners need not be aware of this process or of intentionally influencing each other's actions.

Another operant conditioning concept is *discriminative stimuli*, conditions that are cues that reinforcement or punishment is likely to occur. Thus, members of a couple learn that particular nonverbal cues signal whether or not the other person is likely to be receptive to affectionate behavior. Sometimes partners intentionally exhibit such cues, and some arguments occur when the intended recipient of a cue fails to notice and respond appropriately to it. Because partners mutually provide each other with discriminative stimulus cues and consequences for each other's actions, these mutual influences are consistent with circular causal processes captured in family systems theory.

Because operant conditioning processes involving shaping responses via consequences is an inefficient way of learning complex human behavior such as social skills, social learning theorists (Bandura, 1977; Bandura & Walters, 1963) focused on how an individual can observe a complex behavior modeled by another person and then imitate it. The observer is more likely to imitate the model if the model has high status or has been seen receiving reinforcement for the behavior.

Based on these learning and social exchange principles, initial behavioral approaches to couple therapy focused on interventions to increase partners' positive actions and decrease negative ones, especially contracts in which each individual agreed to enact particular behaviors that the other person desired (Jacobson & Margolin, 1979). In addition, observational learning principles were used to teach partners skills for communication (expressing and listening) and problem solving (see Chapter 4) to increase mutual understanding and the likelihood that they would meet each other's needs (Jacobson & Margolin, 1979; Stuart, 1980). Furthermore, communication behaviors that are foci in skills training have been guided by research that has identified patterns associated with distress and instability in couples' relationships. Researchers (e.g., Gottman, 1979, 1994; Revenstorf, Hahlweg, Schindler, & Vogel, 1984; Weiss et al., 1973) identified behavioral interaction patterns (e.g., escalating reciprocal exchanges of negative behavior, demand–withdraw patterns) that differentiated distressed from relatively happy couples and that predicted dissolution of relationships. Because the interventions were developed on the basis of research primarily on samples from Western societies, therapists need to be mindful of adapting communication and problem-solving training to cultural differences that may contribute to a couple's patterns.

Although approaches to couple problems based on learning theory tended to focus on behavior, Bandura's (1977) social learning model also included a cognitive component involving individuals' *expectancies* regarding the probability that a particular action on their part would lead to particular consequences from their partner. For example, an individual may have developed an expectancy that attempts to discuss issues with a partner will result in the partner withdrawing, which may lead the individual to pursue the partner more strenuously or to give up and withdraw as well. A therapist identifies the negative expectancy and may use coaching in communication skills to reduce the couple's demand–withdraw behavioral pattern *and* the associated expectancy. Thus, understanding and modifying a couple's negative behavioral patterns is improved by taking partners' cognitions into account. However, social learning theory did not provide a fine-grained model of complex forms of cognition that influence relationships, and the development of CBCT depended on integrating behavioral concepts and methods with other models that focus on forms of cognition that influence relationships.

Family Systems Theory

Dattilio (2010) noted that some family systems theorists critiqued behavioral and cognitive therapy models as being dominated by linear causal concepts, but Patterson's (1982) behavioral model of coercive family systems in which children with conduct problems and their parents direct aversive behavior toward each other and the behavioral couple therapy concept of reciprocal behavioral exchanges between partners (Jacobson & Margolin, 1979; Stuart, 1980) clearly focused on mutual influences between significant others. The process identified in CBCT in which partners continuously provide consequences for each other's responses is consistent with the systems concept of feedback. For example, when partners reciprocate each other's verbal aggression, leading to an escalation of the conflict, the concept of positive feedback fits in describing how the members' responses to each other amplify the negative interaction pattern. Even though each member of a couple is considered responsible for their own actions (especially abusive behavior), the CBCT model emphasizes the systemic characteristics of the relationship and interventions that take into account partners' influences on each other.

Epstein and Baucom's enhanced CBCT model (Baucom et al., 2023; Epstein & Baucom, 2002) also applies family systems concepts of boundaries and hierarchy. Boundaries within and around a relationship are defined by who interacts with whom and in what roles. They involve partners' overt behavior and their internal cognitions about what patterns are appropriate. For example, when an individual shares intimate information about the couple's relationship with extended family members, it may violate their partner's standard about an appropriate boundary between the couple and the outside world. Similarly, if a person purchases an expensive item without consulting their partner, this action may reflect skewed power in the couple's relationship, as well as their different standards about decision making.

Finally, Epstein and Baucom's (2002) enhanced CBCT model integrated Bronfenbrenner's (1979) ecological model, which focuses on multiple levels of contextual factors that influence a relationship. The partners must cope with factors such as extended family relationships, friends, schools, and jobs; characteristics of the local community, such as crime; and broad societal-level factors such as immigration stresses, forms of discrimination, and adverse economic conditions. CBCT examines how the demands of these factors influence couple interaction patterns (as when job demands limit a couple's time together) and the types of cognitions, emotional responses, and behavioral responses the partners exhibit in attempting to cope with them.

Social Cognition Theory and Research

Behaviorally oriented couple theorists and therapists have drawn on basic research findings regarding human information processing to identify forms of cognition that can influence partners' behavioral responses to each other. For example, Jacobson and Margolin (1979) labeled the perceptual bias that occurs when partners notice each other's negative behavior and overlook positive behaviors as *negative tracking*. They also noted how members of unhappy couples commonly made seemingly biased negative attributions about the causes of each other's displeasing actions. For example, if a member of a couple intends to behave positively toward a partner, but the partner attributes the other's actions to the partner having negative motives, the partner will be likely to experience negative emotions and behavior in response to the other's actions (Fletcher, Overall, Friesen, & Nicolls, 2018).

Social cognition research has focused on two major categories of thinking: (1) relatively stable *knowledge structures* regarding relationships and (2) *moment-to-moment "online" processing of information* about events currently occurring between partners (Fletcher et al., 2018). A variety of terms have been used to label the relatively stable internalized concepts involved in knowledge structures (e.g., schemas, scripts, working models, mental models). Individuals develop these persistent concepts through their experiences with others beginning very early in life. They provide cognitive templates that provide the individual with explanations for current experiences (e.g., "I get angry easily in close relationships because I grew up in an emotionally volatile family"). In addition, they influence the outcomes that one predicts in interactions with others (e.g., "If I express my opinions, I will be ignored"), and they increase one's ability to exert control over particular aspects of relationships (e.g., "After you compliment a person, they are more likely to comply with a request you make").

These knowledge structures or personal theories vary from global views of relationships with people in general (e.g., how trustworthy one believes that people tend to be) to concepts regarding romantic relationships in particular, to concepts about a specific personal romantic relationship (Fletcher et al., 2018). An individual's knowledge structures or theories about a current relationship become more complex as more experiences with the partner accumulate, and the level of satisfaction with the relationship depends on how closely the actual experiences with the partner match the individual's standards for a close relationship (Baucom, Epstein, Rankin & Burnett, 1996; Campbell & Fletcher, 2015). Research indicates that established knowledge structures tend to be resistant to change and that individuals selectively attend to information that is consistent with their existing beliefs (Meichenbaum, 1985). However, there still is potential for them to be modified through new life experiences that disconfirm them (Fiske & Taylor, 1991; Fletcher et al., 2018; Fletcher, Simpson, Campbell, & Overall, 2013). An example of knowledge structures that exhibit significant stability in adulthood are the "working models" identified in attachment theory (Bowlby, 1969), beliefs that individuals have regarding their own lovability and of the emotional availability of an attachment figure such as a parent or romantic partner. Relatively stable attachment working models have been found to influence more momentary cognitions; for example, individuals with more anxious insecure attachment make more negative attributions about the causes of their partners' negative behavior (Fletcher et al., 2018). Research findings such as these have important implications for clinical assessment and intervention, highlighting the need to identify partners' schemas and how they contribute to negative couple interactions and relationship distress.

Another important aspect of relatively stable knowledge structures that has implications for understanding the role of cognition in close relationships and addressing them in therapy is that individuals commonly access them automatically and unconsciously rather than intentionally (Fletcher et al., 2018). Thus, an individual notices a partner's specific verbal or nonverbal behavior (e.g., a scowling facial expression), attaches meaning to it by comparing it to memories of similar events associated with such behavior (e.g., associates a scowl with a significant other's past violent behavior), and experiences fear and an urge to escape. All of this cognitive processing may occur almost instantaneously, without any intentional analysis, and both members of the couple might be taken by surprise as the individual cannot explain the sudden discomfort. Although individuals' level of awareness of such influential cognitions may vary widely, there is evidence that people shift into more conscious analysis when confronted with negative, upsetting events and unexpected events (Fletcher et al., 2018). For example, upon discovering a partner's infidelity, individuals commonly engage in extensive cognitive analyses, searching for information to explain what occurred, one's failure to identify clues about it sooner, and how to reshape positive beliefs about the partner that have been invalidated (Baucom, Snyder, & Gordon, 2009; Janoff-Bulman, 1992). As we describe later, cognitive assessment in CBCT is designed to access as much as possible partners' schemas that are less conscious.

Baucom, Epstein, Sayers, and Sher (1989) classified two relationally oriented forms of cognition as schemas: relatively stable *assumptions* that individuals hold about characteristics of individuals and relationships (e.g., an attachment working model that one cannot rely on a partner to reliably meet one's emotional needs) and *standards* about characteristics that individuals and relationships "should" have (e.g., "A caring partner should always place the other person's needs above their own"). In contrast to those two forms of knowledge structures, *selective perceptions* of present events occurring between partners, *attributions* about causes of one's own and others' behaviors, and *expectancies* involving predictions about likely responses one's actions will elicit from one's partner are forms of moment-to-moment processing of information (Baucom & Epstein, 1990; Epstein & Baucom, 2002). Although all of these forms of processing information that individuals are exposed to in daily life are normal, they are susceptible to distortion that can lead to inappropriate responses. Distortions in perception and inferences have been found to contribute to a wide range of psychopathology (e.g., depression, anxiety disorders, eating disorders) as well as relationship problems (Dobson & Kendall, 1993). A variety of cognitive distortions (e.g., all-or-nothing thinking, selective abstraction, and personalization) have been identified in the model underlying Beck's cognitive therapy (Dobson, Poole, & Beck, 2018). Studies have indicated that individuals' cognitions about intimate partners, such as negative attributions about the causes of a partner's negative actions, are associated with unhappiness about the relationship *and* the individual's negative behavior toward the partner (Epstein & Baucom, 2002). Using such findings to guide assessment and treatment within a CBCT (or other) model is consistent with Karam and Sprenkle's (2010) *research-informed clinical model*, in which clinicians keep abreast of findings about factors that contribute to types of client problems, as well as regarding the effects of specific interventions. Knowledge about cognitive factors in relationship problems has been important in expanding behavioral models to take into account partners' subjective experiences that influence how they behave toward each other.

Cognitive Therapy Models

During the same period when behavioral models of couple and family therapy were capturing complex behavioral interaction patterns in intimate relationships, cognitive models of individual psychopathology and therapy (Beck, 1976; Ellis, 1962; Meichenbaum, 1977) also were developing as a major alternative to traditional psychodynamic models. Ellis's model focused on relatively stable irrational beliefs that individuals develop while growing up in a social context (e.g., that one must be perfect in order to be a worthwhile person); these beliefs produce emotional distress and dysfunctional behavior when real-life experiences fail to match one's unrealistic standards. Beck's model also included unrealistic stable schemas regarding characteristics of the self and world but differentiated them from much more transitory automatic thoughts regarding one's immediate experiences. In the Beck model, a life event (e.g., taking an exam in school) activates an individual's underlying relevant schema (e.g., perfectionism as a personal standard), leading to stream-of-consciousness automatic thoughts (e.g., "I'm not smart enough to do well on this test. I'm a loser!"; Dobson et al., 2018). The model also includes a variety of cognitive distortions or information processing errors (e.g., all-or-nothing thinking) that contribute to distressing automatic thoughts.

Meichenbaum (1985) presented another useful model focused on cognitions that occur during individuals' responses to stressful life experiences. Similar to the Beck model, Meichenbaum notes that individuals' cognitive processing commonly is fairly automatic and beyond awareness, and that individuals can be coached in developing awareness of distressing cognitions that can be tested for appropriateness and modified. In particular, Meichenbaum emphasizes assisting individuals in developing skills for "stress inoculation" that involves conscious, intentional rehearsal and use of positive "self-statements" about stressors. Positive coping self-statements are developed for preparing for an anticipated stressor (e.g., "Just think about what I can do about it"), confronting and handling it (e.g., "One step at a time"), coping with feelings of being overwhelmed (e.g., "Relax and slow things down"), and evaluating one's coping efforts (e.g., "I can be pleased with the progress I'm making"). Given that members of a couple can be stressors for each other, this stress inoculation model has great relevance.

These cognitive models initially were developed primarily to understand problems with individuals' personal functioning such as depression and anxiety. Increasingly, however, they were applied to address couple and family relationship problems that can be among the most stressful experiences in people's lives (Beck, 1988; Dattilio & Padesky, 1990; Ellis, Sichel, Yeager, DiMattia, & DiGiuseppe, 1989; Epstein, 1982; Epstein, Schlesinger, & Dryden, 1988). In a couple's relationship, each member is a source of life events that the other appraises cognitively, influencing the individual's emotional and behavioral responses to their partner. An individual's appraisals are automatic thoughts shaped by underlying schemas such as beliefs or standards regarding the characteristics that a caring family member "should" possess (Baucom & Epstein, 1990; Epstein & Baucom, 2002).

Some of the initial literature on applications of cognitive therapies to relationships primarily described an extension of individually based Ellis and Beck models, identifying each individual's distorted or unrealistic cognitions and intervening with each person to modify them. However, increasingly writers presented a more integrative *cognitive-behavioral* model that simultaneously attends to a couple's dyadic behavioral interactions and each member's cognitions about them, as well as emotional responses. For example, assessment of a couple that presents with escalating verbal arguments would include an inquiry about each person's thoughts about instances of negative behavior from the other (e.g., "He has no respect for me. I'm not going to let him get away with treating me like that!") and associated emotional responses (e.g., anger).

Models of Emotional Experience and Expression

The absence of the term *emotion* in the title "cognitive-behavioral therapy" (CBT) unfortunately has contributed to an impression among the lay public and some mental health professionals that the concepts of the model and the methods of the treatments pay little attention to people's emotions. In addition, groundbreaking publications by founders Beck, Ellis, Meichenbaum, and others described associations between dysfunctional cognition and disorders such as depression and anxiety. For example, Beck (1976) described associations between particular cognitive themes and emotions, such as depression linked with perceived loss associated with depression, danger with anxiety, and violation of one's rights with anger. This model led some readers to conclude that cognitive approaches only proposed a linear causal link in which disordered thinking produced negative emotions and behavior, but not vice versa. More recent publications have focused more on affective components of CBT models regarding individual and relational functioning, and the pathways through which emotional states can influence cognitions and behavior. Writers have emphasized that emotions are natural responses that have had evolutionary adaptive value and that a wide variety of positive and negative emotions are normal and common aspects of human experience. They have also reported that emotional states influence cognition and behavior; e.g., motivate avoidance behavior, interfere with cognitive and behavioral problem-solving skills, shape selective attention to others' positive or negative actions, and elicit negative interpersonal behavior such as aggression as well as positive acts such as altruism (Leahy, 2015; Linehan, 1993; Nezu, Nezu, & Hays, 2019; Rizvi & King, 2019).

Furthermore, the conceptual model of emotionally focused therapy (EFT; Greenberg & Goldman, 2008; Johnson, 1996; Johnson, Wiebe, & Allan, 2023) proposes that members of a couple continuously regulate each other's emotions. One member's cues of emotion (e.g., tears) signal the other member about the individual's unmet needs and how the individual is likely to respond to the partner's actions (e.g., increased upset if the partner fails to reassure the individual of their love). The EFT model also proposes that individuals commonly hide vulnerable "primary emotions" such as sadness and fear under harder defensive "secondary emotions" such as anger. Consequently, EFT therapists guide partners in identifying and expressing vulnerable feelings, which increases the likelihood that they will elicit caring responses from each other. Thus, increased awareness and communication of emotional responses can alert partners about unmet needs and motivate them to take action to rectify the problem. Goldman and Greenberg (2006) stress that better emotion regulation is needed, either to increase recognition and expression of hidden emotions or to reduce excessive emotional responses. They emphasize how members of a couple "co-regulate" each other's emotions, continuously influencing the degrees of positivity and negativity in the other's emotional experience. The CBCT model that has developed over time overlaps with that of EFT, with both deficits and excesses in emotional awareness and expression considered to be problematic, and with the goals of therapy including increasing partners' awareness of their emotions and developing their skills for communicating their emotional states constructively to each other (Baucom & Epstein, 1990; Baucom et al., 2023; Epstein, Dattilio, & Baucom, 2016; Epstein & Baucom, 2002; Rathus & Sanderson, 1999).

Research on emotions in close relationships has indicated that positive and negative emotions are relatively independent rather than opposite poles of a single dimension (Planalp, Fitness, & Fehr, 2018). Consequently, reducing an individual's experiences of negativity does not automatically result in an increase in positivity. Therefore, CBCT interventions for decreasing negative couple interactions are balanced with interventions to increase positive interactions (Epstein & Baucom, 2002). Gottman (1999) also advocates CBT-like strategies for implementing "repair" attempts for couples to counteract negative with positive interactions (e.g., taking responsibility for a problem, expressing affection).

BEHAVIORAL, COGNITIVE, AND EMOTIONAL DOMAINS ADDRESSED IN CBCT

Based on the integrative CBCT theoretical model that we have described, assessment and interventions target the core domains of behavior, cognition, and emotion. The following are brief summaries of the characteristics addressed in each domain.

Behavioral Domain

Based on social learning principles and social exchange theory, CBCT focuses on the *frequencies of positive and negative verbal and nonverbal behaviors* that members of a couple direct toward each other. It also focuses on their association with each partner's subjective level of satisfaction with the relationship. Commonly, particular types of behavioral deficits or excesses that are linked to a couple's presenting concerns (e.g., deficits in types of shared activities that result in a general sense of limited intimacy) become foci. In a *functional analysis*, events from each individual are identified that elicit the other's specific actions, as well as the behavioral *consequences* that partners provide for each other's actions. Problematic dyadic sequences and patterns (e.g., escalating reciprocation of negative actions; a demand–withdraw pattern) are identified.

Also tied to social learning theory are partners' *behavioral skills* for expression and empathic listening, as well as for systematic, constructive problem solving, which are evaluated for potential intervention. Partners are coached in translating global complaints into specific behaviors that can be increased or decreased. Specialized skills for managing particular roles in couple and family life (e.g., joint parenting, money management, sexual interaction, dyadic coping with a child's chronic illness) also are selected for intervention, as needed. Overall, clinicians attempt to differentiate between *micro-level behaviors* that are limited to specific situations (e.g., a couple argues about differences in their ideas of how to get their young child to go to sleep at a reasonable time) versus macro-level behavioral patterns that occur across a broad range of situations (e.g., a couple exhibits mutual verbal aggression in a variety of situations as they engage in a general power struggle).

Cognitive Domain

The five types of cognition identified by Baucom, Epstein, and colleagues (Baucom & Epstein, 1990; Baucom et al., 1989; Epstein & Baucom, 2002) are foci of CBCT. They include two that are forms of schemas: *assumptions* are beliefs about the characteristics of individuals and close relationships (e.g., a man's assumption that women like to control men; attachment "working models"), whereas *standards* are beliefs about characteristics that individuals and close relationships "should" have (e.g., an individual's standard that intimacy requires that partners disclose all of their innermost thoughts and emotions to each other). The other three types of cognition, which tend to involve relatively transitory automatic thoughts, are *selective attention, attributions*, and *expectancies*. Selective attention (also labeled selective abstraction) involves noticing some aspects of the available information in a situation and overlooking other information. *Attributions* are inferences that individuals make about the factors influencing observed events, including a partner's behavior (e.g., a man's partner failed to act excited when he gave her a surprise gift, and he attributed her lack of enthusiasm to her not appreciating him, an inference that turned out to be inaccurate, as he learned that she had heard earlier that day that her mother was seriously ill). *Expectancies* are predictions about probabilities that particular events will occur in the future (e.g., an individual has an expectancy that telling their partner they are not enjoying the partner's form of sexual touch will hurt the partner's feelings severely, a prediction based on negative experiences from a previous relationship).

In addition to those five types of cognition, CBCT attends to cognitive distortions or errors in information processing that have been described extensively in the cognitive therapy literature (e.g., A. T. Beck, Rush, Shaw, & Emery, 1979; J. S. Beck, 2021; Dobson et al., 2018; Leahy, 1996). Examples are *magnification* (e.g., appraising a negative event as especially severe) and *personalization* (e.g., an individual infers that a partner's bad mood is related to themself rather than to other events in the partner's life). Handout 1.1 (available on the book's web page at *www.guilford.com/epstein-materials*) presents a list and definitions of common cognitive distortions for use by therapists and clients. Cognitive distortions typically are involved in unrealistic or inaccurate assumptions, standards, selective attention, attributions, and expectancies. For example, an attribution that a partner's lateness in arriving home is due to the partner not prioritizing the couple's relationship potentially involves the distortions of *arbitrary inference* and *personalization*.

Other characteristics of partners' relationship cognitions that are foci of CBCT are the extent to which individuals are *conscious* of their cognitive processing, the degree to which they *intentionally engage in cognitive activity* (e.g., self-reflection) rather than it occurring automatically, and how actively they *evaluate the validity or appropriateness* of their cognitions. These characteristics are similar to those commonly included in the concept of *psychological mindedness* (Conte, Ratto, & Karusa, 1996).

Emotion Domain

In the cognitive therapy models that initially were developed to understand and treat individuals' problems with depression, anxiety, anger, and other emotions (Beck, 1976; Ellis, 1962; Meichenbaum, 1977), the emphasis was on how forms of distorted and negative thinking produced dysfunctional emotional responses. That type of causal path became a significant component of CBT approaches to a wide variety of client presenting problems, including couple relationship distress (Baucom & Epstein, 1990; Beck, 1988; Dattilio & Padesky, 1990; Rathus & Sanderson, 1999), and it still is. Consequently, in CBCT, therapists routinely inquire about automatic thoughts that preceded and appear to have elicited individuals' specific emotional responses to their partners. In addition, therapists probe for an individual's underlying schemas that are activated by a partner's behavior, eliciting negative automatic thoughts and emotions. For example, an individual discovers that a partner shared with the partner's family members information about the couple's arguments. This action violated the individual's personal standard that members of a couple should maintain a firm boundary around intimate aspects of their relationship aspects and elicited his automatic thought "My partner is disloyal to me!" and considerable anger.

As we noted previously, however, the basic models underlying cognitive therapy, as well as theory and research on emotional experiences, have not been strictly linear, and emotions also are viewed as influencing cognition and behavior. Moods such as sadness, anxiety, anger, and shame shape individuals' perceptions of events and prime particular behavioral responses. In Beck's model, an individual's depression or anxiety serves as a negative filter that can affect perception and memory ("I've always been a failure." "My partner never shows that she loves me." "I'm too anxious to speak up in class."). Weiss's (1980) concept of *sentiment override* describes how an individual's existing general feelings about a partner (e.g., overall persistent unhappiness and anger) determine their emotional and behavioral response to the partner more than the other's actions in the moment. Shame responses narrow individuals' self-perception and evaluation, and also tend to elicit withdrawal from significant others (Epstein & Falconier, 2017). As we have noted, Goldman and Greenberg (2006) emphasize how members of a couple regulate each other's emotions, sending and receiving verbal and nonverbal information about emotional states that influence the other's moods and actions.

Consequently, CBCT clinicians assess partners' relatively stable emotions (e.g., chronic depression, persistent negative sentiment toward the other person) and momentary shifts in emotional states that are both elicited by and elicit their own and the other's emotions, cognitions, and behavior. They also inquire about other emotions that may underlie those that an individual expresses overtly (e.g., anxiety underlying expressed anger toward a partner) but that the person may fail to mention: a process similar to the search for unstated "primary emotions" in the EFT model. One advantage of conducting conjoint couple therapy sessions is the opportunity to observe first-hand the interpersonal processes between partners in which those emotions operate.

INTERVENTIONS USED TO MODIFY PROBLEMATIC BEHAVIORAL PATTERNS, COGNITIONS, AND EMOTIONAL RESPONSES

This book provides detailed descriptions of CBCT interventions for couples' problematic behavioral interaction patterns, cognitions, and emotional responses in order to assist clinicians in devising treatment plans to address a variety of presenting problems. The following is a brief overview of the variety of interventions used in CBCT. These interventions are summarized in Handout 1.2 (available at *www.guilford.com/epstein-materials*), which can be shared with a couple as a psychoeducational part of the therapist–client collaboration. This book's chapters that focus on specific presenting problems describe particular ways in which therapists use these interventions to alleviate negative patterns and build couple strengths.

Interventions for Behavior

Based on social exchange and learning theory principles, clinicians typically begin with a *systematic assessment* of the presenting problems, their history, and a functional analysis of the behavioral patterns and members' associated cognitions and emotions (Dattilio & Epstein, 2016; Epstein & Baucom, 2002), which we describe in detail in Chapter 3. The functional analysis focuses on the conditions preceding a particular cognitive, emotional, or behavioral response (e.g., an individual arrives home from work and hugs their partner) and the consequences that follow the response (e.g., the partner withdraws behaviorally from the individual's hug), which influence when and how often the individual exhibits the response (hugs occur infrequently). Information about such patterns is derived from the couple's reports about their interactions in daily life and from the therapist's observation of the couple's behavior during therapy sessions.

Based on the assessment, the CBCT clinician may use a number of types of interventions to attempt to modify behavioral components of negative patterns. Overall, interventions focus on (1) improving communication, problem-solving, and dyadic coping skills; (2) replacing negative interaction behavioral patterns (e.g., demand–withdraw, reciprocal verbal aggression) with constructive behavior; and (3) increasing positive, pleasing actions because simply decreasing negative actions does not necessarily result in members of a couple being happy.

Therapists conduct interventions during therapy sessions but also emphasize partners' engagement in homework activities during daily life, such as practicing communication skills, as research has indicated that homework promotes the transfer of changes to daily living (Dattilio, Kazantzis, Shinkfield, & Carr, 2011).

- **Improving communication, problem-solving, and dyadic coping skills.** CBCT clinicians use skills training procedures to enhance partners' skills for expressing themselves clearly and constructively and for listening to each other's expressions empathically. They also teach couples skills for collaborating to solve problems in their relationship. The steps in problem solving include defining the characteristics of a problem in behavioral terms, generating alternative potential solutions, collaborating as a couple in evaluating the advantages and disadvantages of each solution, reaching consensus about a solution, devising a plan to implement that solution, and revising the solution if the results indicate that it was ineffective (Epstein & Baucom, 2002). Furthermore, CBCT includes enhancement of a couple's skills for dyadic coping with various life stressors affecting one or both partners. As described in Chapter 4, the collaborative nature of dyadic coping differs from partners' individual coping styles. All three types of skill training include initial psychoeducation about the importance and methods of using constructive and effective skills with one's partner, didactic presentation and modeling of the desired skills by the therapist, and coaching of the couple as they practice the skills.

- **Replacing negative interaction patterns with constructive behavior.** When the assessment identifies a negative behavioral pattern, the clinician reviews the evidence of its problematic consequences with the couple and works to motivate them to experiment with alternative behaviors. The therapist provides brief psychoeducation regarding research evidence for drawbacks of a pattern such as demand–withdraw or reciprocal verbal attacks, notes how each partner can make a contribution to changing their own part in the pattern, encourages each partner to make a commitment to such changes, collaborates with the couple in specifying the constructive behaviors that they are aiming for, blocks any instances of the negative behavior during sessions, and coaches partners in substituting positive behaviors at those times (Epstein & Baucom, 2002; Epstein & Falconier, 2014). Interventions focused on changing negative behavior commonly are combined with others that address cognitions and emotions that can interfere with behavior change—for example, an individual's expectancy that unless they are verbally aggressive with their partner, the partner will not take them seriously.

- **Increasing positive, pleasing actions.** Because decreasing negative behavior does not ensure an increase in positive behavior, clinicians set a goal of identifying actions that produce pleasure for the couple and developing plans for them to engage in those actions. Couples commonly express relief when their negative interactions decrease but still long for a more pleasing, intimate relationship, so efforts to identify and increase pleasing behavior are very important (Baucom & Epstein, 1990; Epstein & Baucom, 2002). Early forms of behavioral couple therapy (e.g., Jacobson & Margolin, 1979) engaged couples in behavioral contracts in which each member identified pleasing actions they desired from their partner. However, more recent "guided behavior change" procedures (Baucom et al., 2023; Epstein & Baucom, 2002) focus on increasing forms of behavior that address particular needs of a couple. For example, a couple that complains of feeling a lack of intimacy can be coached in interacting in ways that have potential to increase their sense of closeness. Because partners often differ in the actions they find most pleasant, cognitive interventions may be needed to reduce conflict over personal standards about the "best" ways of relating.

Interventions for Cognitions

CBCT addresses partners' automatic thoughts, relatively stable underlying schemas, and the cognitive distortions involved in dysfunctional thinking that cognitive therapists have emphasized (A. T. Beck et al., 1979; J. S. Beck, 2021; Dattilio, 2010; Leahy, 1996). The five types of relational cognitions that Baucom et al. (1989) identified include three that involve automatic thoughts (selective perceptions, attributions, expectancies) and two that are forms of schemas (assumptions and standards). The interventions are similar to those used in individual cognitive therapy, but they are tailored to treating partners jointly. An advantage of joint sessions is that a person's partner is available to introduce information that may modify the person's negative cognitions. However, individuals may be defensive when a therapist coaches them in examining the appropriateness of their thoughts, due to concern of losing face in front of their partner (or giving the partner "ammunition" to use in arguments). Therefore, therapists must be tactful in using "cognitive restructuring" during conjoint sessions.

An additional complication that may arise in couple therapy occurs when the members of a couple share a common problematic cognition, validating each other's perspective (Dattilio, 2010)—for example, when partners both attribute one member's depression symptoms primarily to innate biological causes that are unlikely to change. The major types of therapeutic interventions for cognitions in CBCT are based on traditional cognitive therapy methods, but couple therapists emphasize creating an environment in joint sessions that helps the partners be open to examining their own and shared cognitions, supporting each other's self-examination. They include (1) identifying automatic thoughts and associated emotions and behavior, (2) identifying cognitive distortions, (3) testing and modifying automatic thoughts, (4) testing expectancies with behavioral experiments, (5) using imagery, recollections of past interactions, and role-playing techniques, (6) using the "downward-arrow" technique, and (7) exploring relationship histories to evaluate assumptions and standards.

- **Identifying automatic thoughts and associated emotions and behavior.** In a psychoeducational manner, the therapist introduces the couple to the concept of automatic thoughts and encourages them to monitor their thoughts that are associated with their negative, as well as positive, emotional and behavioral responses to each other. The therapist coaches them in practicing this monitoring during sessions and as homework. A modified version of the Daily Record of Dysfunctional Thoughts (Beck et al., 1979), which was developed initially for use in individual cognitive therapy, is used to collect examples that link partners' automatic thoughts to their emotional and behavioral responses to each other. This is a prerequisite for "cognitive restructuring" methods that guide couples in examining the appropriateness and validity of their thoughts.

- **Identifying cognitive distortions and labeling them.** The therapist also introduces the couple to a typology of common cognitive distortions in a psychoeducational manner by sharing a list of them (Handout 1.1), with definitions, and providing examples. Whenever possible, the therapist uses material from the couple's expressed cognitions to illustrate particular cognitive distortions. The goal is to help the partners become adept at noticing the cognitive distortions in their own stream-of-consciousness automatic thoughts.

- **Testing and modifying automatic thoughts.** The basic process in modifying problematic automatic thoughts involves each member of the couple being open to considering alternative ways of thinking about situations that upset them (e.g., anger over a partner's failure to phone to warn the individual that they would arrive home late from work). The individual is asked to search for information that would support or contradict the negative thought (e.g., memories of other instances when the partner did or did not exhibit thoughtful behavior), to brainstorm alternative reasons that might explain why the partner failed to call, or to examine how reasonable the individual's personal standards regarding attentive behavior are. Challenging core schemas or beliefs about relationships commonly is a gradual process (Dattilio, 2010; Fletcher et al., 2018).

- **Testing expectancies with behavioral experiments.** In CBCT, therapists guide partners in devising "behavioral experiments," to test their expectancies that particular actions will lead to certain responses from each other (Dattilio, 2010; Epstein & Baucom, 2002). For example, a woman may predict that her partner will ignore her suggestions when they are discussing possible solutions to a problem. Their therapist may guide the couple in setting up an experiment in which both members have an opportunity during the therapy session to propose solutions, and both partners observe how their discussion progressed. Even if the woman initially discounts her partner's acknowledgment of her ideas by attributing the partner's openness to an attempt to impress the therapist, the therapist can point to the results of the experiment as some evidence that the initial negative prediction did not "come true."

- **Using imagery, recollections of past interactions, and role-playing techniques.** When members of a couple have difficulty identifying their cognitions (as well as emotions and behaviors) that occurred during past incidents, experiential methods such as imagery and role playing may help to revive memories. Furthermore, these techniques can lead partners to re-experience their initial reactions, so that a role play may transform into a real couple interaction with associated cognitions and emotions. In addition to re-creating experiences that were distressing (but doing so cautiously to avoid retraumatizing victims of abuse), encouraging partners to access early experiences when they felt intimacy can increase their motivation to put effort into therapy sessions.

- **Using the downward-arrow technique.** Cognitive therapists commonly use the downward-arrow technique to uncover "deeper" thoughts underlying an individual's automatic thoughts, which at first seem relatively trivial but are associated with strong emotional and behavioral responses (A. T. Beck et al., 1979; J. S. Beck, 2021). As the therapist asks a series of questions of the form "And if that happened, what would it mean to you?" or "What might that lead to?," the client reveals a chain of thoughts that leads to a clearly nontrivial distressing meaning. Thus, an individual who initially expresses the automatic thought, "My wife's talking to an attractive man makes me very anxious." may ultimately reveal a catastrophic expectancy that "she will find him a lot more interesting than me and leave me." The therapist then can guide the individual and couple in evaluating the validity of the catastrophic automatic thoughts.

- **Exploring relationship histories to evaluate assumptions and standards.** A therapist searches for the origins of partners' assumptions and standards about intimate relationships by asking them to report memories of their experiences in families of origin and other significant relationships. Constructing a genogram depicting each partner's family relationships over generations (McGoldrick, Gerson, & Petry, 2020) can help structure this history taking that serves not only as an assessment but also as a means of increasing partners' insight about the factors that have shaped their cognitions about their current relationship. Individuals may have a "the buck stops here" experience, becoming motivated not to respond in the dysfunctional ways that prior generations exhibited.

 • **Guiding partners in considering the advantages and disadvantages of potentially unrealistic personal standards for their relationship.** Individuals typically enter a relationship with personal standards regarding the characteristics a relationship "should" have. Although many standards may be appropriate and contribute to a mutually satisfying relationship (e.g., partners should treat each other with kindness), others may be extreme or unrealistic (e.g., partners should be able to sense each other's inner feelings and needs without the other person having to tell them explicitly). Individuals commonly do not question the validity of these standards and react negatively when events in their relationship do not meet them, so guiding an individual in modifying an unrealistic one tends to be a gradual process (Dattilio, 2010; Fletcher et al., 2018).

Rather than directly challenging an individual's relationship standard, which may elicit defensiveness, we find it more useful to begin by exploring with the person the advantages they see in conducting their relationship according to the standard and then exploring potential disadvantages. For example, a hypothetical advantage of believing that a caring partner should be able to "mind-read" one's feelings and needs is that one need not experience the discomfort of disclosing unpleasant feelings to one's partner and can cling to an idealized view of being "in-tune soul mates." However, failing to disclose one's experiences is likely to lead to disappointment and frustration when the partner is unable to mind-read. Although relinquishing romantic beliefs about a relationship can be disappointing, individuals gradually may realize that sharing one's feelings and having one's partner demonstrate support outweighs the distress from suffering in silence.

Interventions to Modify Problematic Emotional Responses

As we have described, members of couples may have difficulties either with deficits in awareness and expression of emotions or with excessive experiences and expression of strong emotions such as anger, anxiety, depression, and shame. Consequently, clinicians use a variety of interventions to facilitate clients' awareness and acceptance of a wide range of positive or negative emotions as well as constructive outward expression of one's experiences to other people. Broadly, interventions can be divided into (1) methods for *enhancing* one's awareness, experience, and outward expression of emotions and (2) methods for increasing one's ability to *regulate downward* one's inner experience and outward expression of strong emotions.

 • **Enhancing awareness, subjective experience, and outward expression of emotions.** A variety of interventions are used in CBCT to enhance the emotional experiences of inhibited individuals (Epstein & Baucom, 2002). When a member of a couple describes experiencing little emotion, one possible reason is past experiences (in the family of origin, past couple relationships, or the current relationship) in which self-expression led to negative consequences. To create a safe environment for awareness and expression of feelings, the therapist can set explicit guidelines for the couple's behavior within and outside of sessions, in which partners are not allowed to punish each other for expressing themselves. In addition, when an individual lacks experience in paying attention to inner thoughts and emotions, the therapist can use downward-arrow questioning to inquire about such reactions to particular experiences with a partner. The therapist also can engage the individual in imagery and role plays focused on issues in the couple's relationship that may elicit emotional responses. This process of enhancing self-awareness or "psychological mindedness" can be facilitated by coaching the individual in noticing internal cues to emotional states such as bodily sensations. Because some clients tend to use cognitive and behavioral strategies to avoid experiencing aversive emotions, therapists can refocus their attention on emotionally relevant topics when they attempt to change the topic with their partner, engage in distracting behavior, and the like, while conveying empathy for the person's distress and encouraging gradual exposure to uncomfortable feelings. Because an individual may not disclose their discomfort with their partner's presence in the session, the therapist should monitor nonverbal cues of partners' emotional responses to each other and inquire about them.

• **Increasing regulation of the internal experience and outward expression of strong emotions.** Gottman (1994) identified some couples who have "volatile" but stable relationships, experiencing both positive and negative intense emotional exchanges. However, other couples that include one or both members with degrees of poor emotion regulation are at risk for severe conflict, distress, and partner aggression (Epstein, LaTaillade, & Werlinich, 2023; Fruzzetti & Payne, 2015). Those couples are in need of assistance with managing intense emotional responses. In CBCT, therapists can use a combination of interventions that focus on situational constraints on emotional responses and intrapsychic strategies. Regarding the structuring of situations in which emotions are experienced and expressed, therapists can guide couples in scheduling specific times and places when they will discuss distressing topics, while avoiding such discussions at other times. They also can teach couples how to use a time-out in which either partner is allowed to announce that the tension level between them has risen and to suggest a "cool-down" break. Partners also are taught to use constructive skills for expressing their emotions when they reunite after the time-out. Emotion-regulation strategies that focus on internal experiences can include coaching the couple in self-soothing activities such as progressive muscle relaxation, exercising, taking a warm shower, or talking with a calming person. Acceptance-focused techniques can be used to develop partners' abilities to tolerate distressing feelings. Interventions that target unregulated emotions commonly are integrated with cognitive interventions that improve partners' ability to monitor and modify their thoughts that elicit strong emotions, such as stress inoculation techniques described by Meichenbaum (1977).

APPLICATION OF CBCT TO INDIVIDUAL PHYSICAL AND MENTAL HEALTH ISSUES AND SEVERE RELATIONAL PROBLEMS

CBCT has evolved from its early focus on improving the ratio of pleasing to displeasing behavioral interactions between members of a couple, with enhanced global relationship satisfaction the goal, to a model applied to a variety of complex relational and individual functioning problems. On the one hand, it provides sophisticated concepts and methods for understanding and intervening with each partner's internal cognitive and emotional experiences. On the other hand, its dyadic approach to the mutual influences between the two partners' cognitions, emotional responses, and behaviors makes it a flexible systemic model for treating complex relational problems.

CBCT increasingly has been applied to presenting problems in individual functioning (e.g., alcohol abuse, depression, anxiety disorders, eating disorders) that previously were treated only with individual therapy. Such systemic approaches are based on evidence from both cross-sectional and longitudinal research studies of a bidirectional association between relationship distress and a variety of psychopathology symptoms (Baucom, Whisman, & Paprocki, 2012). In addition, individual therapies for psychopathology commonly do not improve partners' relationship satisfaction (Whisman, 2001). Furthermore, a partner's attempts to be supportive and caring may inadvertently reinforce an individual's maladaptive behavior, as when a partner makes it easier for an agoraphobic individual to avoid feared situations by taking over the individual's tasks that involve going outside the home.

Typically, couple-based treatments integrate traditional interventions for the individual's symptoms with couple therapy interventions to reduce aversive interactions that exacerbate the symptoms and to improve mutual support between partners. For example, programs for alcohol abuse by Birchler, Fals-Stewart, and O'Farrell (2008) and McCrady, Epstein, and Holzhauer (2023) combine interventions for the individual's substance use (e.g., self-help meetings, medication, dealing with urges, drink refusal training) with behavioral couple therapy procedures (e.g., increasing exchanges of pleasing behavior, improving communication and problem-solving skills) to decrease negative couple interactions and enhance mutual emotional support. Couple-based interventions also have been developed for depression (Baucom, Fischer, Corrie, Worrell, & Boeding, 2020; Beach, Dreifuss, Franklin, Kamen, & Gabriel, 2008; Whisman, Beach, & Davila, 2023), anxiety disorders (Chambless, 2012), posttraumatic stress disorder (Monson & Fredman, 2012, 2023), obsessive–compulsive disorder (Abramowitz et al., 2013), and anorexia nervosa (Bulik, Baucom, & Kirby, 2012). In addition, Baucom, Porter, et al. (2009) developed a CBCT-based program for women suffering from breast cancer and their partners that includes training in communication and problem-solving skills that partners use to address cancer-related topics such as medical decisions, sexuality, and fear of mortality. Conjoint interventions can help couples cope with a variety of physical health problems (Baucom, Porter, Kirby, & Hudepohl, 2012).

Protocols that involve partners in the treatment of individuals' psychological problems tend to fall into three categories (Baucom et al., 2023; Epstein & Baucom, 2002). In *partner-assisted intervention*, the partner of a symptomatic individual also receives psychoeducation about the disorder during couple sessions and serves in a supportive, collaborative role in the identified patient's treatment. Thus, in panic disorder cases both members of the couple receive psychoeducation about the disorder (its causes, symptoms, effects on couple relationships, and effective treatments); both receive interoceptive exposure to conditions that simulate panic symptoms (e.g., breathing through a narrow straw to create sensations of suffocation); and the partner accompanies the anxious individual during *in vivo* exposure exercises to provide encouragement and occasional coaching. In *disorder-specific intervention*, the therapist assesses couple interaction patterns associated with the individual's symptoms, increases their awareness of patterns that may maintain the individual's problem, and coaches them in altering such behavior. Thus, in a case of agoraphobia in which the partner has taken over the symptomatic individual's tasks involving trips outside the home, the therapist would show them how their coping pattern maintains the individual's avoidance and would encourage changes that would increase the individual's autonomous functioning. Finally, in *couple therapy* used to address problems in individual functioning, general conflict and stress in a couple's relationship that elicit or exacerbate the individual's symptoms are targeted. These three couple-based approaches to treating problems in individual psychological functioning are described in Chapter 10.

Regarding CBCT that is tailored to treating specific types of *severe relational problems*, generic assessment and intervention methods (e.g., behavioral observation of dysfunctional communication behavior and coaching of couples in constructive communication) are integrated with interventions for particular types of cognitions, emotional responses and behaviors that are associated with a particular relational problem. For example, Snyder, Baucom, and Gordon (2007) developed a CBT-based program to help couples dealing with infidelity. Research has indicated that revelation of an affair commonly elicits trauma symptoms in the betrayed individual (including cognitive disorientation as their core assumptions about security in the relationship were shattered), severely disrupted equilibrium in the emotional and behavioral functioning of the two members and their relational routines, and potential escalation of aversive behavior between partners. Betrayal-specific responses that must be addressed include hurt, anger, the desire to reestablish some sense of control over one's life, and the need to reconceptualize the characteristics of one's unfaithful partner. Couple therapy is used to stabilize the functioning of the partners and their interactions, to gain insight into factors that led to the affair, and to make constructive decisions about the future of the relationship. This approach is covered in Chapter 6.

CBCT also has been used to treat couples experiencing psychological and mild to moderate physical partner aggression (but not cases of physical battering), common in the general population but especially among couples seeking therapy (Epstein, LaTaillade, & Werlinich, 2023). It targets partners' anger management skills and cognitions that influence aggressive behavior (e.g., a belief in retribution toward a partner who was hurtful), as well as dyadic interactions that exacerbate couple conflict, such as negative reciprocity. CBCT and solution-focused couple interventions have been found to be safe and effective (LaTaillade, Epstein, & Werlinich, 2006; O'Leary, 2015; Stith, McCollum, & Rosen, 2011). Chapter 5 describes CBCT for partner aggression.

Cognitive-behavioral concepts and clinical methods have long been core components of sex therapy programs, and CBCT provides a systemic approach to working with couples with a variety of sexual problems (Metz, Epstein, & McCarthy, 2018). It addresses both the intrapsychic components of sexual disorders involving desire, arousal, and orgasm and dyadic couple processes that contribute to conflict and sex dysfunction. CBCT for couple sexual problems is described in Chapter 7 of this book.

Interventions to improve individuals' parenting skills commonly incorporate cognitive-behavioral principles and methods (e.g., Barkley & Benton, 2013; Eyberg et al., 1999; Forgatch, 1994; Kazdin, 2009). However, the parenting role frequently is shared by two or more adults who have responsibility for a child's care and upbringing (McHale & Lindhal, 2011), and the success of co-parenting depends on the quality of the alliance between the caregivers. Chapter 9 describes a CBCT approach to enhancing a couple's co-parenting relationship.

Because financial issues are among the most prevalent challenges that couples face together, couple therapists are highly likely to encounter couples who are experiencing financial stress and conflict. Although financial counseling and money management are specialized areas of expertise that lie outside the domain of couple therapy, partners who are experiencing financial stress and conflict commonly can benefit from intervention with their relational dynamics associated with money. Chapter 8 focuses on CBCT for relational aspects of couples' financial issues.

Finally, the increasing diversity of couple characteristics in clinicians' caseloads includes intercultural couples, who commonly present with some relational dynamics associated with partners' cultural differences. Clinicians need to be prepared to address issues associated with each individual's cultural background (e.g., beliefs and traditions regarding partners' appropriate roles in a relationship, discrimination experiences of minoritized group members), as well as challenges the couple experiences dyadically as they navigate their cultural differences. Chapter 11 describes characteristics of intercultural couples and associated CBCT assessment and treatment planning.

STRUCTURAL CHARACTERISTICS OF CBCT

Cognitive-behavioral therapies in general have been described in the extensive clinical literature as highly structured approaches with clearly defined roles for the therapist and clients. This level of structure was derived in part from the empirical perspective that is prominent in the model, in which the clinician conducts a systematic functional analysis of factors that influence the occurrence of problematic symptoms, designs interventions to modify the controlling conditions, and uses the most objective data available to evaluate the outcomes of treatments. The emphasis on empiricism includes a strong tradition of controlled studies investigating the effects of cognitive-behavioral treatments. High-quality efficacy trials require standardized treatment protocols with manuals of procedures that trained therapists follow in sessions, as well as random assignment of clients to treatment and control groups. Although those types of control strengthen the internal validity of the studies, they minimize clinical flexibility as therapists work with clients presenting diverse problems and personal characteristics.

Consequently, books and journal articles describing empirically supported cognitive-behavioral treatments tend to portray highly structured treatments with little apparent room for the operation of *common factors* involving the characteristics of therapists (e.g., warmth, empathy), clients (e.g., motivation to change), and the therapeutic alliance that have been found to account for a large percentage of variance in client improvement in individual and couple therapies (Sprenkle, Davis, & Lebow, 2009). However, in actual clinical practice, therapists have much more leeway to tailor validated interventions to the needs and characteristics of each individual or couple. Certain structural aspects of sessions are standard procedures in CBCT, beginning with the therapist initiating each session by briefly setting an agenda collaboratively with the couple regarding topics to be covered, and ending with the therapist recapping what was covered during the session, inquiring into what the clients found helpful or unhelpful, and collaborating with the partners to devise one or more homework tasks that they will carry out before the next session. Nevertheless, therapists use their personal styles in relating to their clients and introducing CBCT concepts and methods. We strongly believe in using empirically supported treatments, but we consider common factors to be essential for effective therapy. We always have CBCT concepts in our heads, but we express them in sessions in diverse ways that are designed to meet each person's needs. In Chapter 2, which focuses on how one conducts couple therapy, and throughout this book, we describe concepts and methods that can guide treatment planning. We emphasize the roles of clinical assessment and judgment in establishing strong alliances with couples and in designing individualized treatment plans that will assist them in achieving their personal goals.

INTEGRATING CBCT WITH OTHER COUPLE AND FAMILY THERAPY THEORETICAL ORIENTATIONS

As we noted previously, for decades a large percentage of practicing couple and family therapists have been using CBCT methods (Northey, 2002). The systems theory aspects of CBCT and simultaneous attention to partners' cognitions, emotions, and behavioral interactions make it a highly integrative model that is compatible with a variety of other systems-focused couple and family therapy models that include core concepts involving partners' thoughts, emotional responses, and behavioral patterns (Dattilio, 2010). The attention that CBCT pays to partners' intrapsychic experiences involving cognition and emotion (and roots of current responses in individuals' past experiences in family of origin and other significant relationships), as well as current circular processes in couple behavioral interactions, makes it compatible with a variety of other models. Benson, McGinn, and Christensen (2012) identified core principles or processes that are common to evidence-based couple therapies, and they are closely related to the CBCT domains of cognition, affect, and behavioral interaction. Those processes include altering partners' views of their presenting problems to be more objective and dyadic (in contrast to distressed partners' common global blaming of each other), decreasing emotion-driven dysfunctional behaviors (such as partner aggression), uncovering emotion-based avoided behavior (such as partners' avoidance of intimate interactions based on anxiety), increasing constructive communication, and emphasizing relationship strengths. Given these common elements across models, interventions from a variety of models can be used to produce change in a common aspect of couples' relationships. In the couple therapy field, alternative models may target a similar aspect of a relationship that has been identified as contributing to a presenting problem but may prescribe somewhat different interventions to achieve that goal. For example, a pattern in which one member of a couple aggressively pursues the other while the partner actively withdraws can be addressed with diverse interventions from structural, emotion-focused, solution-focused, cognitive-behavioral, and other couple therapy models. Therapists may use different interventions even though they share a view that members of the couple failed to find a mutually comfortable way of meeting their respective intimacy needs.

Furthermore, a therapist may conceptualize couple problems with constructs from another model but use CBCT interventions to enact change. For example, a structural family therapist likely thinks in terms of boundary issues when hearing that a couple argues about the degree to which one of the members shares information about the couple's relationship with friends. A boundary is a concept that people tend to define in terms of partners' interactions with each other and other people, as well as each individual's standards about the appropriateness of those behaviors. In this case, the couple's conflict was based on the gap between the partners' beliefs about how much information about their relationship should be shared with other people, especially when one person's actions violate the other's standard. Structural interventions could be integrated with CBCT approaches to having partners use constructive communication and problem-solving skills to discuss their conflict. Thus, this book emphasizes a CBCT approach to treatment planning, but we believe that the methods described in each chapter can be useful to therapists from other theoretical orientations in conceptualizing a variety of interventions to achieve therapy goals for their clients. In each chapter on a particular presenting problem, we focus on CBCT assessment and interventions, but we often point out how concepts and methods from other therapy models can be applied.

RESEARCH SUPPORT FOR CBCT

CBCT is a couple therapy model that has been identified as empirically supported from treatment outcome studies (e.g., Baucom et al., 1998; Fischer, Baucom, & Cohen, 2016; Lebow & Snyder, 2022). Most studies have focused primarily on the standard CBCT behavioral interventions of communication skill training, problem-solving training, and some form of planned positive behavior exchanges (e.g., contracts), with much less attention to interventions targeting cognitions and emotional responses. Most outcome studies have examined the *efficacy* of treatment in controlled settings with randomized assignment of couples to treatments, a set number of sessions across treatment and control groups, and training of therapists in the treatment protocols, rather than their *effectiveness* in naturalistic clinical settings. Meta-analyses (e.g., Shadish & Baldwin, 2003, 2005) indicated that, overall, treatments that included interventions for cognitions and those restricted to behavioral interventions have produced large effect sizes for improvement in relationship satisfaction. Shadish and Baldwin's (2005) meta-analysis of 30 studies comparing behavioral couple therapy to no-treatment control groups found an effect size of 0.59 in favor of the therapy. Fischer et al.'s (2016) review indicated that behaviorally based couple therapies, some of which included cognitive interventions, had an average effect size of 0.84, similar to the effects found for other therapy models. Christensen and colleagues' randomized clinical trial (Christensen et al., 2004) compared integrative behavioral couple therapy (IBCT), which combines interventions to increase partners' acceptance of each other with communication and problem-solving training to facilitate change (Christensen, Dimidjian, Martell, & Doss, 2023; Jacobson & Christensen, 1996), and what the investigators label "traditional behavioral couple therapy" (TBCT), which is the model developed by Jacobson and Margolin (1979) and others. The two treatments showed somewhat different rates of improvement in relationship satisfaction, but the outcomes were for the most part similar, with large effect sizes of 0.90 for IBCT and 0.71 for TBCT at the end of treatment, which were not significantly different (Christensen et al., 2004). In a 5-year follow-up, Christensen, Atkins, Baucom, and Yi (2010) found even larger effect sizes for improvement in relationship satisfaction of 1.03 for IBCT and 0.92 for TBCT, with 50.0% of IBCT couples and 45.9% of TBCT couples reaching clinically significant improvement according to the index proposed by Jacobson and Truax (1991).

Two studies conducted by Baucom and colleagues (Baucom & Lester, 1986; Baucom, Sayers, & Sher, 1990) investigated whether adding cognitive restructuring modules to TBCT would enhance the outcomes. However, in order to keep the total number of sessions constant, adding sessions of cognitive restructuring necessitated reducing the number of sessions of behavioral interventions. All treatments increased relationship satisfaction more than a waitlist condition, and the cognitive and behavioral interventions were equally effective. There also was some evidence that cognitively focused interventions tended to produce more cognitive change.

Although no further studies on the overall effects of CBCT for improving relationship satisfaction have been conducted, studies we described earlier that tested CBCT protocols that include cognitive and affective as well as behavioral interventions with specific types of severe relationship problems and individual psychopathology have been promising. For example, cognitive-behavioral programs for treating couples experiencing psychological partner aggression and mild to moderate physical aggression (see Chapter 5) have received support through initial efficacy studies (Epstein et al., 2023; Heyman & Neidig, 1997; LaTaillade et al., 2006). The protocol tested by Epstein and colleagues, which included interventions for cognitions, regulation of anger, and behavior, increased relationship satisfaction, decreased psychological partner aggression, decreased males' use of physical aggression and showed a trend toward a decrease in females' physical aggression, reduced negative attributions about one's partner, increased overall trust in the partner, decreased anxiety and increased positive moods prior to engaging in a conflict resolution discussion with one's partner, and decreased negative communication by both males and females during the couple discussion (Hrapczynski, Epstein, Werlinich, & LaTaillade, 2011; Kahn, Epstein, & Kivlighan, 2015; LaTaillade et al., 2006). Furthermore, Chapter 10 reviews the promising effects of CBCT for forms of individual psychopathology.

Unfortunately, no further outcome studies have been done in isolating the independent effects of interventions focused on modifying partners' negative cognitions and emotional responses, so the existing encouraging results must be considered preliminary. The absence of dismantling studies examining the relative effects of interventions for cognitions, emotional responses, and behaviors likely is due to the complexity and expense of such designs, especially when funding for couple therapy studies is scarce. Furthermore, the vast majority of research has been conducted on Western, middle-class, cisgender, heterosexual couples. Studies with more diverse samples will be essential to fully gauge the breadth of CBCT effectiveness.

KEY POINTS

- CBCT provides therapists a comprehensive and flexible framework for understanding and treating a variety of behavioral, cognitive, and emotional characteristics contributing to problems in intimate relationships.

- CBCT strikes a balance between structure in the assessment and treatment planning process and opportunities for clinicians to use their joining skills creatively to develop a strong collaborative therapeutic alliance with members of the couple to alleviate distressing presenting problems.

- Clinicians who primarily adhere to other theoretical orientations can integrate CBCT concepts and methods into their work with clients.

- Therapists must be attuned to clients' cultural identities, including experiences of discrimination and marginalization that had major impacts on many clients' lives.

- The interplay between two individuals' personal histories and current intrapsychic experiences and the couple's circular behavioral interactions provide opportunities and pathways for intervention. Therapists need expertise both in systemic concepts and methods and in intervention with individual psychological processes.

CHAPTER 2

Conducting Couple Therapy

This book is intended to be useful in the treatment planning process for couple therapists with all levels of experience and expertise. However, individuals who are in the early stages of their clinical training and those who have more extensive experience but primarily with individual therapy may benefit more than veteran couple therapists from this chapter's overview of professional and clinical issues that commonly arise in working with dyads. Yet, we believe that highly experienced therapists will still find it useful to read this chapter, as it sets the stage for the following chapters, which are devoted to treatment planning for specific presenting problems within our CBCT framework. For less experienced clinicians, we intend to draw attention to dynamics that commonly occur when intervening directly as a couple's dynamics unfold in front of the therapist, and to help the therapist feel comfortable making clinical decisions.

WHO SEEKS COUPLE THERAPY?

One of the common issues that motivate people to seek individual therapy is stress associated with their couple and family relationships. The individual therapy context is a setting in which one's hopes, goals, disappointments, and alternative choices for one's intimate relationships can be explored. However, couple therapy is a collaborative treatment available to two individuals who are involved in a romantic relationship and wish to work together in conjoint sessions on making changes in the ways they relate to each other. The focus frequently is on improving the quality of their interactions that have deteriorated from a more mutually satisfying previous state, although some couples primarily seek assistance with coping jointly with one partner's mental or physical health problem. In either case, couple therapy assessment and treatment procedures focus directly on the dyad rather than solely on each individual's experiences in the relationship. As we describe throughout this book, conjoint couple therapy has significant advantages over individual therapy for addressing relationship problems. As initially documented by Gurman and Kniskern (1978), couple therapy is the more effective modality for treating distressed relationships.

Couple therapy does not always begin with an explicit request for such joint services by both members of a couple who have agreed to work on their relationship. The following describes a variety of circumstances that may lead to dyadic treatment.

- **One partner is motivated to engage in couple therapy, but the other is not, or even does not know that the other person is seeking therapy.** In these situations, the therapist can discuss with the requesting partner (during the individual's initial phone inquiry regarding treatment or during an in-person pretherapy assessment session) possible approaches to encourage the other partner to start couple therapy. For example, the therapist could ask the person who called to invite the other partner to contact the therapist so that they could have a conversation about the characteristics of couple therapy. This conversation might be used to identify any concerns that the other partner has about the process of therapy. For example, some individuals fear that the therapist will "dig into" the couple's unresolved issues and worsen their relationship. The therapist also can clarify that the goal of couple therapy is not to press for partners to stay together regardless of the quality of their relationship. Rather, it is to help them explore strategies that may improve the relationship, taking both partners' perspectives and experiences into account and ultimately leaving the decision of whether to stay together with the two individuals. The therapist also can reduce pressure that either partner may feel by suggesting that they meet a few times and then decide whether they are interested in continuing couple therapy.

In some cases, the person who approaches a therapist individually and portrays their partner as unmotivated for couple therapy in fact is uneasy about joint sessions because they fear that the partner may present a negative picture of them to the therapist. This possibility sometimes is apparent when the therapist explores the option of the client or therapist discussing couple therapy with the absent partner and the client balks at the suggestion. The therapist then can inquire about what the individual imagines would occur if the partner joins the sessions, especially if the individual anticipates aversive experiences. Such concerns commonly can be reduced by reassurance from the therapist that they will take responsibility for keeping aversive interactions during sessions under control and will guide the couple toward constructive "teamwork" in improving their relationship.

- **One partner seeks individual therapy, but the presenting issues are partner related.** Sometimes individuals seek therapy solely for themselves because their most prominent symptoms are global emotional distress (e.g., depression, anxiety), and their most immediate goal is to feel better on a daily basis. Even though they may be aware that issues in their couple relationship influence their overall well-being, they may not have thought of couple therapy as an appropriate and realistic pathway to feeling better. Many people have little knowledge about the substantial research evidence regarding the negative impact of relationship problems on partners' psychological well-being. In addition, lay conceptions of "couple counseling" commonly involve a stereotyped notion of a professional listening to partners' complaints about each other, making judgments about who is "right" during disagreements, and giving them detailed instructions for ways to improve their relationship. Consequently, the individuals avoid such an experience by seeking individual therapy, perhaps after receiving a prescription for antidepressant medication from a physician. However, as the therapist conducts an assessment, it becomes clear that intimate relationship issues are contributing to the emotional distress, and couple therapy, either as an adjunct to individual therapy or even as the primary intervention, would be appropriate.

In such situations, therapists may suggest couple therapy, as long as it is deemed safe for both partners, providing the individual psychoeducation about the effects of relationship problems on individual physical and psychological well-being, as well as generic descriptions of goals and methods of couple therapy. As noted in the previous scenario, if the individual voices concerns about that option, their concerns should be discussed thoroughly, and therapists should not pressure anyone into pursuing couple therapy. If the individual agrees to couple therapy, the therapist should plan with the client how to proceed. When the clinician specializes in individual therapy, this involves a discussion of appropriate couple therapist referrals, but if the clinician is skilled at working with couples, the focus can shift to how to involve the other partner. In either case, it is important to explain the ethical issues regarding dual relationships that generally preclude a clinician from serving as both a couple therapist and an individual therapist for a member of the couple. Before proceeding, it is important to explain to the person who initially sought individual treatment how individual and couple therapies differ and how the treatment will change once the other partner joins the sessions.

A common next step is for the client to invite their partner to join a future session, preferably as soon as possible in order to prevent the client from developing a significant individual relationship with the therapist that could unbalance the couple therapy. In the event that the nonattending partner is reluctant to come to therapy, the therapist could discuss approaches to encourage the partner to participate and might even suggest a brief individual phone conversation with that partner to discuss any concerns they may have. Therapists should obtain written consent from the person who initially sought individual treatment that authorizes speaking with their partner.

• **Relationship issues emerge after several individual therapy sessions.** As we have noted, in general it is recommended that individual therapists do not become the couple's therapist, as this may create an imbalance in the therapeutic alliance, including the therapist's ability to understand the two partners' perspectives and experiences equally. Unless the clinician has only seen the individual client for very few sessions (even long ago), it is advisable that the individual therapist makes a referral to a couple therapist. Before exchanging information with the couple therapist, the therapist obtains written consent from the individual client.

• **Couple relationship issues emerge in the context of family therapy.** Sometimes in family therapy sessions, it becomes evident that the parental subsystem may benefit from focused work. Although it is common in family therapy to assist parents in working more collaboratively and effectively in their roles as leaders of the family, therapists also often identify problems in the overall couple relationship that "spill" into their parenting roles.

When parents are motivated to work on their relationship issues, couple therapy can be recommended. They may voice a preference that the family therapist will become their couple therapist rather than beginning all over again with a new person. One advantage of having a therapist work with both the family system and the couple subsystem is that it allows the therapist to develop a more systemic view of the family's dynamics. However, serving as both the family therapist and the couple therapist creates challenges. This is another situation that has the potential to create dual relationship issues for the clinician, and the decision of whether to refer them to someone else for couple therapy will depend on the family therapist discussing with the couple ways in which dual relationship processes can arise, as well as safeguards that the therapist and couple would need to implement to avoid that (e.g., explicit communication about what material from couple sessions can be shared in family sessions). The therapist should try to keep the treatments separate, reflected in the maintenance of two separate case files.

Despite such efforts, the boundary between the treatments can become blurred when the therapist has difficulty identifying what material should be addressed in each treatment modality. For example, issues such as infidelity and limited couple sexual intimacy typically should be addressed in couple therapy sessions. However, even in some such cases the issue might spill into the family system, as when a betrayed individual has attempted to draw the children into an alliance against the unfaithful spouse by divulging the infidelity to them. Although most of the work must be done in couple therapy, it may be necessary to address the alliance and its effects on the children in one or more family sessions. In contrast, when a therapist observes that a power issue between partners affects their parenting, it might seem that this is a family-level issue. However, shielding the children from distressing exposure to couple conflict may require drawing a firm boundary between couple and child subsystems and restricting discussion of power struggles to the couple therapy. Whenever sharing content across modalities is clinically indicated, it cannot take place without explicit discussion with the clients about the associated risks and benefits and obtaining their authorization to share information.

INDIVIDUAL AND CONJOINT SESSIONS IN COUPLE THERAPY

An individual session with each partner (perhaps more than one session, depending on the scope of the material that surfaces regarding each person) usually is recommended in the initial stage of couple therapy as part of the assessment process. These sessions focus on safety, each person's commitment to work on the relationship, and potential individual issues (e.g., substance abuse, psychopathology symptoms, prior traumatic life experiences that influence current functioning, suicidality). The structure of the individual assessment sessions is discussed in detail in Chapter 3. The assessment chapter also addresses the possibility of ad hoc individual meetings with each partner later during treatment whenever there is a need for further assessment of individual issues (e.g., if a current experience in the couple relationship triggered posttraumatic stress disorder [PTSD] symptoms in a member who was traumatized earlier in life) or regarding topics that are safer to address first individually (e.g., ongoing physical aggression and fear of one's partner).

In addition, either partner may request to meet individually with the therapist at any time during the therapy process. Clinical judgment should be involved in deciding when to schedule such a session and how to handle the information provided in those individual meetings. As a general guideline, whenever an individual session is offered or granted to one partner, the possibility for a similar meeting should be offered to the other partner, with the objective of keeping the therapeutic alliance and treatment balanced.

In individual meetings, clients may share information that is unrelated to the couple relationship (e.g., frustration with a co-worker at one's job) or that does not seem to have an impact on the conjoint couple therapy work. However, individual sessions often include the discussion of issues that are related to the couple relationship, either directly (e.g., the individual's sadness about feeling decreased love for the partner) or indirectly (e.g., the individual's grief over the recent death of a parent is affecting their emotional availability to the partner).

Risen (2010) has described an important distinction between *private* information that individuals keep to themselves (e.g., having periodic sexual fantasies about a neighbor) and that has no significant deleterious effect on the couple's relationship, and *secrets* that involve information about the individual (e.g., involvement in an affair) that does detract from the couple's relationship. We concur with Risen that individuals have a right to privacy, and their decision to share what can be considered private information with a couple therapist need not create a dilemma for the clinician. In contrast, because both partners are the therapist's clients and the clinician bears ethical responsibilities toward both individuals, it is important for the therapist not to hold secrets about conditions that, from the secret-keeper's report, are influencing the couple's relationship and the viability of couple therapy significantly. For example, if during a one-on-one session devoted to gaining information about each individual's personal history and psychological functioning (see Chapter 3, on assessment) a member of a married couple reveals periodically fantasizing about a neighbor but expresses strong commitment to the spouse, the therapist likely will feel comfortable briefly exploring whether the attraction reflects a deficit in the couple's relationship that could be addressed by increasing shared activities and communication. In that case, keeping the information private poses no notable barrier to couple therapy. In contrast, if the individual reveals an ongoing affair to the therapist, reports a desire or actual plan to leave the spouse for the other person, and requests that the therapist keep the secret, the individual's implied lack of motivation to try to improve the marriage is highly likely to undercut the couple therapy, creating an ethical dilemma for the therapist regarding maintenance of confidentiality. We discuss the handling of such secrets in Chapter 6 on couple therapy for infidelity. Mark and Schuman (2020) provide further discussion of the couple therapist's task of balancing ethical principles and clinical judgment in making decisions regarding keeping and divulging secrets.

Another important circumstance that raises issues regarding confidentiality for the individual members of a couple occurs when an individual reveals dangerous conditions within the relationship, such as being physically abused by a partner and being at risk for further harm if the partner learns that the individual told the therapist about it. When a therapist learns of partner abuse, the safety of a victimized individual becomes paramount, and conducting joint couple therapy sessions can increase the risk of further harm. Consequently, a traditional stance taken by clinicians who learn about ongoing or past intimate partner violence, either during a joint couple session or during an individual session with a victim, is to refuse to conduct couple therapy. Complicating this issue further, a therapist who declines to work with a couple jointly based on information revealed by a victim during an individual session is faced with protecting the victim by not disclosing to the abuser that the victim revealed the violence. In Chapter 5 on partner aggression, we discuss this ethical issue in more detail and describe strategies that couple therapists can use to minimize risk.

Overall, when a member of a couple has disclosed private or secret information during an individual session, the therapist needs to discuss with that person how the issues are influencing the discloser and the couple relationship. The therapist also needs to evaluate the level of risk, as well as any benefits, that would occur if the discloser raised the topic in a conjoint session with the other partner present. For example, if the individual reveals that they have made a decision to separate from the partner in the near future, the therapist should inquire about what has prevented the client from sharing this major decision with the partner and how this could be addressed in conjoint sessions. Difficult situations such as when there has been a violation of trust (e.g., affairs; hidden financial issues), strong reluctance to be transparent (e.g., regarding sexual orientation, gender identity), or intense feelings of shame (e.g., about past sexual abuse victimization) may require a number of individual meetings to discuss how to best address those issues in front of one's partner. The therapist should never bring up in conjoint sessions content that was revealed in individual sessions without the individual's authorization (preferably in writing) to reveal the information. Furthermore, when it is deemed safe and appropriate for an individual to share private or secret information with the partner, the therapist should always try to facilitate a process in which it is the client who reveals the information.

Partners sometimes request individual sessions only to vent their frustrations, complain about the other person's behaviors, or speak more about how they experience their couple relationship.

In those circumstances the couple therapist explores what prevents the client from sharing such views in the conjoint sessions, encourages the individual to share their experiences and perspectives in front of the other partner, and discusses strategies to do so. Often the individual predicts an aversive response from the partner, so the therapist provides reassurance that they are committed to maintaining a safe and constructive atmosphere during conjoint sessions. During the initial session with any couple, the therapist stresses that it is essential that both partners feel safe in couple therapy, which requires that each person be able to express personal thoughts and emotions without concern that the other will punish them for it during the session or later at home.

THERAPY CONTRACT

Establishing a therapy contract involves providing a written contract and consent document that describes (1) the characteristics, goals, and process of couple therapy; (2) the ethical principles applied to couple therapy such as procedures for maintaining confidentiality; (3) an overview of the clinician's theoretical model and training, (4) policies and expectations regarding fees, payment methods, cancellation policies, billing, and communication outside the session; and (5) guidelines for emergency situations. As is true in the ethical conduct of all forms of therapy, it is crucial that therapists devote sufficient time to discussing the therapy contract, which is sometimes mistakenly viewed only as "paperwork" until a client's misunderstanding or forgetting of a key component such as the therapist's position against holding secrets leads to a serious clinical quagmire. People may decide not to pursue couple therapy after better understanding the characteristics of the service and the rights and responsibilities of each party, including both partners and the therapist. Therapists should ensure that their proposed contract is consistent with state laws and the code of ethics of the therapist's professional affiliation (e.g., American Psychological Association, National Association of Social Workers, American Association for Marriage and Family Therapy, and American Counseling Association).

Handout 2.1 (available on the book's web page at *www.guilford.com/epstein-materials*) is a sample template for a couple therapy contract and consent form. However, the therapist should discuss two additional topics with the couple when contracting for therapy: individual diagnosis in third-party billing and teletherapy services when relevant. When third-party billing is involved, therapists should discuss with clients whether a relationship and/or individual diagnosis will be required. Some insurance companies accept an ICD-10 or DSM-5 relational diagnosis (i.e., relational conflict and distress) without requiring that either partner meet the criteria for an individual diagnosis, but other companies only reimburse for treatment that involves a diagnosed identified patient. It is essential that the therapist discuss these parameters of diagnoses with the couple and with the individual who will qualify as the identified patient.

When therapy services will not be provided in the therapist's office but will be technology assisted, therapists need to ensure that they are compliant with their professional code of ethics and guidelines for the practice of teletherapy (e.g., American Association for Marriage and Family Therapy, 2017) as well as with federal laws and regulations of the states where the therapist is licensed, where the therapist will be physically located when rendering services, and where the client is physically located when receiving services. It is beyond the scope of the present book to cover all aspects related to the practice of online couple therapy, but at a minimum the therapy contract should include a description of the risks and benefits of online therapy, the availability of alternative treatment modes, the appropriateness of teletherapy for treating relationships, and the therapist's electronic systems used to protect clients' privacy and security. The therapist should also make clear in the contract whether such services will be provided when partners are in two different locations and/or when one partner can be in the therapist's office and the other cannot.

The consent procedure should include warnings about potential technology failure and steps to follow for reconnection and continuation or ending of a therapy session. Furthermore, the consent form should raise the possibility of breaches of confidentiality, as well as the impact of such failures on the therapy process. Given those warnings, the therapist should discuss with the couple the steps that would be taken to address such failures if they ever occur. The therapist should explain that the critical role of observing partners' interactions for assessment and intervention in couple therapy is more limited in an online environment. Nevertheless, therapists should inform clients about existing research supporting the effectiveness of telehealth delivery of couple therapy and relationship education programs (Doss, Knopp, Wrape, & Morland, 2023; Falconier, Kim, & Lachowicz, 2023), and group multi-couple therapy for low sexual desire (Kleinplatz, Charest, Paradis, Rosen, & Ramsay, 2022). Therapists should also explain when online services may not be appropriate for couples (e.g., if there is physical and/or severe psychological aggression) and should advise that the therapist may decide to discontinue the online modality if it is not clinically appropriate for the couple. The therapist should also describe expectations regarding clients' conduct and acceptable locations for their participation, to protect their privacy and safety as well as professional boundaries. These expectations may include clients having cameras on at all times so that the therapist can see them, disclosing their locations, choosing locations that are safe and private, and so on. Overall, clients should be informed that their behavior and attire should be comparable to what is expected in in-person therapy sessions.

THE ROLE OF THE COUPLE THERAPIST

The role of the couple therapist is usually to assist clients in working through their presenting issues by assessing their strengths and the challenges they face both within their relationship and from external circumstances, developing treatment goals and plans, and implementing interventions that help them achieve their goals. In couple therapy, the clinician has additional tasks based on working with two individuals who are likely to seek somewhat different changes in their relationship. Those aspects of the couple therapist's role involve:

• **Facilitating understanding between the partners.** The therapist focuses on helping partners understand each other's perspectives, emotions, and experiences. Understanding one's partner (especially their basic human needs and sources of emotional pain) may reduce negative attributions about the other's motives and traits and therefore, hostility toward the partner. It can increase compassion, empathy, and therefore emotional connection and intimacy. Viewing one's partner less as an adversary can increase motivation to make personal changes and/or accept some characteristics of the partner.

• **Maintaining a multipartial position toward the partners.** Multipartiality (Anderson, 2007) is not about bringing neutrality or objectivity into a discussion; rather, it is the therapist's ability to understand both partners' perspectives and experiences as they engage in conflict and to avoid taking sides. This is a major reason why the couple therapist makes the therapy process transparent to the partners, including the stance of not holding secrets.

• **Balancing time so that the partners have similar opportunities to express themselves during conjoint sessions and any individual sessions.** The therapist should explicitly state the goal of maintaining an atmosphere in which neither partner feels that the therapist is biased toward one of them. A concrete way of accomplishing that goal is to balance partners' opportunities to express their thoughts and feelings.

• **Managing partners' interactions in the session in ways that support the therapy process and create a safe atmosphere.** As we described earlier, it is critical to monitor couple interactions during sessions, looking for opportunities to enhance constructive interactions, and blocking and changing harmful exchanges that undermine progress (Epstein & Baucom, 2002). The interventions that promote positive interactions, perceptions, and emotional responses are described in Chapter 3 and in subsequent chapters on specific presenting problems.

ESTABLISHING THE THERAPEUTIC ALLIANCE IN COUPLE THERAPY

As described in Chapter 1, research has shown that the therapeutic alliance plays a critical role in therapy outcomes (e.g., Martin, Garske, & Davis, 2000; Quinn, Dotson, & Jordan, 1997; Raytek, McGrady, Epstein, & Hirsch, 1999; Sprenkle et al., 2009). The therapist's ability to establish and maintain a strong alliance with both partners is fundamental not only for positive outcomes but also for the continuation of treatment (Knobloch-Fedders, Pinsof, & Mann, 2004; Sprenkle et al., 2009). Creating and maintaining a therapeutic alliance can be more challenging than when working with one client, as each partner may try to lead the therapist to side with them against the other. The clinician can facilitate a balanced alliance at the outset of treatment by discussing with the couple the importance of the therapist demonstrating understanding and respect for both partners' needs and perspectives. One can overtly invite the couple to provide feedback about one's degree of success in remaining multipartial ("how well I'm paying adequate attention to your partner as well as to you"), as it may reduce partners' temptation to pressure the therapist to take sides.

Similar to other therapy modalities, couple therapists' own attitudes play a significant role in building a strong therapeutic alliance. Remaining curious, nonjudgmental, respectful, ethical, competent, and culturally sensitive are all important ingredients for joining with couples and sustaining that relationship over time.

SELF OF THE THERAPIST

Therapists are considered to have a professional self and a personal self (Kissil, Carneiro, & Aponte, 2018), and it is expected that training in the profession helps them prevent personal life issues from interfering with their clinical work. Self-of-the-therapist issues may stem from family-of-origin experiences, other historical personal experiences (e.g., the therapist's past couple relationships), and present circumstances, but they may also be related to professional burnout or compassion fatigue (Soloski & Deitz, 2016; Timm & Blow, 1999). Relative to psychodynamic approaches in which countertransference or the therapist's personal responses to the client are a significant focus (Freud, 1910), the therapist's potentially biased cognitions about clients and their experiences, as well as emotional activation from session material, have been discussed less regarding cognitive-behavioral approaches to individual therapy. Safran and Segal (1990) emphasized that ruptures to the therapeutic alliance can be repaired more effectively when therapists are aware of their own contributions to problems in the therapist–client relationship and disclose that information to the client. Freeman and McCloskey (2003) noted that a therapist may have some similar cognitive distortions as those of the client or may hold negative beliefs about the degree to which individual or relational dysfunction is amenable to treatment. Leahy (2007) and Cartwright (2011) have focused on countertransference in which the cognitive therapist's personal schemas or core beliefs affect their responses to clients; for example, a therapist who demands perfectionism from oneself in "curing" clients may become frustrated and angry with clients who make limited progress.

Similarly, with the exception of more psychodynamic approaches such as Bowen's intergenerational systems therapy (Kerr & Bowen, 1988), to some extent the relative inattention to self-of-the-therapist responses to clients also has been true for some time in the couple and family therapy field as a whole. However, Harry Aponte's development of the Person-of-the-Therapist Training model (POTT; Aponte & Carlsen, 2009) provided therapists with tools to identify such core personal issues, understand their potential impact in clinical work, and resolve personal issues as needed (Kissil et al., 2018). This focus resulted in the inclusion of the therapist's ability to monitor internal processes and address personal issues that can have a negative impact on therapy as a core clinical competency in the training of couple and family therapists (Commission on Accreditation for Marriage and Family Education, 2004). However, limited attention to self-of-the-therapist responses to clients has been apparent in literature focused on cognitive-behavioral approaches to couples and families.

Couple therapists have known for a long a time that working with more than one individual in a session increases the likelihood that the therapist will react emotionally. The therapist may have personal reactions not only to each partner's material but also to the interaction in the room. There often are tense moments between partners, involving either uncomfortable silence or escalation of conflict. Observing those interactions easily can elicit reactions from the therapist based on personal relationship history (e.g., exposure to intense arguments between their own parents during childhood) and current couple and family relationship issues. Therapists' emotional and behavioral reactions to these moments are important, as they need to serve the goals of therapy rather than the therapist's own emotional needs. For example, a therapist who learned to escape parental conflict as a child may intervene quickly to interrupt a couple's argument, shifting the topic rather than guiding the partners to express themselves in more constructive ways. Similarly, a therapist who has unresolved personal couple sexual issues may avoid asking clients about sexual intimacy and deflect partners' attempts to initiate discussions about sex (Long, Burnett, & Valorie Thomas, 2006). Some therapists may experience discomfort when working with couples of a different sexual orientation, gender identity, race, religion, and the like (Rutter, Leech, Anderson, & Saunders, 2010).

Because such self-of-the-therapist issues can detract from effective couple therapy, it is important that therapists explore their personal triggering topics and situations, monitor their emotional responses to clients, and develop ways to respond that serve clients' clinical needs. Similar to approaches to countertransference used in individual therapy, couple therapists are encouraged to seek personal therapy and/or clinical supervision to manage their emotional responses to couples' characteristics, relationship material and session dynamics.

CULTURAL SENSITIVITY AND SOCIOCULTURAL ATTUNEMENT

Like other mental health professionals, couple therapists are expected to approach their work with cultural sensitivity by (1) increasing their awareness of their beliefs, values, and biases about characteristics of their own and other cultural groups; (2) learning about different cultural groups' traditions and values; and (3) providing culturally sensitive interventions (Sue & Sue, 2003). When clinicians work with couples from cultural backgrounds with expectations and traditions regarding romantic relationships and family life that are different from theirs, they need to understand and be respectful of the clients' cultural values and norms. Therapists need to be aware not only of their own values and beliefs about couple relationships, but also of the implicit values regarding healthy functioning of couple relationships present in the therapy models they use.

For example, in this book we emphasize a cognitive-behavioral approach that includes a focus on couples' cognitions, which include their assumptions and standards about characteristics of intimate relationships. CBCT was developed primarily within a Western cultural tradition that includes a strong value regarding direct, open communication in relationships. Communication training, which historically has been a core behavioral intervention in CBCT, is intended to increase couples' relationship satisfaction and stability by replacing both hostile and avoidant interactions with constructive exchanges of information and mutual empathy. The advantages of such positive communication and of couple communication training interventions have been supported by research conducted mostly in Western cultures (Epstein & Baucom, 2002; Fischer et al., 2016; Gottman, 1994; Shadish & Baldwin, 2005).

One assumption underlying communication training is that couples need to communicate directly and verbally. However, such open verbal communication may not be valued equally across diverse cultures, particularly in cultures that rely less on verbal messages and more on contextual cues (Falconier, Randall, & Bodenmann, 2016). For example, cultural values in China emphasize maintenance of harmony and the avoidance of loss-of-face in relationships, so individuals commonly use indirect messages in which nonverbal behavior and instances of what is *not* said verbally convey key meanings (Epstein et al., 2012). Consequently, therapists need to be aware of the implicit assumptions about couple relationships that underlie their interventions and discuss those assumptions explicitly with client couples. The therapist can have a discussion with the couple about the cultural appropriateness of the proposed interventions, exploring how well the treatment plan fits the partners' cultural values and how comfortable they feel with it. Thus, the therapist and couple could discuss the extent to which communication training (e.g., making "I" statements, empathically reflecting one's partner's thoughts and emotions, avoiding being judgmental) matches the cultural values that have shaped their existing communication style (e.g., avoidance of disagreement based on attempts to maintain harmony). This does not mean the therapist will abandon efforts to promote more open communication to help the couple resolve long-standing conflicts. Rather, the therapist must tactfully and sensitively convey respect for the couple's cultural values while helping the partners communicate differently without feeling that they are violating highly meaningful beliefs and traditions. The therapist could emphasize that communication skills used in CBCT are designed to convey mutual respect and increase harmony between partners, whereas the couple may have noticed that their avoidance of particular conflict topics has resulted in chronic unresolved issues that unfortunately create an underlying lack of harmony. In this way, the couple's values are included in the therapy process in an empowering way that supports aspects of the therapy model.

In addition to couples from different ethnic or cultural backgrounds, therapists may see clients with minority sexual orientations and gender identities. Unfortunately, many clinical training programs still provide most therapy training with cisgender heterosexual individuals and relationships. As a result, therapists have only limited preparation for work with LGBTQ+ clients on their romantic relationships (Green & Mitchell, 2015). Couple therapists likely need to expand their cultural competence in this area to prevent heteronormative and cisgender identity views from marginalizing the experiences of diverse clients and committing microaggressions toward them. It is beyond the scope of this book to provide culturally relevant interventions for each minority group that therapists may encounter. However, we want to emphasize the importance of therapists' being aware of the values implicit in the interventions they use and the ethical obligation they have to intervene in ways that are culturally sensitive and respectful of their clients' values and lives.

In addition to being culturally sensitive, couple therapists should be socioculturally attuned, in terms of being aware of the social position of one's clients (as well as one's own) and committed to assisting them address inequities in their lives (Knudson-Martin & Kim, 2023). They should be attuned to and understand their clients' experiences and their own within an inequitable world. In other words, they should be aware of the privileges and oppression associated with their own social location and their clients' locations. Those privileges and experiences of oppression commonly are associated with membership in dominant or marginalized/underrepresented/minoritized groups in terms of race, ethnicity, gender identity, sexual orientation, socioeconomic status, age, physical and mental ability, religion, and immigration status/citizenship among others.

A society's dominant discourses (e.g., which characteristics are associated with greater or lesser personal value as a human being) are associated with dynamics of power and oppression. As McDowell, Knudson-Martin, and Bermudez (2022) argue, "power processes in the broader society tend to be reflected in the power dynamics within intimate and family relationships" (p. 215). However, individuals commonly are unaware of the extent to which societal beliefs and values become internalized in their own cognitions (and related behaviors and emotions) about relationships with others. If therapists do not understand individual and relationship distress and the therapeutic relationship within the larger context of power, privilege, and oppression, they run the risk of attributing individual partners' distress to individual and/or relationship deficits. For example, internalized dominant societal messages regarding the role of women as primary caretakers of children and the household may explain why in many heterosexual couples in which both partners work outside the home and both do household and child care tasks, women may still carry a "mental load"—responsibility for knowing which tasks need to be done and planning for them. Both partners may be insufficiently aware of these internalized role demands that may account for the female partner's exhaustion and distressed moods, as well as strained couple communication (McDowell et al., 2022). In addition, a male therapist who does not reflect on gender differences in terms of power and privilege that favor men in society may not only fail to see and address a woman's mental load but also evaluate her behavior as a personal deficit, thus perpetuating gender inequity in the couple's relationship.

The presence of racism, heterosexism, ageism, ableism, sexism, classism, and other "isms" undoubtedly affects clients' lived experiences, and therapists should neither ignore this reality nor miss opportunities to change them through their work. In addition, sociocultural attunement and cultural sensitivity reduce the likelihood that the therapist will commit harmful microaggressions toward their clients and ignore similar behaviors between partners or directed from clients toward the therapist. A full discussion of sociocultural attunement and cultural sensitivity is beyond the scope of this book but can be found in McDowell et al.'s (2022) volume *Socioculturally Attuned Family Therapy.*

PROBLEM DEFINITION AND GOAL SETTING IN COUPLE THERAPY

Even though defining what the problem is and setting treatment goals are part of any therapy, this initial step can be especially challenging in couple therapy. The two individuals commonly have different perceptions of what the issues are in their relationship, the causes of the problems, and what they want to achieve as a result of attending therapy. In fact, in some cases one member of the couple already has decided to leave the relationship and hopes to use therapy as a relatively safe setting for attempting to achieve an amicable separation, whereas the other member is committed to staying together and is motivated to work on repairing problems.

In some cases, the individual who wants to dissolve the relationship has disclosed that goal, but others initially keep it a secret from the partner and therapist, waiting for the "right moment" to reveal their intent. If the therapist senses that a member of a couple is not being forthcoming regarding goals for therapy, it is not in the clinician's best interest to schedule an individual session in the hope of encouraging the person to reveal a secret, as we have noted. However, the therapist might address that individual during a joint couple session with a fairly indirect inquiry that conveys to the client that the therapist is aware that there may be a hidden agenda:

> "Tyler, I've gotten the impression that you have been somewhat uncomfortable during our couple sessions, and you haven't described some specific goals that you have for therapy. I understand that the relationship has been stressful for you for a long time, and having the three of us sit in such close quarters in my office to talk about where to go from here can be difficult in itself. I will do my best to make this a safe place for both of you to talk about your thoughts and feelings, and to make some constructive plans for the future."

Doherty, Harris, and Wilde (2015) use the term *mixed agendas* to describe situations in which one partner is determined to preserve the relationship and is motivated for couple therapy but the other is skeptical about the future of the relationship and ambivalent about couple therapy. In such situations, the therapist does not discuss goals that involve relationship improvement but rather sets "discernment" as a goal, guiding the couple in reaching a decision regarding a direction in which they will move: working on improving the relationship, dissolving the relationship, or not making any change (Doherty et al., 2015). The therapist seeks both partners' commitment to engage in that process and contracts with the couple to meet for a specific number of sessions for that purpose. Whereas individuals who are ambivalent about staying in their couple relationship commonly are uneasy about entering therapy that has an explicit goal of improving the relationship, they may be more willing to engage in discernment sessions that offer other options. Guiding couples in exploring those options requires that therapists themselves are comfortable with those alternative outcomes.

Even when the members of a couple agree on the overall definition of a problem and goal, they may have different views about specific aspects of that goal. For example, partners may agree that they have "communication problems" and that their overall goal is "improving communication," but they may have different definitions of what improving communication entails. One individual may state that the goal of couple therapy should be to talk more often, whereas the other individual may want to communicate differently (e.g., talk more about personal feelings instead of mundane life events) rather than more often. The gap in partners' views of a problem commonly involves a difference in who they view as responsible for a problem, with each person more likely to blame the other than themselves (Epstein & Baucom, 2002). A critical task for the therapist is helping the couple arrive at a shared definition of their problems and goals for treatment. The therapist can work toward an *attributional shift*, away from partners blaming each other for problems and toward each member setting a goal of taking responsibility for engaging in specific constructive actions that can contribute to more positive interactions.

Developing a common understanding of a problem and its causes involves the therapist inquiring about each partner's subjective experience of the relationship issue, facilitating their empathic understanding of each other's experience, and encouraging their acceptance that the problem can be viewed from two different perspectives (their experiences are not mutually exclusive). The initial step involves introducing a *systemic perspective* for the therapy, which contributes to goals that meet both individuals' needs. For example, one person may complain about not having enough autonomy and privacy, whereas the other may complain about having an insufficient connection with the partner. These different needs may contribute to a behavioral pattern in which the more one person seeks the other's company, the more the other person avoids interacting, and vice versa (a circular demand–withdraw pattern). Commonly, each person considers the other's goals and behavior as the cause of their problem, rather than recognizing that it is a dyadic pattern to which both partners contribute.

When the therapist guides the couple in defining a problem in terms of both partners' subjective experiences and the manner in which they are interconnected through their behavioral interactions, this serves as a cognitive intervention as well as a template for setting behavior change goals. The focus of therapy shifts from partner blaming to contributions that both individuals can make to develop mutually satisfying interactions. Thus, a couple with a demand–withdraw pattern may agree on a goal of finding a way of managing their time and interactions that is congruent with both partners' personal needs for connection and independence. Once therapy goals have been established, it is important that the therapist collaborate with the couple regularly in evaluating the extent to which the treatment has been focused appropriately on the goals and whether they have been achieved. As we describe in Chapter 3, assessment is an ongoing process, and the clients may set new goals over the course of treatment.

INTERACTION AND CONSULTATION WITH OTHER PROVIDERS

Couple therapists often work with clients who concurrently see individual therapists, psychiatrists, substance abuse counselors, fertility specialists, probation officers, and social workers, among other professionals. Consistent with an ecological perspective that takes into account multiple influences on a couple's relationship, it is important for the therapist to exchange relevant information with other professionals and at times coordinate interventions. After obtaining authorization from *both* partners to exchange information (a crucial consent issue), it is advisable that the therapist contact these providers at least once, to obtain their perspectives and be aware of life circumstances that are affecting the couple. In some cases, ongoing communication with another professional may be needed. For example, one member of the couple may have been seeing a substance abuse counselor for drinking problems, and the couple therapist may need to communicate more often with that counselor during a period of relapse in order to coordinate treatment. Also, when one or both partners are seeing a psychiatrist or an individual therapist, it is important that the couple therapist talks with such professionals to obtain any information about the individual treatment that may affect the couple's relationship. Knowledge of individual personal history, personality traits, or moderate to severe psychiatric disorders may be critical in understanding challenges facing the couple and the extent to which the issues can be addressed in the context of couple treatment. When receiving information from providers that are working with only one of the partners, the couple therapist should not share that information in conjoint sessions without prior authorization from that partner.

Furthermore, mental health providers who treat individuals typically only hear the client's perspective on the partner and relationship, so couple therapists often help them develop a more systemic conceptualization of the client's issues. We personally have experienced instances of partners' individual therapists often welcoming this information and finding it helpful.

As we described in Chapter 1, one of the relatively recent developments in the couple therapy field has been the use of conjoint treatment to address presenting problems that involve an individual partner's psychological or physical health problems. However, when one of the partners is also involved in individual therapy to address personal issues, this raises the question of whether and how the couple therapy also should target those issues. Because there is substantial research evidence that individual psychopathology commonly is influenced by both intrapsychic and interpersonal factors, there is a strong rationale for an integrated treatment that addresses both realms, using modalities designed for maximal impact. Whereas individual therapy provides a consistent focus on the individual's history and current functioning, couple therapy offers direct access (observation and intervention) to the couple's dyadic patterns. In a coordinated treatment approach, an individual therapist or psychiatrist can intervene with intrapersonal factors contributing to symptoms, while a couple therapist can guide the partners in coping as a team with the individual's symptoms and reducing sources of stress in their relationship that elicit or exacerbate those symptoms (Baucom et al., 2012; Fischer et al., 2016). The likelihood that such an integrative "team" approach will work may depend on discussions between the professionals to establish a shared model of factors influencing the clients and a boundary between the two treatments.

Individual therapy can enhance the process of couple therapy, particularly when it provides a partner with space to address individual issues (e.g., substance abuse, trauma, severe mood or anxiety disorders) that otherwise would not be addressed sufficiently in couple therapy. Nevertheless, partners commonly describe their relationship problems to their individual therapists, and based on what may be a skewed perspective that the therapist develops from the individual's descriptions, the therapist may offer the individual evaluations of that unseen partner, which the individual then brings into the couple therapy sessions (perhaps accurately conveyed but perhaps not). Sometimes the person uses their therapist's comments to blame their partner and legitimize a request for the partner to change. Although the couple therapist needs to refrain from criticizing the individual therapist who offered an evaluation of the other partner, they can refocus the discussion on the individual's own distress about the relationship and wishes for improvement. For example, the therapist might state:

> "I can see that you told your individual therapist how unhappy you are about your relationship and aspects of your partner's behavior, and the therapist seems concerned about your well-being, as I would expect. An advantage of our couple therapy is that the three of us can take a close look at the patterns in your relationship and can work on changes that can make both of you feel better about it. Let's look more at the concerns you shared with your therapist that we can work on together here."

TERMINATION OF COUPLE THERAPY

Ideally, couple therapy concludes when both partners believe their relationship goals have been achieved and they predict they will be able to maintain the changes. However, in some cases, even though both partners perceive progress, one desires some additional sessions either to achieve further progress on those goals or to work on a new goal. In those situations, the therapist can return to the same process that was used initially to reach agreement between partners on therapy goals and preferred length of treatment to establish a new therapy contract, with a specified number of additional sessions before termination.

There are other scenarios in which couple therapy may be discontinued. For a variety of reasons (e.g., an impasse in the therapy process, hopelessness about the other partner's willingness or ability to change, a decision to terminate the relationship, problems in the therapeutic alliance among the clinician and members of the couple), one partner may no longer be motivated to participate in sessions. When this happens, couple therapy cannot continue. However, the therapist should explore with that partner the reasons for wanting to discontinue treatment because sometimes it may reflect frustration or hopelessness regarding the potential for change rather than a true desire to end the treatment or relationship. An empathic and supportive response from the therapist, combined with a discussion with the couple regarding the importance of some collaboration to produce some noticeable change in chronic negative interaction patterns, may be sufficient to keep the reluctant partner engaged in treatment for a mutually agreed upon number of sessions. Nevertheless, in some cases a partner who has expressed the intent to withdraw from therapy will have reached a firm decision, and the conjoint treatment will end.

The therapist may initiate discontinuation of therapy when continuing sessions is judged to be contraindicated. These situations typically include but are not limited to relationships in which there appear to be risks to the safety and well-being of one or both partners, untreated moderate to severe substance abuse or mental health conditions that are interfering with couple therapy, or when one member is not willing to share with the other partner information that affects the relationship and/or the other partner, such as infidelity or an unacknowledged difference in sexual orientation or gender identity (Wolska, 2011).

As discussed in Chapter 5, in situations in which one or both partners engage in physical violence or severe psychological partner aggression (e.g., preventing one's partner access to essential needs, controlling and monitoring the partner's behavior, demeaning and shaming the partner), the clinician should discontinue couple therapy. The clinician should explicitly explain to the couple the purpose of protecting both partners' emotional and physical well-being, until the physical violence and/or psychological aggression stops and there are processes in place to prevent them from recurring. As described in Chapter 3 on assessment, couple therapy usually should not be *initiated* when one or both partners are abusing alcohol or other substances, which will likely interfere with their abilities to internalize changes in therapy. There also are situations during the course of therapy in which an abstinent partner relapses or a pattern of substance abuse develops. In such circumstances, the therapist may discontinue the couple therapy until the substance abuse is treated in a formal way (i.e., involvement with professionals rather than a stated personal commitment to stop using). Similarly, the clinician may discontinue therapy if there is a mental health condition (e.g., psychotic episode, severe eating disorder, significant suicidal risk) that requires individual treatment before couple therapy can be feasible and resumed.

KEY POINTS

- Some individual sessions with each partner take place in couple therapy. Whereas the therapist honors each partner's right to privacy, clear guidelines are set to avoid keeping secrets regarding conditions such as affairs that directly affect the relationship and process of conjoint treatment.

- The therapist's role in couple therapy involves unique challenges. It requires taking a multipartial but not a neutral perspective.

- Couple therapists need to focus on cultural sensitivity and sociocultural attunement when working with diverse clients, particularly from marginalized groups.

- Consultation with other providers treating the individual partners helps develop an integrative and systemic intervention plan.

- Couple therapy may be initiated by one or both partners, or may be recommended to an individual who has sought individual treatment primarily for relationship problems. In turn, the therapist may discontinue couple therapy based on concerns about partners' safety, well-being, or an individual's secrets that can affect the other partner.

CHAPTER 3

Assessment

Assessment involves identifying a couple's presenting problem(s) and factors in their lives that may be influencing the issues that brought them to therapy. Even though some interventions may be helpful in a generic way for many different problems, each couple and the challenges they face likely have a unique combination of characteristics to which treatment must be tailored. Furthermore, a systemic approach to couple relationships requires that the clinician consider multiple levels of factors influencing a relationship. Those range from each partner's personal history and current psychological functioning to interaction patterns within the dyad, to relationships with other family members and friends, to influences of broader systems within which the couple is embedded (e.g., jobs, community violence, discrimination, racism, economic conditions and inequities in society, legal barriers such as abortion bans, and cultural practices).

Although the treatment plan is derived from the initial assessment sessions, the clinician continues to be on the lookout for additional information that may surface in subsequent sessions and may modify the treatment plan accordingly. Because the therapist is a stranger to the couple during initial assessment, which limits the quality of the therapeutic alliance, clients often will hesitate to reveal some personal information until they become more comfortable and trusting of the therapist. This is particularly the case when there are significant differences in social location between clients and therapists regarding race, ethnicity, socioeconomic status, gender identity, sexual orientation, and/or religion, among others. In such instances, clients are unsure whether the therapist can fully and fairly understand their experience and situation and, understandably so, may be cautious about opening up completely to avoid being misunderstood, judged, or even recipients of microaggression from the therapist. As discussed in Chapter 2, it is critical for therapists to be socioculturally attuned and inform themselves about the past and current sociopolitical, legal, and economic conditions that may have discriminated against or privileged the groups of which their clients are part.

When clients reveal relational and individual functioning problems after several (or even many) sessions, it is important that the therapist conveys empathy for the discomfort that made them censor that information and appreciation for their willingness to share the information at this point. The therapist then discusses with the couple how the new information may suggest the need to adjust therapy goals to some extent. Because this is a collaborative process, if the clients state that they do not feel ready to take on the new issue that was revealed, it is best for the therapist to support their preference but state a plan to check with them later to see whether spending some time on it seems appropriate at that point.

41

This chapter describes several aspects of the assessment process that provide the information needed to develop a treatment plan tailored to the characteristics and needs of each couple. These include:

- A contextual ecological framework for assessment of couples
- Sociocultural sensitivity and attunement in assessment
- Individual and relational developmental processes
- Assessment of partners' behavioral interactions, cognitions, and emotions
- Interview, questionnaire, and behavioral observation assessment methods

A CONTEXTUAL ECOLOGICAL FRAMEWORK FOR ASSESSMENT OF COUPLES

Epstein and Baucom (2002) describe a contextual model for assessing and treating distressed couples, in which a couple is faced with coping with a variety of demands or stressors associated with the characteristics of the individual partners (e.g., depression or chronic physical illness), the dyad (e.g., differences in partners' values and goals), and their social and physical environment (e.g., financial strain, racism, socioeconomic inequities, caretaking for an ill extended family member, discrimination, legal constraints on freedoms). Such a contextual approach, which is consistent with Bronfenbrenner's (1979) ecological model of multilayered influences on intimate relationships, guides the clinician in developing a relatively comprehensive view of factors that should be included in the treatment goals. It is tempting for couple therapists to focus on the complex and often emotionally intense interaction patterns between the partners, especially when those patterns play out during sessions. However, it is crucial to understand various contextual factors that influence the pair's functioning and to plan appropriate interventions. For example, demands from the couple's jobs, children, extended family, and other circumstances commonly interfere with couple intimacy, as can stress from discrimination experiences outside the home. Consequently, interventions focused on increasing the time that the partners engage in intimate experiences together will be hampered unless the therapist helps the couple devise strategies to cope with their external stressors together while protecting some time for their relationship.

Thus, the assessment must gather information systematically about levels of contextual factors influencing the couple's relationship in general, as well as specifically affecting their presenting problems. Consistent with Epstein and Baucom's (2002) model, that means inquiring about each individual's functioning (e.g., chronic personality characteristics such as low self-esteem, psychopathology symptoms, residual effects from prior life trauma), sources of stress within the dyad (e.g., different beliefs about the qualities of a close relationship, different ways of coping with racial discrimination), and demands from their physical and social environment (e.g., a child with school problems, job stress, an ill extended family member, language barriers facing many immigrants, an unsafe neighborhood, discrimination based on race, sexual orientation). All of the assessment methods we describe in this chapter (interviews, questionnaires, behavioral observation) can be used to gather information about contextual factors that may be targeted in the treatment plan. Given the collaborative relationship that CBCT clinicians attempt to foster with clients, discussions of assessment findings that identify contextual factors influencing a presenting problem also often increase clients' understanding of their problems and their motivation to implement specific changes.

SOCIOCULTURAL SENSITIVITY
AND ATTUNEMENT IN ASSESSMENT

As we discussed in Chapter 2, *sociocultural sensitivity and attunement* are crucial in assessment as well as in the treatment process. On the one hand, therapists need to be aware of the values and traditions associated with their social location and cultural background. These influence what therapists notice about clients and what they are unaware of or tend to ignore. This is especially the case when the therapist's social location and cultural background involve belonging to dominant groups in society.

On the other hand, therapists must be aware of their assumptions about characteristics of the cultural groups to which their clients belong, in terms of gender, race, ethnicity, sexual orientation, gender identity, disabilities, religion, political views, immigration status, marital status, parenthood, and the like. Stereotyped beliefs about the groups one belongs to and that one's clients belong to can influence a therapist's assessment of clients' functioning and factors that affect that functioning. For example, if one learns that a couple has an intentional nonmonogamous relationship, which is counter to what the therapist considers appropriate, that might influence the therapist's identification of treatment goals. As another example, an immigrant couple may report a high level of emotional distress and difficulty adjusting to their new community in the United States. If a therapist attempts to focus them on efforts toward assimilation such as taking classes to improve their English fluency but fails to explore experiences that the couple has had with discrimination from neighbors and teachers at their children's schools, this lack of sociocultural sensitivity in the assessment and treatment plan is likely to lead to inadequate clinical practice. Therapist self-awareness promotes cultural sensitivity, respect, and humility, as do efforts to learn about clients' social identities, cultures, and stressors linked to social location during the initial assessment and throughout therapy.

A number of factors often vary across groups depending on race, ethnicity/country of origin, gender identity, sexual orientation, religion, ability/disability, and body characteristics, among others. These factors should be addressed in the assessment of each couple, as they influence both the characteristics of clients' intimate relationships and the appropriate way of conducting therapy (Epstein, Falconier, & Dattilio, 2020). The factors include:

- *Views prevalent in a group regarding causes of mental health problems and relationship problems* (e.g., as due to biological versus psychological and interpersonal processes) *and acceptable treatment methods* (e.g., psychotherapy, consultation with local indigenous healers, Western or Eastern medical treatments).
- *Collectivist versus individualistic values* (whether the top priority is the relationship/group or individual self-actualization).
- *Standards and expectations about gender and family roles and boundaries* (e.g., division of household labor, breadwinning, parenting, relationship with extended family).

- *Sexual practices and intimacy standards and expectations* (e.g., birth control, open relationships).
- *Developmental standards and expectations* (e.g., when to start dating and the degree to which family members influence mate choices; how important procreation is considered for couples; involvement of grandparents in child rearing).
- *Reproductive methods* (e.g., natural birth, reproductive technologies, adoption, surrogate pregnancy).
- *Conceptions of the role of a therapist* (e.g., as revered and directive expert versus almost a family friend).
- *Communication styles* in close relationships and with a therapist (e.g., direct versus tactful and indirect).
- *Ethical standards* (e.g., whether it is appropriate for a therapist to accept gifts from clients).

Therapists' understanding of clients' social location, cultural background, and preferred identities is crucial in therapy for various reasons. First, identification of clients' social location and cultural background inform the therapist about the presence or absence of privileges in the clients' lives and how such conditions can create opportunities or constraints and marginalization in systems of oppression. Second, it helps the therapist be mindful of differences from their own social location and avoid actions toward clients that perpetuate inequities and marginalization of their personal experiences. Third, it helps therapists validate their clients' experiences and address discrimination and marginalization. Fourth, it contributes to therapy being a safe place where aspects of the couple's external context that influence their relationship negatively can be addressed. Fifth, it allows therapists to engage in affirming practices that honor and celebrate the identities embraced by their clients.

Couple therapists can learn about clients' social location and cultural background by asking interview questions or through written surveys. Questions should address at a minimum self-identification of race, ethnicity/country of origin, immigration status, gender identity, sexual orientation, religion, disabilities, education, income level, native language and proficiency in English, and other identities that clients consider significant to them. Our interview guide for individual members of a couple (see Figure 3.2, below) includes questions that tap various aspects of social identity. Questions regarding immigration should be addressed carefully because of circumstances (e.g., documentation, changes in visa status) that may raise client fears of deportation. Before asking any questions, therapists should be familiar with the extent to which such information can remain confidential according to federal and state laws, and they should share those guidelines with the clients. It is important to invite clients to share what they want us to know about their identities and cultures. Therapists can invite clients to do so by saying:

"Before discussing the issues that brought you to therapy, I'd like to get to know you better, so I would like to ask you some questions I routinely ask my clients. How would you describe who you are in terms of characteristics and cultures that are important to you and define who you are. I would also like to know why those identities are important and if you want to comment on any privileges you experience in your life, or lack of them, associated with those identities."

If clients struggle with the question, the therapist may provide an example regarding their own identity. It is our experience that clients value therapists who are open to hearing their worldviews, traditions, and realities, and who affirm and value their preferred identities. However, therapists should not burden clients with the task of having to educate them. Therapists should take an active role in learning about the history, values, and traditions of the groups their clients identify with, as well as about the impact of socioeconomic, political, and legal contexts on their clients' lives.

ASSESSMENT OF INDIVIDUAL AND RELATIONAL DEVELOPMENTAL PROCESSES

Epstein and Baucom's (2002) contextual model of factors that influence the functioning of a couple's relationship and Bronfenbrenner's (1979) ecological model also emphasize developmental changes that occur over time in partners and their relationship, potentially presenting challenges for the couple. As members of a couple age, they may mature emotionally, shift their core life values and priorities, pursue different career paths, develop health problems, among other things. Areas in which partners initially were similar and felt connected may become sources of conflict. At the same time, a couple's relationship, including the roles they play, is likely to change over time as they experience changes such as births of children, adult children balancing visits with them and in-laws, caregiving for their aging parents, and changes in time together that occur with retirement. Developmental changes at the individual and relational level often are "double-edged," bringing advantages and disadvantages. It is important that the assessment of a couple include information about developmental changes, what they have meant to the partners, and how the couple has adapted to them. The most efficient way to gather this information is during the initial interviews with the couple and individual partners we describe in this chapter.

The initial pretreatment assessment typically involves one or more joint interviews with the couple and preferably at least one separate interview with each partner (Epstein & Baucom, 2002). Figures 3.1 and 3.2 include outlines of the joint and individual interviews, respectively. We include individual interviews in order to provide each person a comfortable setting for revealing personal characteristics (e.g., abuse by a previous partner, chronic low self-esteem) without the partner observing. It is important that couple therapists be well versed in identifying symptoms of problems in individual functioning (psychological disorders, residual effects of prior negative life experiences such as abuse by a former partner). However, the couple therapist's ability to conduct a thorough diagnostic assessment with each partner is limited, compared to the typical assessment in individual therapy. When one or both partners have been in individual therapy with other clinicians and/or have been seeing a psychiatrist specifically for medication, obtaining assessment data and treatment information from those providers with the individuals' consent can be very helpful. As described in Chapter 2, we establish clear guidelines for keeping information confidential that is shared during the individual interviews and avoiding secret-keeping regarding issues such as ongoing infidelity that are likely to interfere with couple therapy. Information about each partner's history and current functioning also can be gathered during subsequent joint therapy sessions.

(text resumes on page 50)

Initial Meeting and Interactions

- How did the two of you meet? When and where?
- If any other people were involved in your meeting, how were they involved? *(This question can address arranged marriages, and if the couple indicates that is how their relationship began, the therapist should modify subsequent questions accordingly.)*
- At that time, to what extent were you actually interested in meeting someone you could develop an ongoing relationship with?
- Each of you, please describe anything going on in your life at that time that may have influenced your level of interest in starting a couple relationship.
- What characteristics of the other person attracted you initially?
- In what ways would you say the two of you are similar, in terms of your personal characteristics, such as personality, temperament, energy level, and interests, and in what ways are you different?
- What social identities (race, ethnicity, immigration/citizenship, gender, sexual orientation, religion, ability, SES, etc.) do you have in common, and which are different?
- What roles did those differences and similarities in your personal characteristics and social identities play in the beginning of your relationship?
- Describe any events or situations that occurred at the beginning of your relationship that you think shaped your relationship long-term? How?
- Please describe any aspects about how your relationship formed that you think are important for me to understand if my social identity and yours are not the same in some ways?
- How did you spend your time together in the early days of your relationship? Are there aspects of things you enjoyed doing together back then that the two of you still like to do together now?

Deeper Involvement in the Relationship

- Please describe how your relationship progressed from being new and casual to a more serious relationship. To what extent did you have similar ideas about where your relationship was going (such as how committed to each other you were ready to be)?
- How involved were you as a couple with your families and friends?
- How supportive (or not) of your relationship were your families and friends? What seemed to influence how those other people felt about your relationship?
- Were you involved in any communities based on social identity characteristics (e.g., race, ethnicity, gender, sexual orientation, religion) individually and/or as a couple? If so, which ones and how? How supportive were such communities of your couple relationship?
- During the process of becoming a more serious/committed relationship, what events occurred that you think had either a positive or a negative influence on your relationship?
- How did you deal with any stressful events individually and as a couple?
- Have you had any experiences of discrimination as individuals or as a couple, based on any of your social identities? If so, please describe them and how they have affected you individually and as a couple?
- To what extent have the two of you discussed goals for the future, as individuals and as a couple, and how similar or different do your goals seem to be?
- In what ways have your personal social identities influenced your goals and preferences for your couple relationship?
- As your relationship was developing, how did you communicate when you had disagreements?
- If you have children, how has being parents affected your lives individually and as a couple?

(continued)

FIGURE 3.1. Couple assessment interview regarding relationship history and current functioning.

Relationship Characteristics over the Years

- Over the years, what types of activities have you shared that brought you pleasure and/or brought you closer together. How have you gone about choosing things to do together?
- What new experiences would you like to share together in the future?
- Please describe any stressful experiences you have experienced over the years (for example, from jobs, relationships with extended family members, finances, children, health issues, disabilities, discrimination against you as individuals or as a couple based on your social identities) and how you dealt with them together.
- If your experiences and social identities (e.g., culture, ethnicity, race) are different, how have the differences been positives in your relationship or sources of stress? How have you related to each other regarding the differences?
- Besides each other, who else do you have available to turn to when you are facing stresses in your life? How comfortable are you with asking for help from those people?
- To what degree do the characteristics that you found attractive in each other originally still exist today?
- What signs did each of you notice that the concerns that led you to seek couple therapy had developed? When you noticed those signs, how did the two of you communicate about them?
- What have you done to improve the issues that you are concerned about, other than couple therapy? What was successful and what was not? Why?
- Please tell me about any previous couple therapy the two of you have had. What was helpful about it? Describe anything about it that did not seem helpful.
- When you disagree about something, how do you tend to communicate with each other about it? How similar or different are your communication styles? How well does your communication help in resolving your disagreement?
- Over the years, how have you expressed your positive feelings for each other? When each of you becomes upset during discussions of issues in your relationship, how well does each of you keep your emotions from becoming intense or even feeling out of control? What works for each of you in helping you calm down when you begin to get upset about something?
- Over the time you have been together, what have you come to admire or respect the most about your partner?
- Over the time you have been together, what have you come to appreciate the most about your relationship?
- It is normal for members of a couple to have some different memories of the development of their relationship over the months and years. As you think back to the time you have been in a relationship together, what times do you both identify as the most satisfying/happy for you? What about that time makes it stand out for you?
- What changes would you like to see happen in your relationship?
- What else would you like me to know about your relationship, past or present, so I can understand your life as much as possible?

Expectations Regarding Couple Therapy

- What characteristics are you looking for in a couple therapist, in terms of their personal characteristics, social identities, and style, as well as methods of conducting therapy?
- How important is it to you that the therapist has social identities similar to yours, such as culture, religion, race, gender, and sexual orientation? Why?
- To what degrees do you hope the therapy will focus on insight into aspects of partners' pasts that influence their way of relating to each other now?

(continued)

FIGURE 3.1. *(continued)*

- To what degrees do you hope the therapy will focus on changing specific ways that partners behave toward each other?
- To what degree do you have concerns that discussions during couple therapy will "open a can of worms" and make your relationship worse?
- Please describe any other goals or concerns you have about beginning couple therapy.

FIGURE 3.1. *(continued)*

Demographic Information and Family of Origin

- What is your date of birth? Where were you born?
- *If the individual reports a place of birth other than the current country, ask about birth countries of parents, any other places the individual lived between their original country of origin and the current country (sometimes this involves more than one relocation), and information about immigration. Questions regarding immigration may include: Their age when they arrived, why they left their country of origin, how much they were able to choose to immigrate, with whom they immigrated, whether immigration resulted in them reuniting with friends/family members, how long they have been in the present country, whether any close family members remain in their country of origin and whether they remain in touch with them, whether they have ever returned to their country(ies) of origin, whether they have plans to return to their country(ies) of origin permanently, and so on.*
- Who were the people in your family of origin? If any of the members of your family of origin have died, who was it, when, and how?
- Where does each living member of your family of origin live now? How would you describe your relationship with each person in your family of origin in the past? How do you get along with each living member now?
- When you were a child and when you were an adolescent, who lived in your home?
- How do you define your social identities in terms of gender, sexual orientation, race, ethnicity/culture, religion, socioeconomic status, ability, or any other characteristics? Which are the more important/relevant identities for you? Why?
- How do your social identities shape your values and lifestyle? *(Understanding some of the individual's social identities may require follow-up questions. For example, regarding gender identity and sexual orientation, the therapist can ask when they came out, to whom, and how those people responded to their disclosure; when a transgender individual began transitioning, and experiences associated with that process; for an individual with a disability, when and how it developed. For all of these social identities, one also should ask about acceptance and support versus rejection from family and friends, other sources of support, and whether the individual thinks their social identities have influenced their couple relationship. Have these always been their social identities, or have there been changes in their abandoning, adopting, or redefining their social identities? If so, ask for a brief explanation of the changes.)*

Health History

- Beginning with childhood, describe any physical health problems that affected your daily life, school work, job performance, or relationships with other people.
- What, if any, types of treatment have you had for those physical health problems, and how much did the treatments help?

(continued)

FIGURE 3.2. Interview with individual partners.

- How much are those physical health problems affecting you now?
- Beginning with childhood, describe any psychological/mental health problems that affected your daily life, school work, job performance, or relationships with other people. What, if any diagnoses have you received?
- What, if any, types of treatment have you had for psychological/mental health problems, and how much did the treatments help?
- How much are those psychological/mental health problems affecting you now?
- Please describe anything that occurs in your couple relationship that seems to affect your personal psychological/mental health problems.
- Please describe your use of tobacco, caffeine, marijuana, and other substances, beginning in childhood and up to the present. If any substance use has resulted in problems in your life, please describe that, and any treatment you received.
- If you currently use any substances, describe any issues or conflict that it has caused in your relationship with your partner.
- What medications do you presently take for any physical or mental health problem? Who prescribes them? Do they have any side effects that concern you?
- How much do you exercise? What types of exercise do you engage in?
- How would you describe your present overall physical health? Your overall mental health?

Developmental History and Current Functioning

- What is the highest level of education you received?
- Were you ever diagnosed with a learning disability or any other condition that affected your performance in school? If so, what was it? What help, if any, did you receive for it from your school, parents, doctors, or others?
- What were your relationships like with peers as a child? How about during adolescence and as you got older?
- In the present, how are your friendships—number and quality?·
- What leisure activities have you enjoyed as a child, adolescent, young adult, and so on?
- How much time do you devote now to leisure activities that you enjoy?
- If you had more free time, what would you most like to do with it?
- To what extent have you experienced and been affected by discrimination, harassment, bullying based on your race, ethnicity, religion, sexual orientation, age, gender, physical disabilities, and so on. How have you dealt with being treated in those ways?
- To what extent have the communities in which you have lived, worked, and studied been supportive of your social identities? In what ways? How?
- Have you experienced any traumatic experiences during your life, such as being in a serious car accident, experiencing one's own or witnessing another person's abuse or neglect as a child, losing a loved one suddenly, being abandoned by someone important in your life, being a victim of physical or sexual abuse as an adult, being a victim of or witnessing a hate crime or bullying, not having basic needs met, or experiencing a natural disaster, war, and so on? I want you to feel free to tell me if it would be too upsetting to give me details now about your experience, and that would be fine.
- If you did have any of those experiences, what help, if any, did you receive for them? *(Regarding child abuse and neglect, it is essential that the therapist inform clients beforehand via the therapy consent form and again verbally when introducing the couple and individual assessment procedures, about local requirements for mandating reporting, so the clients can judge what information they want to share.)*

(continued)

FIGURE 3.2. *(continued)*

- Have there been any other major life stressors in your life that we have not covered so far? If so, what are they?
- When you have experienced stress (large or small) from any events in your life, how have you coped with the stress? How well did your ways of coping work?
- If you have a personal problem, who are you comfortable talking to about it? Who would you be comfortable accepting help from for a problem?
- Briefly tell me about your work history—types of jobs held, how well you did in them.
- How satisfied have you been with your work? Are there any changes you would like to have?
- Please describe any dating and more serious relationships you had before the relationship with your current partner.
- How satisfying or unsatisfying were those prior relationships, and why?
- Did you seek any couple therapy for any previous relationship? What led you and a partner to seek couple therapy? If so, to what degree was it helpful.
- In your current relationship with your partner, please describe any differences that exist between the two of you (for example, personality characteristics, cultural background, goals in life) that have been sources of any stress or conflict.
- If you have experienced some stress or conflict regarding a difference between you, how have the two of you dealt with it? How does each of you behave toward the other person?
- On the Partner Aggression Questionnaire, you indicated that there has been some aggressive behavior in your couple relationship. Please tell me when that has occurred, what led to it, and what effects it has had on you.
- How safe do you feel living with your partner?
- How safe do you feel participating in couple therapy with your partner?
- What are your personal goals for this couple therapy?

If the therapist wishes to ask individual partners questions during these private interviews regarding sensitive topics such as personal involvement in infidelity, it is important that the therapist reiterate their policy regarding management of client secrets that are described in their consent form. Clearly there are advantages to knowing as much as possible about individuals' actions that have influenced their couple relationship, but therapists' inquiries about sensitive topics must adhere to professional confidentiality ethical standards. Further discussion of professional issues in assessment and treatment of partner aggression is covered in Chapter 5, and Chapter 6 focuses on infidelity.

FIGURE 3.2. (*continued*)

ASSESSMENT OF PARTNERS' BEHAVIORAL INTERACTIONS, COGNITIONS, AND EMOTIONS

In addition to assessing the multiple contextual levels and developmental changes influencing a couple's presenting problem(s), the clinician who is guided by a CBCT model (which as we noted previously is relevant to other couple therapy models) needs to collect information at each systemic level about the couple's behavioral interactions, how they think about the circumstances, and what emotional responses they experience. For example, a couple may report financial strain (i.e., difficulties paying bills; worry about paying for children's education; insufficient savings for retirement) (Falconier & Epstein, 2011). The assessment would include identifying how the partners *behave* toward each other regarding the financial concerns (e.g., whether they avoid discussing finances rather than trying to brainstorm possible solutions), how they *think* about the issue (e.g., they each ruminate about what they consider financial mistakes that each other has made), and what *emotions* they experience (e.g., anxiety, anger).

Thus, the clinician seeks information about partners' *behaviors*, *cognitions*, and *emotions* that are associated with each contextual level of influences on their relationship: (1) characteristics of the two individuals; (2) the dyad; (3) family members and friends; (4) organizations within the community such as schools and jobs; (5) community conditions such as the availability of culturally sensitive social service agencies and sources of affordable food, medical care, transportation, housing, and other basic needs; and (6) broader societal conditions such as racism, discrimination on the basis of gender, sexual minority status, legal restrictions, segregation, community violence, and adverse economic conditions such as high costs due to inflation. Figure 3.3 summarizes this assessment framework.

The process of collecting information need not be complex and time-consuming. Once a clinician becomes accustomed to the idea of being sure to gather information about behaviors, cognitions, and emotions about each contextual level, this assessment framework is not cumbersome and helps one feel confident that one has achieved a comprehensive view of factors that should be included in the treatment plan. For a given couple and presenting problem, the clinician will be able to rule out the relevance of many characteristics relatively quickly and focus on a few key factors that need attention. Thus, a couple may report no environmental stressors from their extended family, jobs, and community, whereas they may experience frequent conflict regarding one partner's alcohol use, and the therapist can focus on their behavioral interactions, cognitions, and emotions associated with that partner's drinking. Of course, some couples experience multiple life stressors, but the assessment may indicate that their distress is exacerbated by similar negative ways they cope with all of the problems (e.g., escalating arguments, catastrophic expectancies about dire outcomes). Consequently, interventions that target those negative responses to stressors can have broad positive effects on the couple's joint coping with a variety of current as well as future stressors (Bodenmann, Randall, & Falconier, 2016).

ASSESSMENT METHODS: INTERVIEWS, QUESTIONNAIRES, AND BEHAVIORAL OBSERVATION

The three major modes of assessment in couple therapy are (Epstein & Baucom, 2002):

1. *Interviews* with the couple as a dyad as well as with the individual partners
2. *Questionnaires* that efficiently survey specific areas of individual and relational functioning
3. *Direct observation of the couple's interactions*

Therapists can ask partners to complete a brief set of questionnaires during the first appointment, preferably in separate rooms to protect confidentiality for each person. As we describe below, there are a few brief questionnaires that can be useful for quick screening purposes, but in clinical practice more extensive forms are time consuming and inefficient for treatment planning. In the following chapters, we describe specific questionnaires that are relevant for assessing initial levels of a particular presenting problem (e.g., partner aggression) and for monitoring improvement

Individual Partners

- *Behavioral tendencies*, such as coping with unpleasant experiences by withdrawing; using verbal aggression when others make requests; responding altruistically to others in need.
- *Cognitions*, such as personal standards for characteristics of a relationship; negative attributions about a partner's intentions; selective attention to a new partner's positive characteristics while overlooking signs of relationship conflict.
- *Emotions*, such as chronic depression; generalized anxiety; poorly regulated anger; infatuation with a new partner.

The Couple as a Dyad

- *Behavioral tendencies*, such as mutual escalation of arguing; mutual withdrawal from conflict; constructive dyadic coping with life stresses.
- *Cognitions*, such as shared values and life goals; mutual hopelessness about the future of a relationship after chronic arguments.
- *Emotions*, such as partners' up-regulation or fueling of each other's anger when they are in conflict; an individual reducing their partner's emotional distress from stressors through dyadic coping involving provision of empathy and soothing behavior.

Family Members and Friends

- *Behavioral tendencies*, such as others' behavioral intrusions into the couple's daily lives, disrupting their routines and interfering with partners' collaboration; family members assisting the couple with stressful tasks.
- *Cognitions*, such as partners' concern about their awareness that aspects of their relationship are in conflict with cultural values of their families of origin; perceiving validation regarding their parenting style from friends.
- *Emotions*, such as anxiety about parents possibly rejecting them for their selection of their partner with particular characteristics (e.g., race, sexual orientation, social class); warm feelings from friends' helpful actions when the couple experienced a stressful event.

Daily Interactions with Specific Organizations within the Community (e.g., schools, jobs, religious organizations)

- *Behavioral tendencies*, such as spending excessive time working due to job demands; enhanced solving of life problems through supportive actions from members of the couple's church, mosque, synagogue, and the like.
- *Cognitions*, such as perfectionistic standards for their children's academic performance due to stringent norms for academic excellence in the local school; improved sense of personal acceptance of their religious intermarriage through membership in a religious organization that welcomes diverse couples.

(continued)

FIGURE 3.3. Assessment of positive and negative behavior, cognition, and emotion across contextual levels.

- *Emotions*, such as pervasive anxiety due to role strain in attempting to balance work and family responsibilities; anxiety due to discrimination at one's job based on one's social location (e.g., race, gender); joy as individuals and as a couple in participating in a local parent group education and skills enhancement program.

Community Conditions Addressing Basic Needs

- *Behavioral tendencies*, such as a couple's frustrated attempts to find affordable medical care and housing; demands on parents' time spent in childrearing activities due to limited community resources such as recreation centers with youth programs; support for maintaining one's cultural traditions from existence of local shops selling culturally diverse food and goods.
- *Cognitions*, such as immigrants' frustration and hopelessness from the absence of English for Speakers of Other Languages (ESOL) services in the community for learning English; worry about family safety based on community violence; through contacts with similar minoritized couples in one's community, an expectancy that with perseverance the couple can develop a satisfying life there.
- *Emotions*, such as depression from a sense of isolation from living in a community that lacks resources for meeting needs associated with one's social identity; fear based on local legal restrictions on abortion; positive emotion from living in a community known for values similar to those of the couple.

FIGURE 3.3. *(continued)*

over time. Interviews with the couple and each partner provide rich details about individual and relational functioning. Finally, observations of the partners' interaction patterns during the initial joint assessment session and in subsequent therapy sessions can provide rich data about ways in which the two individuals influence each other.

Although some assessments evaluate the couple at a global level (e.g., the partners' overall level of satisfaction with their relationship; how the partners communicate when discussing areas of conflict in their relationship or when trying to provide each other support), others are tailored to particular presenting problems (e.g., co-parenting issues). The clinician's choice of which assessment measures to use is influenced not only by clients' types of presenting problems, but also by the time and resources available. For example, collecting communication samples from couples is easier for those who work in an outpatient clinic that has video recording equipment, and it likely is easier to motivate clients to fill out a battery of self-report questionnaires if one works in a university clinic known for conducting research. In this chapter we describe several self-report forms that we consider helpful in gathering information about couples' general functioning, and in the following chapters we focus on measures that are specific to treatment planning for specific presenting problems.

ASSESSMENT OF PRESENTING PROBLEMS

Before exploring the couple's behavioral interactions, cognitions, and emotional responses associated with particular presenting problems, the clinician needs to inquire about the presenting problems themselves. As we have noted, they may involve characteristics of individual partners (e.g., depression), the relationship between partners (e.g., differences in life goals), or aspects of the couple's interpersonal or physical environment (e.g., a child with special needs, financial problems). Couples vary in the number and severity of the stressors they face, and for many couples a pile-up of stressors taxes their individual and joint coping abilities more than any single problem (Epstein & Baucom, 2002; Schlesinger & Epstein, 2007). Because clients initially may focus on problems that recently affected them most, it is important to survey a variety of possible problems they may have failed to mention. Questionnaires and interviews are the primary methods for systematically inquiring about the range and severity of problems.

WRITTEN SURVEYS OF PRESENTING PROBLEMS

An efficient method for assessing a variety of presenting problems is a brief survey that asks the individual to identify which problems from a list are occurring in the couple's relationship and how much conflict or distress results from each one. As an example, in our Center for Healthy Families couple and family therapy clinic at the University of Maryland, we developed a Relationship Issues Survey (RIS; Epstein & Werlinich, 1999) that lists problems couples may experience and asks each partner to independently rate how much each topic currently is a source of disagreement or conflict. The respondent rates each topic on a 4-point scale, ranging from 0 ("not at all") to 3 ("very much"). The RIS has been revised to include more items that address client diversity. Some couples may experience problems not included in the RIS, so the form includes an "other" option for describing such issues. The revised RIS can be found in Handout 3.1 (available on the book's web page at *www.guilford.com/epstein-materials*). When the therapist reviews the couple's responses with them during a joint session, further inquiry can be conducted regarding the specific characteristics of the problems they identify, such as how often each one occurs, in what circumstances, and who responds in what ways behaviorally, cognitively, and emotionally. Regarding stressors external to the couple, it is important to inquire about their impact on each partner and the relationship. Differences in partners' perceptions about problems can be explored, although the therapist must be cautious about pursuing details if a person responds defensively when blamed by their partner for a problem.

INTERVIEW SURVEY OF PRESENTING PROBLEMS

It is important to supplement a written survey of problems with an interview. We have already noted that an interview allows one to probe for details about the occurrence of each presenting problem. For example, a couple may identify sexual problems as a source of conflict, and subsequent inquiry may reveal that this became an issue after the couple began to experience a problem with infertility. Similarly, an interview may reveal that conflict over finances began after one of the partners lost a job. The therapist also can ask about strategies that the couple used to manage any similar stressors in the past. The therapist also can broaden the assessment beyond the topics covered by the RIS by asking open-ended questions about any issues regarding the individuals' relationship and environment. The outlines for pretherapy assessment interviews with the couple and individual partners that are presented in Figures 3.1 and 3.2, respectively, include a section for inquiring about presenting problems in those three domains.

ASSESSMENT OF COUPLE BEHAVIORAL INTERACTION PATTERNS

Information about a couple's dyadic behavioral patterns can be obtained through interviews, questionnaires, and behavioral observation. Each method has advantages and disadvantages, so, when possible, it is advisable to use more than one. Because partners provide subjective perceptions and memories in their interview and questionnaire responses, it is valuable to observe their communication within one's office as well. On the other hand, the small samples of behavior couples provide while the therapist is watching likely differ from their behavior at home, so their self-reports about daily life can reveal key patterns.

What types of behavioral interactions should be assessed? As described in Chapter 1, positive and negative verbal and nonverbal acts that each member of a couple exhibits toward the other, which commonly form circular dyadic patterns, are of central interest. Because we value the strong empirical tradition in CBCT, we tend to focus on forms of behavior that have been identified as problematic in research on relationships. The studies typically have been conducted in laboratory settings in which couples are asked to hold brief discussions, often regarding topics that have been sources of conflict. Video recordings of the discussions are coded by research assistants with extensive training in identifying specific types of positive and negative communication behavior.

Prime examples of this microbehavioral coding approach are the Marital Interaction Coding System (MICS), initially developed by Weiss, Hops, and Patterson (1973) and later refined (Heyman, 2004); the Kategoriensystem für Partnerschaftliche Interaktion (KPI; Hahlweg, 2004; Hahlweg et al., 1984); and the Couples Interaction Scoring System (CISS; Gottman, 1979). Those systems have identified some common dyadic patterns (e.g., one partner making demands and the other withdrawing) that are associated with relationship distress. Those coding systems have been invaluable in identifying constructive and problematic forms of communication and in measuring improvement during therapy outcome studies (Epstein & Baucom, 2002; Kerig & Baucom, 2004). However, they tend to be impractical for clinical practice. Nevertheless, if clinicians become familiar with the types of positive and negative behavior included in them, they will be attuned to them during therapy sessions. Our own use of behavioral coding in our research has increased our skill for tracking couples' interactions, and students we trained as coders commonly reported that they now notice such patterns in couples they observe in daily life.

Therapists also have the option of asking a couple to engage in a discussion of a conflict topic during a session and to use their familiarity with coding systems to observe how they behave when they disagree. One also can pay attention to how quickly negative interactions intensify during therapy sessions (often within seconds), how partners react (e.g., reciprocating criticisms, withdrawing from each other, with one partner pressuring while the other person "shuts down") and can point this out to the couple. It is our experience that even when couples are aware that negative interactions erupt quickly, they often are unaware of how that process unfolds, and a therapist can coach them in developing better self-regulation. This focus on a couple's interaction process is consistent with a systemic framework and can help identify patterns that can be foci of the treatment plan.

Questionnaires that ask members of a couple to describe their typical communication behavior have been limited in number and scope. A measure that has been used widely in research and is brief enough to apply in clinical practice is Christensen and colleagues' Communication Patterns Questionnaire (CPQ; Christensen, 1987; Crenshaw, Christensen, Baucom, Epstein, & Baucom,

2017). The CPQ asks each member of a couple to report how the couple as a dyad behaves when a problem arises in their relationship, when discussing a problem, and after such a discussion. It includes 35 items, but less than half have been used to form four subscales assessing constructive communication (e.g., "Both suggest solutions and compromises"), self-demand/partner withdraw (e.g., "I start discussion, my partner avoids"), partner demand/self-withdraw (e.g., "My partner starts discussion, I avoid"), and mutual avoidance (e.g., "Both avoid discussing"). Given inadequate psychometric qualities of those original subscales, Crenshaw et al. (2017) conducted further analyses, resulting in the constructive communication and both of the demand–withdraw subscales having much improved psychometrics and dropping the mutual avoidance subscale. Although a clinician may be able to elicit partners' reports of those patterns during interviews, the CPQ offers an opportunity for each person to recall the couple's general pattern and report it without the other person monitoring and perhaps interfering. The therapist can examine the partners' CPQ responses, point out areas of agreement, and initiate a discussion of any differences. We also have constructed a screening questionnaire (Handout 3.2) (available on the book's web page at *www.guilford.com/epstein-materials*) that asks each member of a couple questions about a variety of dyadic communication patterns in their relationship, such as mutual arguing, mutual avoidance, pursue–withdraw, diverging into complaints about other past or present issues, and verbal aggression.

Because partner aggression is prevalent among couples seeking therapy and there is a risk that participating in conjoint sessions might result in increased harmful aggression, it is very important that clinicians screen for it before beginning treatment. Questionnaires such as Straus, Hamby, Boney-McCoy and Sugarman's (1996) Revised Conflict Tactics Scales (CTS2) ask individuals to report privately about the frequencies of occurrence of specific forms of physical, psychological and sexual partner aggression, perpetrated by one's partner and by oneself. In addition, Murphy and Hoover's (1999) Multidimensional Measure of Emotional Abuse (MMEA) questionnaire focuses on four major forms of psychological partner aggression: denigration (verbal attacks on the partner's characteristics); domination/intimidation (control through threats); restrictive engulfment (limiting the partner's independence and access to resources); and hostile withdrawal (refusal to interact with the partner). Handout 3.3 (Partner Aggression Scale; available on the book's web page at *www.guilford.com/epstein-materials*) provides a similar type of instrument for brief screening of physical, psychological, and sexual forms of partner aggression. The questions for assessment interviews with individual partners (Figure 3.2) include inquiries about partners' reports of aggression on Handout 3.3.

Therapists also can use interviews to inquire about how the members of the couple behave in particular situations that are relevant to their presenting problems. For example, when a couple has identified conflict regarding parenting as a problem, the therapist can inquire about specific challenges they face with their child(ren), how they each behave toward the child at such times, and how they interact with each other. This *functional analysis* inquiry about the sequence of events reveals when the negative interaction tends to take place, such as when one of them interrupts the other's attempts to manage child behavior, how the conflict tends to escalate (e.g., the person who was interrupted vents anger), and what occurs subsequently (e.g., the child begins crying and both parents storm out of the room). If a couple reports commonly escalating their conflict, the therapist can ask how they finally stop the escalation; if conflict typically results in their avoiding each other, the therapist can ask how they reengage. Members of couples commonly have a perceptual bias in which they focus on the other person's contributions to negative interactions (Epstein & Baucom, 2002), but a functional analysis assists the therapist in identifying instances in which the influences are mutual. This in no way blames victims of partner aggression for the behavior they receive, as each individual is responsible for their own actions, but it captures a common tendency for partners to retaliate.

Behavioral couple therapists such as Jacobson and Margolin (1979) have described the process of *negative reciprocity* in which members of a couple respond to each other's negative behavior by reciprocating negativity. Although a therapist may identify some of a couple's behavioral sequences by observing their interactions during sessions, and couples may report some patterns on a questionnaire, interviews with the couple in which the therapist conducts a functional analysis each time the partners report a recent negative interaction tend to yield the richest information about behavioral interactions, including ways in which partners mutually influence each other's responses. Even when two partners describe different perceptions of the events that occurred, the therapist can emphasize collaboration on identifying any alternative responses each person could try that would lead to a more positive outcome in the future.

In addition to assessment of a couple's exchanges of positive and negative verbal and nonverbal acts that contribute to or detract from their relationship satisfaction, the behavioral assessment examines the partners' *communication and problem-solving skills*. Skills for expressing oneself clearly and constructively, as well as skills for listening empathically to the other's expressions of thoughts and emotions, are crucial for the fulfillment of partners' needs within the relationship. Behavioral coding systems such as the MICS and KPI include codes for positive expression, empathic listening, and problem-solving behaviors that can help guide therapists in evaluating the quality of partners' skills. The clinician also can observe the degrees to which the couple adheres to basic communication and problem-solving guidelines—for example, the extent to which they define the characteristics of a problem in behavioral terms, generate potential solutions, collaborate in evaluating the advantages and disadvantages of each solution, reach consensus about a solution they are willing to try, and devise a plan to implement it. The therapist can supplement these observations with questions to the couple such as:

- "When one of you brings up a complaint about your relationship, how does the other person tend to respond verbally and nonverbally?"
- "How do you communicate to each other that you are interested to know about the other's ideas and feelings?"
- "When you are discussing a problem in your relationship, how do you still demonstrate your caring for each other through your words and actions?"

Related to problem solving, another area of behavioral assessment focuses on the *couple's patterns of coping* both individually and as a dyad. Partners may bring different personal coping styles to their life together, which may interfere with solving the problems they face (Bodenmann et al., 2016). For example, when Samantha is faced with a life stressor, she prefers to gather information about potential solutions, set specific goals, and systematically work toward those goals. In contrast, her partner Andrea often distracts herself from upsetting problems and reduces her emotional distress through exercise, watching movies, and socializing with friends. Their different individual coping styles result in conflict when they are faced with a joint problem, such as credit card debt.

A second (and more systemic) perspective on couples coping with life stressors that has developed a strong research base and clinical applications is *dyadic coping*. It is based on the premise that a stressor that one member of a couple experiences likely affects the other member too, as do the partners' resources for coping. A framework for conceptualizing and measuring dyadic coping is Bodenmann's systemic transactional model (STM; Bodenmann, 1995; Bodenmann et al., 2016). As members of a couple experience stressors and communicate their distress verbally or nonverbally to each other, one partner can ignore or dismiss the other's signs of distress, communicate their own distress, or offer a form of dyadic coping, which can involve positive forms that reduce disruption from the stressor for the individual and couple, or negative forms that are intended to reduce one's own stress via negativity (Bodenmann et al., 2016).

There are three forms of positive partner-oriented dyadic coping in which one member of the couple acts to help the other cope with a stressor. The first two fall under the term *supportive dyadic coping*, which involves either emotion-focused actions to help one's partner reduce emotional distress (e.g., expressing affection, engaging the partner in distracting pleasant activities) or problem-focused actions that are intended to reduce or remove the stressors themselves. A third form of positive partner-oriented dyadic coping is *delegated dyadic coping*, in which the partner takes on some of the person's tasks to reduce the load. In contrast, forms of negative dyadic coping occur when the partner also is experiencing stress or lacks motivation or the ability to support the stressed individual. They include *hostile dyadic coping* (e.g., blaming one's partner for creating the problem), *ambivalent dyadic coping* (e.g., providing support but communicating that doing so is a burden), and *superficial dyadic coping* (e.g., providing support in a manner that conveys a lack of empathy for the other's feelings). Finally, *common dyadic coping* involves the two members of the couple sharing the coping process (e.g., reframing the stressor together as less threatening, engaging in joint activities to reduce emotional distress, jointly seeking information to solve the problem). When coping conjointly, partners can do so in a complementary way (e.g., one partner seeks information about their problem and the other evaluates whether the information is relevant for changing the situation) or in a symmetrically way (e.g., sharing a relaxing moment together).

Regarding assessment of a couple's dyadic coping behavioral patterns, the three modes of interviews, questionnaires, and behavioral observation can be used. However, although Bodenmann (2000) developed a system for coding dyadic coping behavior when observing a couple discussing a shared stressor, the complexity of using the system makes it impractical for clinical practice (Nussbeck & Jackson, 2016). Nevertheless, clinicians can become familiar with common dyadic coping patterns so they will notice them during sessions. For example, when an individual during a couple session has described feeling stress about her unpaid student loans from college, the therapist might observe that her partner responds with supportive dyadic coping (e.g., pointing out that she has reduced the debt considerably in recent years) and delegated dyadic coping (e.g., offering to pay more of their joint bills so she can make larger loan payments) versus hostile dyadic coping (e.g., blaming her for spending too much on personal items rather than making larger loan payments). Questionnaires assessing dyadic coping are a more user-friendly alternative. As is true of self-report measures in general, they rely on the validity of respondents' memories of typical behavior in their relationship, so clinicians need to keep an eye out for corroborating information, such as when partners' descriptions of their dyadic pattern are similar. Bodenmann's (2008) 37-item Dyadic Coping Inventory (DCI) has strong evidence of reliability and validity, and is the most widely used dyadic coping scale (Nussbeck & Jackson, 2016). It has a subscale assessing the degree to which a stressed member of a couple communicates with their partner about the problem, a subscale regarding how the partner responds to the individual's request for help in coping, and subscales assessing the eight dimensions of dyadic coping included in Bodenmann's STM model. Six of the dyadic coping subscales involve an individual's response to a partner's stress, and two tap shared coping between partners. There are three dyadic coping subscales assessing an individual's positive responses to a partner's stress: (1) *emotion-focused supportive coping* (e.g., expressing emotional caring); (2) *problem-focused supportive coping* (giving the partner advice in solving their stressful problem); and (3) delegated coping (e.g., taking over some of a partner's tasks in order to allow the partner to use personal time and resources to focus on the stressors). Two other DCI subscales assess joint coping: (4) *emotion-focused common coping* (e.g., mutual efforts to reduce emotional distress) and (5) problem-solving common coping (e.g., joint brainstorming of possible solutions to a problem). In contrast to constructive dyadic coping, there are three DCI subscales that assess negative forms, involving an individual's responses to the partner's expressions of stress: (6) *hostile coping* (e.g., explicitly communicating disinterest in the partner's distress); (7) *ambivalent coping* (e.g., providing support to the partner but also communicating a lack of motivation to do so); and (8) *superficial coping* (e.g., failing to listen and empathize actively with the distressed partner). Nussbeck and Jackson (2016) note that the DCI also contributes to a systemic view of coping within the relationship by measuring each member's perceptions of both their own and their partner's coping behavior.

Whether or not the therapist uses a questionnaire such as the DCI to collect information about a couple's dyadic coping, familiarity with the coping dimensions is useful for conducting an inquiry about coping patterns during joint and individual interviews with the partners. After conducting a brief oral survey about past and current stressors that the clients have experienced over the course of their relationship (guided by the ecological model we described earlier that covers multiple levels of life stressors), the therapist can ask open-ended questions about how a stressor affected each member of the couple individually and their relationship, how they communicate to each other about their experienced stress, how they identify when their partner is stressed, and how they have coped as a couple with individual and dyadic stressors. Figure 3.4 is a guide for interviewing the members of a couple about ways they communicate their stress to each other and the dyadic strategies they use to cope with stressors affecting them individually or as a couple. The therapist can listen for each person's individual emotion-focused and problem-focused coping responses, as well as forms of dyadic coping. If the clients fail to describe forms of dyadic coping, the clinician can use follow-up questions to inquire about them.

SUMMARY REGARDING BEHAVIORAL ASSESSMENT

Assessment of a couple's behavioral interaction patterns can include questionnaires but typically focuses on interviews and observation of the couple's interactions in the clinician's office. The therapist seeks concrete data regarding the partners' verbal and nonverbal actions toward each other, conducting a functional analysis to identify ways in which the partners influence each other. In addition to obtaining information about the frequency and sequences of particular actions that influence partners' overall levels of satisfaction with their relationship, the therapist assesses their communication and joint problem-solving skills. Although this chapter describes a variety of behavioral assessment strategies and methods, the therapist must use clinical judgment to collect sufficient information about each couple's behavioral patterns to develop appropriate treatment goals for them. Furthermore, in each of the following chapters that focuses on treatment planning for a particular presenting problem, we describe the assessment of specific types of behavior that are especially relevant to understanding and treating the problem, including communication,

Introduction: I will be asking you some questions about how you cope with stress individually and with your partner. I will be asking each question to each of you individually. Even though you may disagree with some of the responses that your partner gives, it is important not to interrupt because it is important for me to understand how each of you experiences moments of stress that affect you or your partner. At the end I will ask some questions to both of you together.

A. Questions for Partner A

1. What strategies do you use to cope with stress (for example, try to solve the stressful issue, try not to think about it, focus on thinking positively, pray, express your feelings to someone who cares)?

2. Which ways of coping with stress are effective in reducing the level of stress you feel? Which ways are not effective?

3. Do any of those coping strategies have a positive impact on your couple relationship? If so, which ones?

4. Do any of those coping strategies have a negative impact on your couple relationship? If so, which ones?

5. How much do you let your partner know when you are stressed? If you do let your partner know, how do you do it? Do you also let your partner know the type of response or help that you need from them?

6. How does your partner respond to your communication of stress if you let them know about it? What does your partner do/say?

7. What do you find helpful about your partner's responses? Why?

8. What do you find less helpful or even unhelpful about your partner's responses? Why?

B. Questions for Partner B

1. How much do you become aware of it when your partner is stressed? If you are aware, how do you know?

2. What do you think and feel when you know or notice that your partner is experiencing stress?

3. How do you respond to your partner's stress? For example, do you talk with them about it? Do you try to help them reduce their stress? If so, how?

4. Which of your responses to your partner do you think are helpful for them? Why?

5. Which of your responses to your partner do you think are less helpful or even unhelpful for them? Why?

C. Questions for Partner B

1. What strategies do you use to cope with stress (for example, try to solve the stressful issue, try not to think about it, focus on thinking positively, pray, express your feelings to someone cares)?

2. Which ways of coping with stress are effective in reducing the level of stress you feel? Which ways are not effective?

3. Do any of those coping strategies have a positive impact on your couple relationship? If so, which ones?

4. Do any of those coping strategies have a negative impact on your couple relationship? If so, which ones?

(continued)

FIGURE 3.4. Dyadic Coping Interview.

5. How much do you let your partner know when you are stressed? If you do let your partner know, how do you do it? Do you also let your partner know the type of response or help that you need from them?

6. How does your partner respond to your communication of stress if you let them know about it? What does your partner do/say?

7. What do you find helpful about your partner's responses? Why?

8. What do you find less helpful or even unhelpful about your partner's responses? Why?

D. Questions for Partner A

1. How much do you become aware of it when your partner is stressed? If you are aware, how do you know?

2. What do you think and feel when you know or notice that your partner is experiencing stress?

3. How do you respond to your partner's stress? For example, do you talk with them about it? Do you try to help them reduce their stress? If so, how?

4. Which of your responses to your partner do you think are helpful for them? Why?

5. Which of your responses to your partner do you think are less helpful or even unhelpful for them? Why?

E. Questions for Partners A and B together

1. How do you cope when you are both stressed?

2. What do you find helpful for you personally about the way the two of you respond when you are both stressed? Why?

3. What do you find less helpful for you personally about the way the two of you respond when you are both stressed? Why?

4. Overall, how satisfied are you with the way you and your partner communicate with each other that you're stressed?

5. Overall, how satisfied are you with the way you and your partner help each other cope with stress?

6. Overall, how satisfied are you with the way you and your partner cope with stress together as a team?

FIGURE 3.4. (*continued*)

problem solving, and stress-coping patterns. The data from that assessment contribute to goals that involve changing specific aspects of partners' behavior patterns. The behavioral assessment is conducted in conjunction with assessment of partners' cognitions and emotional responses that also contribute to the presenting problem.

ASSESSMENT OF COGNITIONS ASSOCIATED WITH A PRESENTING PROBLEM

As described in Chapter 1, five types of cognition have been identified as influencing the quality of couple relationships: assumptions, standards, selective perception, attributions, and expectancies (Baucom et al., 1989; Epstein & Baucom, 2002). It is important to gather information about partners' cognitions that influence their relationship *in general*—for example, an individual's standard that one should demonstrate caring for a partner by expressing it verbally. In addition, it is crucial to identify cognitions associated with a particular presenting problem (e.g., attributing a partner's decreased sexual desire to decreased love for oneself).

Information about partners' cognitions regarding their relationship in general and about particular presenting problems can be gathered through questionnaires, interviews, and observation of the couple during sessions. As with measures of behavioral patterns, a limited number of questionnaires have been developed to tap types of relationship cognitions that have been useful in research. For example, Eidelson and Epstein (1982) developed the Relationship Belief Inventory (RBI), which assesses several assumptions and standards that tend to be unrealistic (e.g., the belief that partners should be able to "mind-read" each other's thoughts and feelings). A copy of the RBI can be found in Baucom and Epstein's (1990) text. Similarly, the Inventory of Specific Relationship Standards (ISRS; Baucom et al., 1996) and the Inventory of General Relationship Standards (IGRS; Epstein, Baucom, Burnett, & Rankin, 1990; Epstein, Chen, & Beyder-Kamjou, 2005) measure individuals' personal standards for several core dimensions of couple relationships—notably, the degree to which partners should focus on togetherness versus personal autonomy, in terms of sharing time, activities, personal thoughts, and the like; how decision-making power should be distributed between partners; the degree to which partners should invest time and energy in the relationship. The ISRS items ask about those dimensions of relationship standards regarding specific relationship topics (e.g., relations with friends, child rearing, finances, the sexual relationship, expression of positive and negative emotions). An example of an investment item regarding friends is "Each of us should put a great deal of effort and energy into developing good relationships with our partner's friends." In contrast, the IGRS asks about the standards regarding the core dimensions as they apply more broadly to one's couple relationship; for example, a sample investment item is "We should spend a lot of time doing things to benefit our relationship." All three of those questionnaires have been used primarily in research investigating how assumptions and standards are associated with partners' levels of relationship satisfaction and their communication patterns. However, given their length, they can be less efficient measures for clinical practice in comparison to clinical interviews. Handout 3.4 (available on the book's web page at *www.guilford.com/epstein-materials*) is a shortened version of the IGRS that can be used in clinical practice for identifying partners' overall standards. We also suggest that therapists be familiar with the types of assumptions and standards measured by the questionnaires, so that they can keep them in mind when interviewing a couple regarding their beliefs about the issues for which they are seeking help.

As described in Chapter 1, forms of relational cognitive schemas that are emphasized by attachment theorists are an individual's "working models" about the lovability of the self and the emotional availability of significant others (Bowlby, 1969; Fletcher et al., 2018). In Bowlby's model, these schemas tend to develop in childhood and can be fairly stable; they persist into adulthood unless the individual has new relational experiences that counteract them. In anxious insecure attachment, the individual's working model involves a strong need for intimacy paired with anticipated abandonment, leading to hypervigilance for possible signs that a significant other is unavailable and to efforts to keep the needed person close. In avoidant insecure attachment, the working model involves a belief that intimacy and dependence on unreliable others should be avoided (Mikulincer & Shaver, 2016). Such schemas may be influencing a couple's presenting problems, as when an insecure male who has a self-schema of being unlovable uses psychological and physical aggression to control his female partner when she exhibits any independence, given his schema that her independence is an aspect of her unavailability to meet his emotional needs. Consequently, couple therapists may find it useful to include a questionnaire that measures each partner's attachment style in the pretreatment assessment. For example, the 12-item version of the Experiences in Close Relationships scale (ECR; Wei, Russell, Mallinckrodt, & Vogel, 2007) measures anxious attachment (e.g., "I'm afraid that I will lose my partner's love") and avoidant attachment (e.g., "I prefer not to be too close to romantic partners"). The ECR has demonstrated good reliability and validity, and its brevity makes it easy to use in clinical practice.

Similar circumstances exist regarding questionnaires developed to measure partners' attributions about factors influencing presenting problems. For example, Pretzer, Epstein, and Fleming's (1991) Marital Attitude Survey (MAS) asks individuals to rate the degrees to which they agree with statements regarding causes of problems in their couple relationship. The MAS includes subscales for attributions of problems to one's own behavior, one's own personality, the partner's behavior, the partner's personality, the partner's lack of love, and the partner's malicious intent. It also includes subscales assessing expectancies that the couple has the ability to improve problems in their relationship and actually will accomplish that goal. Studies with the MAS have demonstrated how negative (blaming) attributions are associated with relationship conflict and distress, so clinicians could administer it as a screening measure. But its utility for treatment planning, especially for specific presenting problems, is limited. Consequently, therapists can be aware of the types of attributions that can be problematic and probe for them during interviews with clients.

During the initial joint interview, each partner's individual interview, and subsequent joint therapy sessions, the two primary ways to gather information about cognitions are to listen for spontaneous expressions of thoughts and to probe for particular types of cognition (Epstein & Baucom, 2002). Sometimes an individual will explicitly describe a cognition while interacting with the partner and therapist. For example, as an individual is complaining about a partner's failure to follow through on a household task, he may state, "It's just another example of how our home and life together are a low priority for you." This statement reflects the individual's attribution that the partner's actions (or lack thereof) were caused by a lack of care and motivation. The therapist has an opportunity to explore that cognition by reflecting back what the client stated and asking them to say more about the meaning they attached to the partner's behavior. In other instances, members of a couple spontaneously voice their assumptions (e.g., "Your mother taught you that you can do no wrong!"), standards (e.g., "Telling me you love me doesn't count when you don't spend much time with me"), expectancies (e.g., "If I disagree with you, you won't listen to my ideas"), and selective perceptions (e.g., "You never agree with my ideas about child rearing").

In addition to waiting for partners' spontaneous expressions of their cognitions, a therapist can probe for them. For example, the therapist may notice nonverbal cues that an individual seemed to have an emotional response to something their partner just said. The therapist could state, "Samin, you seemed to have a reaction to something Tenzin just said. What emotion were you feeling?" After Samin responds, "I was really irritated by his statement that we don't pay enough attention to our finances," the therapist then asks, "What was it about Tenzin's statement that irritated you?" Samin responds, "I took it to mean that he was saying *I* don't pay enough attention to finances, and he thinks I'm irresponsible with money." The therapist has uncovered Samin's *attribution* that Tenzin's comment was caused by his having a negative view of her, which angered her.

Similarly, therapists can probe for individuals' *expectancies* about the likelihood that particular events will occur in the near or distant future. When Gloria expressed concern that Marco is inattentive to the couple's finances and gave as an example Marco's tendency to purchase expensive gifts for friends and relatives, the therapist reflected, "Gloria, it sounds like you think Marco's approach to purchases could lead to a problem for the two of you. What do you picture happening?" Gloria responded, "I'm worried that over time we are going to build up significant debt that will hurt us financially in the long run." The therapist then asked Gloria. "On a scale of 0% to 100%, what's your estimate of the chance that Marco's spending will lead to a problematic level of debt for the two of you?" Gloria replied, "When he hasn't bought anything for a while, I probably estimate it as 40%, but around holiday gift-giving time, I think it's 90%."

A therapist also can probe for individuals' *standards* for themselves, their partners, and their relationship. For example, when a couple was relating the history of their relationship during their initial interview with their therapist, Carl stated, "I always thought being really close with your partner meant sharing personal feelings on a regular basis, but it turns out that John is a private person, and it's frustrating that I have to pry information from him, and he quickly seems bored when I'm telling him about things going on in my life." The therapist then inquired, "Carl, it sounds like there's a level of sharing of personal thoughts and emotions that you want in your relationship with John, and what actually happens in daily life hasn't been matching that." Carl responded by elaborating on his personal standard for communication in an intimate relationship.

A similar approach can be used to tap partners' *assumptions* about the characteristics of relationships and the people who comprise them. For example, a therapist may hear hints that an individual holds an assumption that one's childhood experiences with parents significantly determine (and limit) one's personality and capacity to be a good partner as an adult.

Finally, information about partners' *selective perceptions* of events in their relationship can be elicited through specific questions about what each person has noticed over time, including the frequency of particular events and the conditions in which they have occurred. Thus, Cheryl stated with an exasperated tone, "I'm tired of being in charge of getting things done around our house!" The therapist asked her for some specific examples of her being in charge, and she said that unless she initiated times and plans for paying bills, budgeting, and savings, James failed to take the lead, and nothing was accomplished. The therapist asked her what percentage of the time she noticed that James did initiate tasks, and she replied, "I really can't think of any. I think I'd faint if he did it." The accuracy of Cheryl's perception can be explored by asking her to think about any exceptions that she has noticed, even small ones, because that would be important information. In addition, James may respond to Cheryl's depiction of him by identifying instances in which he took the lead, and the therapist can explore whether Cheryl had overlooked those events or discounted them as legitimate initiation on his part.

COGNITIONS ABOUT THE PARTNER, SELF, AND RELATIONSHIP

In order to identify the core cognitions influencing a couple's presenting problems, it is important to assess each partner's cognitions about the self, as well as the other person and relationship. Some individuals are more likely to reveal their cognitions about their partner, in the context of blaming the partner for the relationship issues, but cognitions about the self and relationship also can have significant effects. For example, individuals commonly make *attributions* about the causes of their emotional responses to their partner and relationship, which influence their evaluation of the status and future of the relationship. Thus, Angela noticed that she increasingly felt sad in Maya's presence, and in addition had low motivation to express affection toward her. Angela developed an attribution that the shift from positive to negative emotions toward Maya might indicate that she was falling out of love with her, an inference that was alarming to her. The couple therapist concluded that the treatment plan should include interventions to help Angela examine the validity of her distressing inference about her changed emotions.

Similarly, an individual's personal *standards* about couple relationships may influence their satisfaction with the current relationship. For example, Minh was frustrated and anxious that he and Mai had not achieved what he judged to be a secure future for their children 10 years after immigrating from Vietnam to the United States. Both had worked hard to overcome language barriers, held two jobs each, purchased a home, raised two children, and obtained American citizenship. However, Minh believed he and Mai had *failed* in their dream of providing their children a great education because they could not afford top colleges with expensive tuition that some of their children's friends would be able to attend. His high (and potentially unrealistic) standard regarding achievement as a couple caused him significant distress and contributed to conflict between him and Mai.

SELF-REGULATION OF COGNITION

In Beck's cognitive therapy model (e.g., Beck et al., 1979), an individual's stream-of-consciousness thoughts are referred to as "automatic thoughts" because they seem to be spontaneous, unplanned, and beyond the person's control. Thus, whenever Marisa did not pay attention to something Esteban said, he immediately had thoughts such as, "She doesn't care about me." In that moment his cognition became his reality, triggering anxiety, anger, and sarcastic comments toward Marisa. Similarly, individuals' limited ability to self-regulate by employing *executive functions* involving cognitive problem solving has been implicated in a wide variety of psychological problems such as anxiety, depression, suicidal ideation and behavior, posttraumatic stress disorder, and relationship problems, as well as academic and vocational difficulties (Diamond, 2013; Epstein & Baucom, 2002; Epstein, Baucom, Kirby, & LaTaillade, 2019; Fruzzetti & Payne, 2015; Murray, Rosanbalm, & Christopoulos, 2016; Newman, 2018; Nezu et al., 2019; Pronk, Finkenauer, & Kuijer, 2017; Resick, 2018). Types of executive functions include *inhibition* (resisting acting impulsively, delaying gratification, staying on task), *working memory* (holding information in mind and using it to problem-solve), *cognitive flexibility* (seeing various perspectives and adapting to changes in circumstances), *fluid intelligence* (being able to reason logically through inductive and deductive thinking, seeing patterns or relations among things), and *planning* (Diamond, 2013). Diamond's extensive review of research indicates that life experiences that negatively affect children's social, emotional or physical health interfere with the development of executive functions, but they can be improved through training.

Given the complexities of two partners understanding and meeting each other's needs, as well as accomplishing tasks of daily living and solving problems, it is important that therapists get a sense of partners' executive functioning. A widely used questionnaire is Roth, Isquith, and Gioia's (2005) Behavior Rating Inventory of Executive Functioning—Adult Version (BRIEF-A), which includes inhibit, shift, emotional control, initiate, working memory, organization of materials, task monitor, plan/organize, and self-monitor subscales. During interviews with the couple and individual partners, the clinician can use knowledge of the types of executive functions to ask them how they attempt to solve problems individually and together. When clients spontaneously describe difficulties such as impulsive verbal aggression, the therapist can probe for more examples of how the individual responds to frustrating actions on their partner's part. To observe a couple directly, the therapist can ask them to discuss and work on resolving a problem in their relationship, and watch how they attend to information from each other, inhibit impulsive responses, and integrate their ideas to formulate solutions.

SUMMARY REGARDING COGNITIVE ASSESSMENT

In sum, the goal of cognitive assessment is to collect information about cognitions that contribute to a couple's presenting problems, which should be included as foci of the treatment plan. Questionnaire responses, spontaneous expressions of cognitions during interviews, and responses to the therapist's inquiries about each partner's thoughts all can uncover assumptions, standards, selective perceptions, attributions and expectancies that contribute to relationship problems by being unrealistic or inappropriate. Based on the cognitive assessment, the therapist needs to consider including in the treatment plan interventions that focus on (1) altering cognitions directly (e.g., modifying a negative attribution by exploring alternative explanations for a partner's upsetting behavior); (2) creating behavior change that shifts cognitions (e.g., improving an individual's empathic listening skills so that a partner is less likely to view the individual as uncaring); (3) directly modifying emotional responses that trigger negative cognitions (e.g., using self-soothing exercises that reduce anger toward a partner and the associated tendency to focus on the partner's displeasing actions); and (4) guiding partners in practicing effective forms of executive functioning. The following chapters include assessment of cognitions that commonly arise with particular presenting problems, with implications for treatment.

ASSESSMENT OF EMOTIONAL RESPONSES IN COUPLE INTERACTIONS

As described in Chapter 1, in a CBCT model individuals' emotional experiences can be either causes or consequences of the partners' behavioral interactions and cognitions. Members of couples may exhibit *excesses* in their emotional states (e.g., poor emotion regulation in which they quickly become enraged when their partner frustrates them) or *deficits* in emotional responses or awareness of their emotional states, which interferes with joint problem solving and intimacy (Epstein & Baucom, 2002).

Assessment of emotions takes place within the therapist's *functional analysis* of couple dynamics, identifying the frequency and intensity of each partner's emotional responses and the contextual factors (stimuli and consequences) that influence them. Because many people experience their emotional responses as being out of their control, identifying links among behaviors, thoughts and emotions can help clients make sense of confusing emotional experiences and increase their belief that they can increase conscious control over them. Interventions, including those in couple therapy (Pronk et al., 2017), can improve emotion regulation and other aspects of executive function (Diamond, 2013; Murray et al., 2016).

It is important that the therapist validate that it is normal to experience a variety of emotions as a human being, but that it is crucial for each person to have the ability to regulate the intensity of those emotional responses and express them constructively. For example, noticing that one feels anger in response to a partner's behavior is important information, in that it may be associated with perceiving some inequity in the relationship that should be discussed. However, if the individual's anger rapidly escalates and is vented through aggressive behavior toward the partner, it likely will contribute to increased couple conflict and distract the couple from the underlying issue of equity.

It also is important to differentiate between *affective states*, in which an individual's moods fluctuate from one situation to another and over time, and *affective traits or disorders* characterized by relatively stable moods. Rodney presented an example of affective states when he and Tom both described his anger outbursts at home, and they agreed that he rarely vented anger with co-workers, friends, or strangers. In contrast, an individual with persistent depressive disorder (dysthymia) tends to exhibit depressed moods across time and situations for years (American Psychiatric Association, 2022). Similarly, individuals with generalized anxiety disorder tend to experience excessive anxiety, associated with worry, across time and various life situations (American Psychiatric Association, 2022), which may manifest in frequent expressions of anxiety in discussions with the partner about finances, jobs, children, and so on. Determining the degree to which individuals' emotional responses are a function of conditions within the couple relationship versus manifestations of trait-like personality characteristics or temperament has implications for treatment planning. Whereas situational affective states may be addressed more directly with couple-based interventions, trait-like emotions are more likely to require concurrent interventions for the individual. Figure 3.5 presents a Guide for Individual Interview Assessing Emotional Responses. It is intended to be administered to partners separately, to identify traits and state aspects of partners' emotional responses.

Often individuals' emotional responses are based on a combination of dispositional and situational factors. Thus, Tanisha's anxious insecure attachment style led her to be hypervigilant for signs in any situation that suggested to her that Naeem was unavailable to her emotionally. Schachner, Shaver, and Mikulincer (2003) note that attachment systems of anxious insecure individuals tend to be activated often and for long periods of time, as these individuals are more easily threatened than most people by the potential that their partner is unavailable. However, the couple's therapist also determined that Tanisha's trait-like tendency to experience anxiety often was triggered by Naeem's tendency to communicate vaguely about his daily plans or how he had spent time while away from her. His evasiveness appeared to be based on his distaste for "being micromanaged" by Tanisha and his tendency to cope with his anger by withdrawing from her. The couple was locked in a pursue–withdraw cycle in which each person's behavior elicited negative emotion and problematic behavior from the other. In such a case, the treatment plan may include interventions to modify the negative dyadic pattern, plus interventions (including possible referrals for individual therapy) intended to reduce each person's reactivity to the other's actions.

The therapist also has opportunities to observe samples of partners' *in vivo* emotional responses to each other during joint sessions, conducting a functional analysis of the conditions preceding and following them. Interviews regarding each partner's personal history can reveal relevant information regarding the development of relatively stable cognitive-affective traits, such as an individual's pattern of perceiving the self as unlovable and feeling anxious in close relationships since childhood.

Finally, clinicians can use a small number of brief questionnaires when relevant to assess dispositional emotional responses. For example, the Difficulties in Emotion Regulation Scale

I would like to ask you a series of questions regarding your experiences of emotions within your couple relationship, especially emotions that you tend to experience when you are interacting with your partner. You are an expert on what you feel inside, so please answer my questions by thinking about emotions you have felt in particular situations, whether or not you told your partner about them at the time.

First, I would like to get a sense of emotions that you feel pretty often in your life, in a variety of situations, not just in your couple relationship. For example, I am interested in learning whether you have a general tendency to feel anxiety in your daily life, not just associated with your interactions with your partner. If there are particular life situations that create negative or positive emotions for you, it will be helpful for me to know about them. The first set of questions is about those emotional responses.

1. How often do you experience anxiety in your daily life—symptoms of tension, shakiness, difficulty concentrating, worry about negative things happening, and so on? When you do feel symptoms of anxiety, how mild to strong are they?
2. In what situations in your life do you experience anxiety? What other people, if any, are present? What thoughts are you aware of having at times when you become anxious?
3. How do you tend to behave when you are feeling anxiety? How does your partner tend to behave when you become anxious?
4. When you feel anxiety, what seems to help you reduce it?
5. How often do you experience depression in your daily life–symptoms of low mood with deep sadness, low motivation, lack of energy, a sense of hopelessness, a desire to isolate yourself from other people? When you do feel symptoms of depression, how mild to strong are they?
6. In what situations in your life do you experience depression? What other people, if any, are present? What thoughts are you aware of having at times when you feel depressed?
7. How do you tend to behave when you are feeling depressed? How does your partner tend to behave when you become depressed?
8. When you feel depressed, what seems to help you reduce it?
9. People commonly feel a variety of other emotions in daily life and in their couple relationships. Please tell me about other positive and negative emotions you tend to experience, such as happiness/joy, warmth toward someone, anger, shame, and jealousy.
10. Often people experience a mixture of emotions in a situation; for example, feeling angry, but also sad. In that example, an individual may be most aware of feeling angry at a partner who has been paying little attention to the individual, and may mostly express anger to the partner. However, underneath the anger the person also may feel lonely and sad. Please tell me about experiences with your partner when you are aware of having mixed emotions.

For each emotion that the individual identifies, ask about frequency, intensity, and situational factors associated with its occurrence (people present, the person's cognitions), and how the individual and partner tend to respond when the individual is experiencing that emotion.

Next, I would like you to focus on emotions you experience with your partner. For each of them, please tell me how often you tend to feel it, how strong the emotion is, and what specific things are going on between you and your partner when you feel that emotion.
Inquire about positive emotions of happiness/joy and warmth, as well as negative emotions of anxiety, fear, depression, anger, shame, or jealousy. Give the individual an opportunity to add any other emotion that they experience.

FIGURE 3.5. Interview guide for individual interviews assessing emotional responses.

(DERS; Gratz & Roemer, 2004) has six subscales that assess problems with affect regulation: *awareness* (inability to identify one's emotional states), *clarity* (difficulty differentiating types of emotion), *goals* (interference of emotions with goal-directed behavior), *impulse control* (lack of behavioral control when upset), *nonacceptance* (failure to accept emotions as normal or appropriate), and *strategies* (limited strategies for regulating emotions). The original 36-item DERS (Gratz & Roemer, 2004) and a revised 18-item short form (Kaufman, Xia, Fosco, Yaptangco, Skidmore, & Crowell, 2016) have demonstrated good reliability and validity. The clinician also can administer brief measures of psychopathology symptoms, such as the Beck Depression Inventory–II (BDI-II; Beck, Steer, & Brown, 1996), the Beck Anxiety Inventory (BAI; Beck, Epstein, Brown & Steer, 1988), and the Generalized Anxiety Disorder–7 (GAD-7; Spitzer, Kroenke, Williams, & Lowe, 2006) scale, which can be accessed free online.

It also is important to measure each partner's *overall level of satisfaction* with the couple relationship. Spanier's (1976) 32-item Dyadic Adjustment Scale (DAS) has been used extensively, with substantial evidence that it taps individuals' overall sentiment regarding their relationships. However, it assesses a number of related aspects of relationship "adjustment" in addition to global satisfaction, such as consensus between partners on a variety of topics (e.g., finances, religious matters, household tasks). Snyder's (1997) 150-item Marital Satisfaction Inventory—Revised (MSI-R) is a well-validated multidimensional measure of how well the individual perceives the functioning of the relationship. For clinical practice, Funk and Rogge's (2007) 16-item version of their Couples Satisfaction Index (CSI-16) is a concise and psychometrically sound instrument that assesses global relationship satisfaction and is available free online.

In the prior section on assessment of cognition, we described how one's ability to regulate emotions is one of several components of executive function, many of which involve intentional cognitive processes (e.g., delaying gratification). Consequently, when a clinician identifies that an individual has difficulty regulating negative emotions, it is important to explore other aspects of executive function that may be influencing problematic emotional responses. This could include administering Roth et al.'s (2005) BRIEF-A, but it primarily can involve probing for the person's thought processes that occur in conjunction with poorly regulated emotional responses. For example, when Will described his "short fuse" in becoming angry and venting it at Sharon quickly, the therapist explored the automatic thoughts he was aware of at such times. Will reported experiencing anger as a full-body response of intense arousal and tension, and he had no sense of anything he could do to reduce it before venting it. He had never done any problem-solving thinking to try to identify anger management strategies he might try.

Thus, it is important to inquire about each person's *cognitions about emotions*, as well as their experienced emotional states and ways of expressing them behaviorally. For example, based on growing up with parents who routinely vented emotions in an unbridled manner, Will developed an *assumption* that emotions are spontaneous and uncontrollable. An individual also may have developed a *standard* that one should vent emotions such as anger in order to be true to oneself; that is, it serves what seems to be a useful function. In some relationships, individuals have developed an *expectancy* that one's partner will ignore calm expressions of upset feelings but will pay attention if one vents anger. In turn, reliance on venting may lead the person's partner to develop a *selective perception* that "he *always* yells at me." Finally, as noted previously, individuals often make *attributions* about the causes of their emotions, such as attributing decreased affectionate feelings to a loss of love for one's partner. Given that at present there are no standardized questionnaires that measure those cognitions regarding emotional experiences, the primary methods for tapping them are clinical interviews with the couple and individual partners. In addition, verbal and non-verbal signs of partners' emotional responses to each other during sessions provide opportunities for a therapist to inquire about the emotional response and the individual's associated cognitions.

In contrast to instances in which members of a couple display overt signs of poorly regulated emotional responses during sessions or describe such occurrences with each other during their daily life, the therapist needs to explore the degree to which each individual may inhibit emotional responses. As is true in individual therapy, it is important that the therapist form hypotheses about emotions that are not being expressed directly but not ask leading questions that may bias the client's responses. Thus, as Isaac described how the heavy workload at his job made it impossible to set aside much time to spend with Ruth, the therapist noticed that Ruth was grimacing and shifting in her chair. The therapist turned to her, said that he noticed her nonverbal behavior, and asked her what feelings she was experiencing in response to what Isaac said. Ruth responded, "I'm frustrated and angry, because he always has excuses for not spending time with me." The therapist reflected back the feelings that Ruth had described, and she acknowledged his understanding of what she had said. However, based on the couple's initial presenting problem of a long-standing difference in their needs for intimacy (Ruth's were considerably higher) and information from her individual assessment interview, the therapist hypothesized that more vulnerable emotions might underlie her expressed anger. As we described in Chapter 1, the CBCT model shares with emotionally focused therapy (EFT) an assumption that when individuals express anger toward significant others there commonly are vulnerable underlying emotions such as sadness and anxiety. Epstein and Baucom (2002) note that individuals may focus on anger in order to protect themselves from experiencing the vulnerability. In this case, the therapist conducted a "downward-arrow" line of inquiry with Ruth to explore thoughts and emotions beneath her frustration and anger at Isaac's unavailability:

> THERAPIST: Ruth, I'd like to be sure I fully understand your experience when Isaac is too busy to spend time with you. What does it mean to you about your relationship when he says he's too busy?
>
> RUTH: I married him because he was really interested in me, and we had a good time together. Now it seems all of that is gone.
>
> THERAPIST: If those positive experiences you used to have are all gone, what would that be like for you?
>
> RUTH: It means I'm alone in this world. Sure, I have friends, but the person I thought would always be there for me, to be really close to, is gone.
>
> THERAPIST: What emotions do you feel when you think about being alone like that?
>
> RUTH: (*tearful*) "Lonely and sad . . . very sad.

A variety of cognitions can influence individuals' inhibition of emotional responses, and they need to be taken into account in treatment planning. For example, an individual may hold an *assumption* that becoming emotional is harmful to one's health, or a *standard* that a strong, competent person does not allow themself to experience (and especially express) "weak" emotions such as anxiety and depression. An individual who grew up in a family in which the expression of emotion generally was ignored may have developed a coping strategy of "tuning out" emotions, engaging in *selective perception*. Similarly, that individual may hold an *expectancy* that giving in to one's urge to express feelings to the partner will be futile. Finally, an individual may fail to notice a link between uncomfortable emotions and current interactions with a partner, instead *attributing* the feelings to job stress. The therapist can include interventions for such cognitive factors in the treatment plan.

SUMMARY REGARDING ASSESSMENT OF EMOTIONS

In order to devise an appropriate treatment plan, the assessment of partners' emotional experiences within their relationship needs to differentiate between emotional states that vary across situations and time, versus relatively persistent trait-like emotions that may be associated with temperament, executive function problems, or specific psychological disorders. Interventions to modify distressing couple interactions can be the focus for addressing emotional states, whereas referrals for individual therapy may be appropriate when one or both partners exhibit chronic difficulties with poor regulation of negative emotions or severe inhibition of emotion. It also is important to assess cognitions that influence emotional responses and to include them in the treatment plan.

KEY POINTS

- Couple therapists need to be competent in assessing both the systemic aspects of a couple's dyadic interactions and the personal functioning of each partner.

- Assessment includes behavioral interaction patterns, as well as each partner's cognitions and emotional responses, looking for influences among the three domains. A functional analysis of antecedents and consequences for each response reveals those patterns.

- Therapists can use questionnaires, interviews, and observation of couple interactions to tap behavioral, cognitive, and emotional domains. Familiarity with questionnaires and behavioral coding systems aids the clinician in interviewing couples about the three domains.

- Partners' cultural beliefs and traditions that influence their relationship and their level of comfort with couple therapy methods need to be assessed and incorporated into the treatment plan.

CHAPTER 4

Interventions in Cognitive–Behavioral Couple Therapy

This chapter describes a variety of interventions used in CBCT to modify aspects of a relationship that are contributing to the presenting problems. Based on assessment of the couple, the therapist plans interventions that focus on their *behavior* toward each other; their *cognitions* about each other and aspects of their environment (extended family, jobs, etc.) that influence each of them and the characteristics of their relationship; and their *emotional responses* to each other and other life experiences (Baucom & Epstein, 1990; Baucom et al., 2023; Epstein & Baucom, 2002; Epstein et al., 2019).

For clarity, we present separate sections for interventions regarding behavior, cognition, and emotion. However, because partners' behaviors, cognitions, and emotional responses continuously influence one another, the therapist pays attention to how intervening with one of these three domains is likely to influence the other two. Often, the success of intervening with one domain depends on some interventions with the other domains. For example, improving an individual's behavioral skills for empathic listening may lead the person's partner to perceive the individual as caring more, resulting in the partner feeling and expressing more affection. However, if the partner attributes the individual's past lack of empathic communication to a negative trait such as self-centeredness, the partner may discount the new demonstration of empathic listening, interpreting it as an attempt to look good in front of the therapist. Unless the therapist guides the partner in considering a more positive reason for the individual's empathic communication, the work on improving communication skills may be ineffective. Similarly, if the partner has difficulty regulating anger, they may experience anger as the individual struggles a bit to use empathic listening skills, which may override the partner's ability to see that the individual is making a sincere attempt to improve.

Because success with interventions for behavior, cognitions, or emotions often depends on paying attention to all three domains, therapists need to consider ways to integrate the three types of interventions. There is no "one-size-fits-all" way to sequence the interventions. For example, by the time couples find their way to a therapist, they commonly have developed ingrained negative cognitions about each other's motives and behavioral tendencies (e.g., a man states about his wife, "I've known her for years, and if I try to do something my own way, she'll just criticize me"). The therapist may be tempted to begin with an intervention designed to produce more positive couple behavior by coaching the couple in collaborative problem-solving skills. However, the partners' cognitions and emotional responses may undermine their attempts at problem solving. Thus, if an individual has an expectancy that their partner will criticize any idea they offer, the individual may communicate irritation nonverbally when making suggestions. The therapist would need to coach the individual in noticing how their negative expectancy results in anger and defensiveness toward their partner and explore their willingness to give the partner an opportunity to show support for their attempt to collaborate. On the other hand, when working to reduce a couple's mutual verbal aggression, it commonly is important to integrate interventions for regulation of emotions (e.g., self-soothing exercises), for cognition (e.g., self-talk focused on not taking a partner's provocative statements personally), and for behavior (e.g., agreeing to take a temporary "time-out" break from each other in order to avoid escalation and calm down).

Regarding the sequencing of interventions, to some extent behavior changes are needed early on to change couples' negative views of their relationship (i.e., seeing is believing). Couples commonly need to gain hope from some concrete evidence that their negative patterns can be changed. However, partners' willingness and ability to change their behavior depend on favorable conditions, including both individuals' *commitment* to the collaborative process of therapy (willingness to cooperate with their partner), as well as their ability to follow the therapist's guidance in refraining from negative escalation. When conditions favorable to behavioral change are lacking, interventions for problematic cognitions and emotional responses are needed early in therapy.

Commitment involves a cognitive process of deciding that it is worth investing one's time and effort into the relationship rather than disengaging. Often, individuals enter couple therapy feeling frustrated that their partner has not seemed to put sufficient effort into making changes, so they are "standing on ceremony," waiting to see effort by the partner before committing to make changes themselves. Therapists express empathy for their frustration but emphasize the value of each person making a contribution to change in the couple's negative patterns, operating with good will. We tell them that one aspect of our job as therapist is to monitor their efforts, providing support when making changes is uncomfortable but also providing feedback and encouragement for them to take some risks in changing behavior before knowing what the other person will do.

Other cognitions that often require intervention early in therapy are negative assumptions and expectancies about one's partner. From interacting with a partner over a period of time (sometimes fairly quickly), a person commonly develops a "frame" (Beck, 1988) or trait attributions (Baucom & Epstein, 1990; Epstein & Baucom, 2002) that their partner possesses relatively broad, stable personality characteristics. Although members of happy couples typically view their partners as possessing a number of positive traits, distressed partners commonly make inferences that each other has negative traits (e.g., dishonest, manipulative, controlling). Individuals who hold negative views of a partner are likely to be pessimistic about the partner's ability to make positive changes. When a therapist's assessment indicates that partners hold rigid negative views of each other, it may be essential to intervene early to broaden the "frame" so that each individual can see positive characteristics in the other person and some potential for change.

When members of a couple have difficulty making even small behavior changes due to flare-ups of emotions such as anger, it is important to intervene early to assist them with emotion regulation. Later in this chapter, we describe those interventions, which involve behavioral strategies such as taking an agreed upon "time-out" to calm down before continuing their interaction, cognitive strategies such as self-talk to counteract inflammatory thoughts, and strategies that directly focus on soothing emotional arousal.

In the following sections of this chapter, we describe interventions for behavior, cognition, and emotion and show how a therapist can conduct them in sessions as well as via homework. We also illustrate how one integrates interventions from the three domains.

INTERVENTIONS FOR MODIFYING BEHAVIOR

Interventions for behavioral patterns focus on the *process* of how the couple interacts regarding aspects of their relationship, such as maintaining emotional intimacy, fulfilling partners' needs and life goals, coping with life stressors, and resolving conflicts. Based on assessment of the couple's patterns (e.g., a tendency to avoid each other when conflict arises), the therapist draws attention to the patterns and discusses their advantages and disadvantages. For example, avoidance may reduce arguments temporarily, but the problems fester. This feedback is a cognitive intervention involving *psychoeducation* that paves the way for developing behavioral changes. It is based on the therapist's understanding that partners will be willing to try behaving differently if they believe that their old pattern has drawbacks and that the proposed new pattern will be better. Psychoeducation is an important method for increasing partners' beliefs in the value of experimenting with new ways of behaving with each other. During discussions of the benefits and drawbacks to the existing patterns, it is important that the therapist is sensitive to aspects of patterns that are based on the partners' social locations and cultural context regarding acceptable behavior within relationships (e.g., regarding gender roles). A therapist must consider differences between their social identities and cultural backgrounds and those of their clients, allowing partners to take the lead in identifying patterns they consider problematic in their relationship. For example, a therapist who grew up in a relatively individualistic society initially may consider it problematic that a couple's parents are highly involved in rearing their children, whereas the couple may consider it normative and acceptable within their collectivist culture.

Therefore, the therapist collaborates with the couple in planning behavior changes that will help them improve their presenting problems, such as reducing stress and conflict regarding financial matters and improving their lack of emotional and sexual intimacy. Although interventions in this section focus on observable behavior changes, the therapist continuously looks for cognitions and emotional responses that contribute to the problematic behavior. For example, after identifying that partners avoid talking about relationship problems, the therapist may inquire about each person's decision to not discuss the issues; both may reveal that they have an expectancy that focusing on problems will result in them breaking up, accompanied by anxiety. At that point, the therapist adds interventions for those cognitions and emotional responses to the treatment plan to produce more open communication and problem-solving behavior. The major types of interventions that focus directly on changing partners' behavior are (1) skills-based interventions and (2) guided behavior change.

In the following chapters, we describe treatment planning for a variety of couple presenting problems. Within a CBCT approach, the skills-based and guided behavior change strategies we cover can be applied to help couples reduce negative interaction patterns and solve those diverse presenting problems. In each chapter, we identify ways in which these behavioral interventions are part of the treatment plan.

The two types of behavioral interventions are similar in some ways. For example, in both skills-based and guided behavior change interventions, the therapist guides the couple in learning and practicing new behavioral patterns. Furthermore, both are designed to shift the couple away from negative interactions toward working as a team to meet each other's needs and deal with life stressors. The basic difference between them is that skills-based interventions help the partners develop specific behavioral skills for clear, effective communication and problem solving that they can apply to a wide variety of relationship issues, whereas guided behavior change focuses on increasing the frequency of particular types of behavior that fulfill partners' needs, such as actions that convey caring.

Skills–Based Interventions

These interventions focus on teaching behavioral skills that promote mutual understanding of each person's internal thoughts and emotions, as well as collaboration in solving problems and coping with life stressors. The therapist typically begins by providing *instruction* and *modeling* of the skills via didactic presentations (psychoeducation): descriptions of the skills (commonly aided by handouts the couple can take home), therapist demonstrations of how to enact each skill, brief readings about the skills the couple can complete as homework, and video demonstrations that show couples using the skills. The therapist then guides the couple as they practice the skills during sessions, giving them feedback and encouragement to shape desired behavior.

Because many couples lack confidence that they can interact more positively, it is crucial that the therapist be supportive when they experience frustration in trying to use the behavioral skills. It is essential that the therapist monitor any cues that they are upset and that the therapist intervene promptly to support their efforts. Therapists who may have learned either through personal upbringing in their families of origin or through professional training to sit back and observe without interrupting other people may need to adjust to this role of active intervention to guide couples toward changing their behavior.

Therapists also need to be aware of cues that individuals' cognitions and emotional responses are interfering with their ability to use new skills. As we have noted previously, some individuals believe that their partner has negative traits (e.g., selfishness) and will respond poorly to the partner's expression of vulnerable thoughts and emotions such as feeling ignored and unloved. Unless the therapist identifies these inhibiting thoughts and addresses them, they are likely to continue to be barriers to good communication skills. If an individual holds an expectancy that a partner will respond negatively to any self-disclosure (e.g., ignore the individual's feelings), the therapist can thank the individual for sharing that concern and then intervene in a way that conveys fairness rather than taking sides. For example, the therapist might first address the individual who described the expectancy of having their feelings ignored, asking what kind of response from their partner would feel good at such times. The therapist then could turn to the partner and say, "Well, Sarah, I have not been in your home and have not observed how you respond to Mark when he expresses vulnerable feelings to you, but it definitely sounds like he'd feel especially good if you would respond to him by saying something like. . . . " Thus, the therapist avoids any debate about whether Sarah's behavior has matched Mark's negative description, and shifts the focus toward increasing a behavior that Mark states he would like. The therapist also has modeled collaborative behavior in which the clinician and members of the couple work together to identify behavior changes that will reduce conflict and increase satisfaction.

Although the communication, problem-solving, and coping skills emphasized in couple therapy are congruent with values and practices of Western cultures in which they were developed, therapists should be aware and sensitive to cultural differences when working with non-Western couples. They should inform themselves about the couple's cultural traditions and openly discuss with a couple any potential cultural factors before asking couples to engage in the practice of skills based on different traditions. The therapist can provide psychoeducation about the skills that will be introduced and the values inherent in them, ask whether there are any specific aspects that are not congruent with their cultural values and practices, and explore the extent to which the partners want to try using the skills. For example, a therapist raised with Western values who is working with an immigrant Asian couple dealing with a chronic stressor (e.g., financial difficulties) might propose to teach the couple dyadic coping skills. Given that one of the skills involves disclosing verbally to one's partner when one is stressed and asking for help, the therapist should be aware that members of Asian cultures may be less reliant on explicit verbal communication and may feel uncomfortable requesting help (for a review on this topic, see Falconier et al., 2016). The therapist could explore these cultural differences with the couple and modify the intervention so that it is more congruent with their values and traditions (e.g., focus more on nonverbal communication of stress and a collectivist view that providing coping support to each other benefits their marriage and even their extended family).

The types of behavioral skills commonly covered in CBCT are:

- Expressive and listening communication skills
- Problem-solving skills
- Dyadic coping skills

Expressive and Listening Communication Skills

Improving couples' abilities to communicate their thoughts and emotions clearly and constructively has been a cornerstone of CBCT and has become popular among couple therapists from a variety of therapy theoretical orientations. Goals include decreased misunderstandings between partners, increased empathy for each other's needs and desires, and increased perception of caring and respect. Clear communication regarding each person's perspective also is a prerequisite for effective joint problem solving (Epstein & Baucom, 2002). We emphasize to clients that even though couples would not be expected to talk in this manner all the time, it would be reassuring for them to know they have skills when needed to enhance their mutual understanding.

As we have noted, communication skills training begins with the therapist providing psychoeducation regarding the goals and procedures, commonly by giving the partners copies of a handout (see Handout 4.1) (available on the book's web page at *www.guilford.com/epstein-materials*) that describes guidelines for being an expresser and a good listener, and demonstrating the skills. The therapist tends to introduce communication skills when the couple exhibits negative communication during a session and has reported that they have trouble communicating. The therapist can state that communication difficulties are among the most common complaints that couples bring to therapy, and therapists have well-tested approaches to helping them talk in a more effective and satisfying way. The in-session psychoeducation can be supplemented by assigning couples self-help books such as Markman et al.'s (2010) widely used *Fighting for Your Marriage* text, which includes a video with didactic material and examples of couples modeling expressive and listening skills.

After providing guidelines for expressive and listening skills and modeling them, the therapist guides the couple in selecting benign topics to begin their practice, emphasizing that starting with upsetting conflict topics could make it difficult to concentrate on changing the way they communicate. Thus, a member might select a topic to discuss regarding a frustrating experience at her job that has no negative implications for the couple's relationship. Her role as expresser is to convey her thoughts and emotions regarding her job experience, and her partner's role is to focus on understanding her subjective experiences and reflect that empathic understanding to her. After the listener has successfully provided empathic feedback to the expresser, the couple switches roles: the other member expresses thoughts and emotions about a personal experience, and the partner takes on the empathic listener role.

While the couple practices expressive and listening skills, the therapist serves as a consultant/moderator, gently providing corrective feedback as well as encouragement. When a couple demonstrates good ability to communicate about benign topics, the therapist guides them in discussing topics that involve issues in their relationship. Some couples quickly grasp the communication guidelines and are adept at using them with minimal intervention, but therapists must be prepared to intervene actively with some other couples, whose performance is compromised by individual and relational factors.

Successful use of expressive and listening skills is influenced by the partners' cognitions and emotions, as well as past experiences with each other. For example, self-disclosure may be inhibited by an individual's low self-esteem, a belief that expressing one's feelings is selfish or inappropriate, anticipation (often based on the couple's history) that the partner will react negatively to it, depression, and so on. In contrast, a speaker who has a negative view of the listener's motives and has difficulty regulating anger may vent negative thoughts and emotions, punishing the listener.

A listener's ability to focus on understanding the speaker's thoughts and emotions also may be impeded by negative cognitions and emotions. For example, an individual who has developed a belief that their partner "always needs to be right" may immediately think of defensive counterarguments while the partner is speaking, rather than listening actively to the partner. Thus, the therapist needs to assess the potential that the partners' cognitions and emotions will interfere with their use of communication skills and may need to use some interventions that address those risk factors. Furthermore, the therapist must intervene with any *circular interaction process* between partners that contributes to poor communication. For example, the therapist may point out:

> "I've noticed that the two of you are locked into a pattern in which the more you see Latoya as tuning you out, James, the more you try to get your points across, and the more you see James pushing for his ideas, the more you want to stop listening and get away, Latoya. How much have you noticed that? Let's all think about ways in which the two of you could use the expressive and listening skills we've been discussing in order to decrease those frustrating experiences."

Problem-Solving Skills

The goal of joint problem-solving skills is to strengthen collaboration between partners in developing mutually acceptable solutions to life stressors and sources of conflict. Many distressed couples report that discussions of problems across a variety of domains (e.g., finances, relationships with extended family, dealing with discrimination) deteriorate quickly and become adversarial. Problem-solving skills focus on teamwork in the service of designing solutions that are feasible and palatable to both people. It requires a collaborative attitude (a cognitive component) and collaborative behavior.

Similar to communication skills, problem-solving training begins with the therapist providing psychoeducation about ways in which the steps can free the couple from their existing pattern of unproductive, frustrating arguments. The therapist gives the partners a handout (see Handout 4.2; available on the book's web page at *www.guilford.com/epstein-materials*), which describes goals and steps of joint problem solving, models examples of how a couple moves through the steps, and emphasizes how that process could help the couple devise solutions to their personal problems. The steps in Handout 4.2 are widely used in CBCT, as well as other couple therapy models (e.g., the solution-focused approach of Stith et al., 2011). Another useful source of psychoeducation is self-help books such as Markman et al.'s (2010) text, which includes a section on problem solving.

Following the psychoeducation, the therapist gives the couple Handout 4.3 (Problem-Solving Steps and Worksheet, available on the book's web page at *www.guilford.com/epstein-materials*). The therapist guides them in selecting a real but relatively low-conflict problem to begin their practice, again because diving prematurely into a problem that arouses strong emotion can interfere with focusing on collaboration. The therapist guides the couple in reaching consensus about a problem they face together that is observable, so it will be possible to monitor potential progress. For example, a couple may focus on nightly difficulty in getting their young children to go to sleep at a reasonable time. The therapist coaches the couple in brainstorming a variety of possible solutions to the problem, without evaluating them, in order to maximize creativity and minimize criticism of each other's ideas. A list is made of possible solutions, with each solution described in terms of concrete actions required of each partner. It is crucial that the therapist guide the couple tactfully through this process, gently interrupting with corrective feedback when they stray from the desired behavior and praising good efforts.

Once the couple has compiled their list of possible solutions on the Handout 4.3 worksheet, the therapist guides them in thinking about and writing the advantages and disadvantages of each solution. The therapist emphasizes that the couple should be respectful of each other's ideas, while trying to be realistic about how feasible each solution would be in their daily life and how comfortable they would be in carrying it out. The goal of this step is to eliminate alternatives from the list based on their relative ratio of disadvantages to advantages, arriving at a solution the couple agrees is feasible and attractive.

The next step is for the couple to decide specifically when they will attempt to carry out the proposed solution at home, taking into account potential barriers such as job demands and family obligations. The therapist emphasizes that this should be considered an experimental trial of the solution, and no matter how effective it is, much will be learned from the attempt. During the next therapy session, the couple reports how they enacted the solution and how well it worked. Any difficulties they encountered are discussed, and further brainstorming focuses on ways in which the solution could be improved, or another solution from the couple's list might be substituted.

As is the case with expressive and listening skills, partners' abilities to collaborate on problem solving often is influenced by each person's cognitions and emotional responses that also may require intervention. For example, emotion-regulation skills are likely to be important when a couple becomes frustrated and angry when their attempts to implement a solution are not going smoothly. It also is important that the therapist directly address any chronic adversarial behavior a couple has exhibited in the past, emphasizing that problem solving will be effective and satisfying to the extent that the partners can realize the advantages of collaborating as a team. Some couples benefit from being asked to think about their experiences in collaborating with people at their jobs, even though they had personal conflicts with them, by staying focused on accomplishing a task. We also point out to couples that solving problems together can increase positive feelings between partners.

As with expressive and listening skills, problem-solving skills are relevant in treatment plans for a variety of presenting problems. Therefore, we include their role in treatment plans for the presenting problems covered in the following chapters.

Dyadic Coping Skills

Closely related to problem solving is dyadic coping, which involves strategies that members of couples use when various life stressors affect one or both partners. Beginning in the 1990s, scholars began to apply systems concepts to understanding how stressors affecting a member of a couple also influence the other member's functioning and well-being (Bodenmann et al., 2016; Falconier et al., 2016). Even though each individual tends to have preferred personal strategies for coping with stressors (Lazarus & Folkman, 1984), partners commonly participate in each other's coping in ways that can enhance or detract from the outcomes. As described in Chapter 3, Bodenmann's (1997, 2005) systemic transactional model (STM) of stress and coping within couples focuses on the interdependence of partners' experiences with life stressors and ways of coping. The model includes the critical first step of verbally communicating to one's partner about one's stress. Then the nonstressed partner can provide emotional and/or instrumental support to the stressed partner, or the two of them can cope jointly when a stressor affects both of them (e.g., their child's illness). As described in Chapter 3, the therapist can use Bodenmann's (2008) Dyadic Coping Inventory or systematic interviewing of the couple to determine the extent to which partners are able to communicate to each other when they experience stress, as well as the extent to which they engage in each type of assisting the other person's efforts to cope with stress, joint coping, or responding negatively to the partner's need for support (see Chapter 3 for descriptions of those forms of coping).

As with procedures for improving couples' communication and problem-solving behavioral skills, the therapist can begin with psychoeducation, providing partners with copies of Handout 4.4 (Guidelines for Dyadic Coping Skills; available on the book's web page at *www.guilford.com/epstein-materials*) and describing examples of the types of dyadic coping and their benefits or drawbacks. The therapist can emphasize that members of a couple have a potential major resource for facing life's challenges with each other's support, and that research has shown that partners who communicate to each other when they are stressed and who help each other cope are more satisfied and have better mental health. Next, the therapist can review instances the couple can remember in which they used forms of positive or negative dyadic coping, and the partners can discuss whether they have preferences for particular types. When the couple is dealing with complex environmental stressors, the therapist may include psychoeducation regarding potential resources for coping with those stressors. The therapist then can coach them in preparing to access those resources (e.g., a financial counselor; help with dealing with a child or elderly parent's need for special care; legal resources for hate crimes and discrimination in the workplace, school, or health care system).

The therapist needs to monitor how the members of the couple are processing the psychoeducation information. Individuals may find it difficult to shift from their existing beliefs about life stresses and their partner's characteristics as a potential ally, and to adopt some of the dyadic coping concepts. We avoid lecturing the clients and routinely check with them regarding their thoughts and level of comfort with the material. This is particularly important when working with couples whose cultural values and practices may not be fully congruent with this model of dyadic coping.

Following the initial psychoeducation, the therapist should focus on the first stage of dyadic coping: *stress communication*. It includes being able to identify cues of stress in oneself and in one's partner, and one's willingness to disclose your stress to your partner. Therapists can ask members of a couple what verbal and nonverbal behaviors seem to be indicators of their own stress or signs that their partner is experiencing stress. Each person can add to what their partner has identified. The therapist can emphasize observing cues of stress in oneself as well as in one's partner, and talking about them.

Regarding self-disclosure of stress, the therapist should explain the importance of letting one's partner know about one's internal experience of stress so that the partner can provide needed support. Couples can be guided in practicing communication about stress through role plays during sessions. Each person takes a turn describing a current stressor, what it is about the situation that is stressful, and the emotions that are elicited. Each individual's ability to notice and describe the link between stressor events and internal thoughts and emotions is critical. For example, an individual may describe sadness about an argument with their mother, but the description limits the partner's ability to provide support if the individual does not explain the cognitions that elicited the sadness (e.g., an expectancy that the mother will never accept their life choices). Once an individual has communicated stress, the partner is invited to describe what they understood, using empathic listening skills and, if needed, ask the individual open-ended questions to understand the stress experience better. Many couples need practice before they can communicate well about their stress experiences.

Because the capacity to communicate about one's stress requires awareness of one's thoughts and emotions, ability to differentiate various emotions, acceptance of them as legitimate experiences, and willingness to express them, some partners may have difficulty during this stage of dyadic coping. Therapists need to be prepared to identify and intervene with individuals' cognitions that are barriers (e.g., a belief that feeling emotions is a sign of weakness), as well as prepared to coach partners in emotion regulation as described later in this chapter.

Following the practice of communication about stress experiences, the therapist can guide the couple in the role-playing use of dyadic coping to deal with hypothetical or real circumstances in which one of them faces a stressor or the couple faces a joint stressor. The therapist coaches as they practice stress communication and forms of dyadic coping, and then debriefs them about how each person experienced the coping process. In order to maximize the couple's familiarity with all forms of dyadic coping, the therapist can coach them in describing how each positive form could be applied to a particular life stressor. For example, after one member describes feeling anxiety regarding an increased workload at their job, the therapist can coach the partner in role-playing alternative positive ways of helping the individual cope with their stress. Emotion-focused supportive coping might involve the partner expressing caring; problem-focused supportive coping could involve the partner suggesting actions the individual might try to reduce their workload; and delegated coping might involve the partner offering to take over some of their household chores to give the partner more time for work tasks. The therapist and couple also can discuss how the stressed individual's experience would have been worse if the partner had used any negative forms of dyadic coping (e.g., ambivalent coping, with an obviously half-hearted attempt to take over one of the individual's chores).

As with other behavioral interventions, we have described how it is important to monitor the need for interventions focused on partners' cognitions and emotional responses that are influencing the dyadic coping process. If the therapist notices verbal or nonverbal cues that either person is responding negatively to the other's actions, the therapist should interrupt and probe for each person's thoughts and emotional responses. For example, an individual whose partner is attempting problem-focused supportive coping by recommending particular actions may show nonverbal cues of discomfort. The therapist asks the partner what their goal was in using this strategy and also asks about the recipient's reactions (thoughts and emotions). Perhaps the partner describes trying to motivate the individual to try a new approach in order to reduce their stress as quickly as possible. The therapist acknowledges the partner's positive intent and then turns to the stressed person, who reports being irritated because it seemed that their partner thinks they know better how to solve problems. The therapist can guide the couple in reviewing forms of dyadic coping and discussing which approaches by their partner they would prefer. The therapist could coach the couple in role-playing, using a form of dyadic coping that the stressed individual reported preferring. This exchange also might uncover a broader issue in which one member perceives the other as harboring feelings of superiority, which is interfering with dyadic coping and may need attention in therapy.

Because coping with stressors requires that partners regulate negative emotions, therapists need to monitor and intervene with poor emotion regulation during the work on dyadic coping. On the one hand, a person who is experiencing a stressor will benefit when able to manage emotional arousal individually. On the other hand, a partner who is attempting to provide forms of dyadic coping for the person is more likely to be effective when able to manage their own emotional arousal triggered either by the stressors themselves or by the distressed individual's behavior. When an individual attempts to provide dyadic coping, the other person may behave in frustrating ways (e.g., debating, engaging in self-defeating coping behaviors such as drinking alcohol). Therefore, it is important that therapists assist partners in monitoring their own cognitions and emotions toward the other person as they try to help and in using forms of personal coping to regulate them.

Guided Behavior Change

These interventions focus on partners agreeing to engage in particular types of positive behavior that will benefit each other's personal needs and the quality of their relationship. Each person agrees to enact particular types of behavior regardless of the other person's actions (i.e., it is not a contingency contract). Some such agreements (e.g., "caring days") focus on improving the overall atmosphere of the relationship, so anything each person can do that they know will please the other person is relevant. However, some agreements focus on a specific type of behavior associated with improving a particular aspect of the relationship, such as connection and intimacy. Identification of the behavior exchanges that are needed is based on assessment of the partners' presenting complaints (e.g., "We don't feel as close to each other as we did before").

As with skills-based behavioral interventions, the therapist can begin with psychoeducation that presents a rationale for engaging in these types of behavior, linking them to the couple's presenting complaints. The therapist should ensure that the proposed changes are congruent with each partner's beliefs and practices by directly asking them how those behaviors fit with their identity and cultural values, behaviors, and traditions. The therapist then can adapt behavioral interventions to be more palatable for the clients. Pressuring couples to meet a therapist's prescribed "one-size-fits-all" standards for appropriate behavior is counterproductive.

As described in Chapter 3, our initial assessment interview with the couple includes an inquiry about ways the partners interacted as they initially developed their bond, including joint activities they enjoyed and acts that conveyed their caring and respect for each other. A core theme in the introductory psychoeducation is that beyond physical attraction, characteristics that draw people to each other are pleasing ways that they behave with each other (e.g., "He really listened to me." "Her sense of humor and way of getting excited by little things in life brightened my days"). Although this process can differ for couples from cultures with arranged marriages, partners may report pleasing experiences with each other in daily life as they got to know each other better.

When members of a couple relate memories of pleasant earlier experiences together, even currently distressed individuals may relive at least "twinges" of pleasure, evident through smiles. This is an opportunity for the therapist to suggest that it may be bittersweet to remember happier times that seem lost and that one of the goals of therapy is to collaborate on establishing new patterns that can restore positive feelings. Thus, the therapist appeals to any motivation partners still may have to get their needs met with each other and sets the stage for guided behavior changes that will address those needs.

The therapist can explain that daily interactions play a significant role in what people often refer to as the "chemistry" between them, and it is common for pleasing interactions to decrease over time as the couple becomes busier with the demands of life. The therapist's goals are to (1) increase partners' awareness of how their behavioral interactions are associated with their internal thoughts and emotional experiences, and (2) introduce the idea that actions designed to meet each other's needs for affection, validation, security, and respect can rebuild the bond they feel. Although these goals are more obviously consistent with the experiences of couples who chose to be together based on romantic love than for those whose unions were founded on fulfilling social roles (as in arranged marriages), the principle still applies that humans will be happier in relationships when daily interactions fulfill their basic needs.

If the therapist determines that partners are motivated to use insight into their own and each other's personal needs to plan more satisfying interactions, the therapist describes steps they could follow and coaches them in making a plan. Enactment of the planned behaviors can be facilitated by building in cues/reminders, such as a note on the refrigerator or on their cell phones. The plan involves specific types of behavior each member commits to enacting in the coming week, cues to remind them, and a method for keeping track of the new behavior so that they can share results with the therapist.

In contrast to guided behavior changes that increase positive interaction between partners, when partners have a pattern of negative escalation (which may lead to aggressive behavior or hostile withdrawal), it is helpful to guide them in using constructive, mutually agreed-upon "time-outs." The steps for engaging the couple in using time-outs are described in Chapter 5.

Throughout the process of guided behavior change, the therapist pays attention to the partners' cognitions and emotional responses that may act as barriers to planning and carrying out the changes. For example, some individuals believe that only spontaneous positive behavior is "real" and meaningful, so they discount the validity of a partner's planned actions that were intended to create greater intimacy. Furthermore, therapists may need to intervene with some individuals' tendencies to "stand on ceremony" for a partner to change first. In addition, as we noted in Chapter 1, individuals who are unhappy with their partner tend to notice the partner's negative actions and overlook their positive behavior, so therapists need to guide couples in objectively monitoring each other's behaviors intended to meet core needs.

The value of balancing desired behavior changes with increased *acceptance* of existing conditions has become a major concept in the psychotherapy field, both in individual therapy and couple therapy (Fruzzetti, McLean, & Erikson, 2019). Gottman (1999) noted that many couple conflicts cannot be resolved through negotiating mutually preferred behavior changes. In addition, integrative behavioral couple therapy (IBCT; Christensen et al., 2023; Jacobson & Christensen,

1996) combines traditional behavioral interventions (communication and problem-solving training) with interventions to increase partners' acceptance of each other's characteristics.

Within CBCT, acceptance is considered a *cognitive process* in which an individual develops *personal standards* for evaluating conditions in their life as satisfactory, even if not what they consider ideal. When individuals are unhappy that a partner's characteristics and behavior fail to meet their ideals, they commonly make efforts to induce the partner to change in the direction of the standards. Although some requests for behavior change can be reasonable, there is a limit to what is possible and even what both parties are likely to perceive as just. Therefore, the therapist guides the partners in thinking about advantages and disadvantages of their personal standards for each other, and in considering whether they could accept more flexible standards. The goal is a belief that "in the best of all worlds, my partner would [insert desired best behavior], but if instead my partner [insert behavior that is a milder version of the ideal] I can accept that as good too, and I can be satisfied with our relationship." We view increasing acceptance as primarily a cognitive process that involves shifting individuals toward blaming their partners less for relationship problems, inferring more benign motives and personality characteristics in each other, and developing greater empathy for each other's unmet needs. The acceptance interventions in IBCT, such as the therapist modeling empathic understanding of motives underlying each partner's behavior that has upset the other person and coaching partners in taking a "unified detachment" perspective in perceiving nonblaming causes of each other's behavior (Christensen et al., 2023; Jacobson & Christensen, 1996), are intended to increase each person's acceptance of the other's actions. We concur with the IBCT perspective that the cognitive aspect of acceptance tends to be associated with greater emotional tranquility (and potential happiness) about the partner and relationship.

INTERVENTIONS FOR COGNITION

Individuals' cognitions are core aspects of their intrapsychic life, shaped from birth through multiple experiences with caretakers and other people. Research has identified relatively stable cognitive structures that shape how children and adults perceive experiences, categorize objects and events, make predictions about future outcomes such as responses from significant others. In addition to *knowledge structures* (e.g., schemas, working models) such as those regarding relationships, social cognition research has focused on *moment-to-moment "online" processing of information* (Fletcher et al., 2018), as individuals perceive and interpret events that occur in the moment.

In CBCT, the goals of interventions for cognitions are:

• To create a balanced, minimally biased perspective by both partners regarding each other, their relationship, and aspects of their social and physical environment (reducing distorted or extreme thinking).

• To enhance partners' understanding of their own and each other's internal thoughts, emotions, motives, and needs, so that they will be more empathic and validating of each other's experiences, even when they disagree with each other.

The therapist avoids imposing views on a couple or judging them, but rather guides them in becoming more attuned to aspects of their thinking that may contribute to problematic behavioral interactions, poorly regulated emotions, and overall unhappiness with their relationship. As described in Chapter 2, the therapist's positive alliance with the partners facilitates their openness to input from the therapist in examining their thinking and its effects. The therapist's efforts to be culturally sensitive to aspects of clients' lives that shape their cognitions play an important role in that alliance.

Broadly speaking, interventions for cognitions can be categorized as primarily involving *Socratic questioning* and *guided discovery*. Particular interventions tend to emphasize one of these or the other, but some may involve aspects of both.

Socratic Questioning

The therapist guides clients in considering the *logic* of their thoughts and any *available evidence* regarding their appropriateness or validity. The goal is to help the client reevaluate thoughts associated with relationship problems. In individual cognitive therapy, clients commonly are receptive to such input from a therapist they perceive as supportive. In couple therapy, however, it can be more complicated. The therapist needs to be cautious when drawing an individual's attention to possible illogical or extreme aspects of their thoughts in front of their partner. The danger that arises is that one or both members of the couple will view the therapist as suggesting the person's negative thoughts are invalid and that the partner's views are more realistic. Sometimes when a therapist challenges an individual's cognitions during a session, the person's partner uses it to criticize the person as being irrational. Therapists must emphasize to the couple that they assume all people need to be cautious about negative thoughts they have about themselves and other people, explaining the concept of *automatic thoughts* that people naturally take for granted as being true. The therapist will be listening for possible instances when either member of the couple may be "jumping to conclusions" without examining their thoughts sufficiently, and so the therapist will coach them to check their thinking. The therapist will not assume any negative thought is inappropriate but will stress that it is important to examine the evidence.

Some interventions involved in Socratic questioning are:

• **Psychoeducation such as teaching the couple about the characteristics of automatic thoughts and the major types of cognitive distortions.** Because the term *cognitive distortions* can be experienced as pejorative, we do use that standard cognitive therapy term with clients. However, we emphasize that they are common errors in logic that everyone is likely to make from time to time, such as arbitrary inferences, all-or-nothing thinking, selective abstraction, and overgeneralization. It is not assumed that these ways of thinking are always inaccurate, but they have the potential to be so and should be evaluated. The therapist can give each member of a couple Handout 1.1 with definitions and examples of the distortions and can ask each person to think about instances in which they remember engaging in any of them in the past and to try to catch themselves if they engage in them in the present. It can be tempting to point out instances in which one's partner seemed to exhibit logic errors from the list, but in order to avoid mutual criticism and maximize learning about oneself, the goal is to focus on one's own thinking.

• **Guiding the individuals in evaluating the logic supporting or inconsistent with a cognition.** This type of intervention involves encouraging the individual to generate alternative ways of thinking about the partner, self, or relationship. For example, when an individual has attributed a partner's displeasing behavior to a negative trait (e.g., "He disagreed with me in front of our friends because he doesn't respect me"), the therapist can comment, "That might be the reason why he behaved that way, and if it is, then we have some important issues to discuss in our sessions, regarding respect between partners. However, in case there may have been another reason, what other possible explanations can you think of?" If the client has difficulty thinking of an alternative attribution, the therapist can propose one or more to consider. Because the partner also is present in the session, the therapist can guide the upset individual in asking the partner to describe factors that contributed to disagreeing with the individual in front of friends.

A therapist also can guide individuals in examining the logic involved in other forms of their cognitions, such as personal standards. For example, an individual might voice a standard such as: "If you cry in front of your partner (or other people), it is a sign of weakness." First, the therapist may inquire where and how the person remembers developing that standard, to promote reflecting on the belief rather than just automatically living according to it. Individuals often describe how they developed a standard in their family of origin ("My parents avoided showing what they considered weak emotions and expected my siblings and me to do the same"). The therapist might reply, "Looking back, what do you think about the way your parents approached life, regarding people's experiences of emotions such as sadness and anxiety?" "In what ways do you think letting another person know you are sad would be a sign of weakness?" "Can you think of ways in which it might be a sign of strength?" These probes are intended to broaden the individual's thinking about emotions and what constitutes weakness versus strength.

• **Weighing advantages and disadvantages of a cognition.** In CBCT it is assumed that individuals adhere to particular ways of thinking not only because they learned to think that way early in life and simply continue in a habitual manner. Consistent with social learning theory, people also engage in responses when they result in rewarding consequences. Thus, an individual may try to live according to a particular standard because they view its advantages as outweighing any disadvantages.

Regarding the individual who holds a standard "If you cry in front of your partner (or other people), it is a sign of weakness," the therapist can state: "I assume your parents saw some advantages to living according to that standard and wanted to pass it down to you and your siblings. What advantages do you see in not revealing emotions such as sadness or anxiety?" However, the therapist then proposes, "Any standard that people live by also may have some disadvantages. What possible disadvantages do you think could be associated with living by the standard that crying and showing feelings to others is a sign of weakness?" This process is intended to help individuals evaluate their thinking actively, producing a broader perspective.

Weighing the advantages and disadvantages of cognitions may also be particularly useful when the therapist discusses with the couple some of their assumptions and standards that have been shaped by their cultures of origin (e.g., regarding appropriate gender role behavior). Some partners may decide to continue adhering to those cognitions, whereas others may find themselves questioning and modifying some of them as they develop more pleasing ways of thinking about their relationship.

Guided Discovery

In contrast to Socratic questioning, which focuses clients' attention on logical analysis of their cognitions, in guided discovery the therapist creates experiences for the couple that provide direct data relevant to evaluating the logic or validity of their cognitions. This emphasis on experiential exercises, homework, and so on emphasizes partners taking responsibility for observing what actually happens between them when they behave in ways about which they currently have negative expectancies. For example, a couple may share a negative expectancy that trying to communicate about issues will result in greater anger and distancing; that is, it will make things worse. Although their prediction may have some basis in past experiences, their pessimism does not take into account the possibility of making improvements in their behavior. In fact, by expecting each other to behave negatively, they may be producing a self-fulfilling prophecy by entering discussions when they are already on the defensive.

In such cases, the therapist can begin with psychoeducation, describing how couples who have upsetting experiences with each other commonly lose faith that they can have positive experiences together, but by avoiding communication they lose any opportunities to solve their problems. The therapist can note that it is natural to try to protect oneself from further upsetting interactions, but making an effort to use positive communication skills can result in new evidence that satisfying discussions are possible. The goal is to engage the couple in a *behavioral experiment*, using expressive and empathic listening skills and observing how interacting that way influences how much they feel understood by each other. Their *in vivo* experiences may help them question their overall pessimistic thinking (Epstein & Baucom, 2002).

Some other interventions that can be used in guided discovery are the following:

• **Identifying experiences in past relationships** (e.g., betrayal, psychological and physical aggression) that influence how a person thinks about a current partner's behavior, and examining ways in which the past conditions are similar or different from the present ones. The person's partner may resent being compared to a past partner, but if the partner responds defensively rather than demonstrating some empathy for the person's residual pain from past wounds, the couple is likely to remain in conflict. A therapist can use psychoeducation to normalize the individual's residual trauma symptoms (e.g., flashbacks to prior painful experiences, a sense of insecurity in close relationships, hypervigilance regarding possible dangers). The therapist can balance demonstrating empathy for the traumatized individual with sympathy for the partner who feels unfairly judged. This balanced approach can be expressed with statements such as:

"On the one hand, it is natural for you to still be uneasy Vivian, based on your very painful past experiences, even though you feel much better in your present relationship with Carol and care a lot about her. On the other hand, I see that you feel frustrated, Carol, when Vivian reacts with such anxiety when you show any emotional intensity when the two of you disagree about an issue. Unfortunately, Vivian, when you become anxious when Carol shows negative emotion, that seems to frustrate you further, Carol. However, when you tell Vivian she should get over her old problems by now, that seems to fuel your insecurity more, Vivian. The two of you seem stuck in a loop that reinforces your shared view that Vivian's past casts a big shadow on your present relationship, and you feel helpless to get out of that loop. I suggest that a first step toward getting out of that dark shadow of the past will be our having a detailed discussion of specific ways in which your relationship is different from Vivian's relationship with Sue, as well as any ways in which they are similar. As each of you expresses your thoughts about that, the other can use empathic listening skills that you have practiced previously to demonstrate your understanding. Then, the two of you can use the problem-solving steps that we also have practiced, to think of ways you can interact that allow Vivian's sense of security in your relationship to grow and Carol's sense of being trusted to grow as well."

- **Increasing the partners' relational circular thinking** by drawing their attention to repetitive cycles in couple interaction, including each partner's contribution. This includes engaging each of them in thinking of points at which they personally have the option of responding in a different way that would change the pattern. The above description of drawing Vivian and Carol's attention to their negative circular pattern that developed from Vivian's past trauma experiences is an example of increasing a couple's relational thinking. As described in Chapter 1, members of couples commonly think in linear causal terms, focusing on ways in which their partner's actions trigger responses in them and overlooking their own contributions to negative interactions. The therapist's role is to increase partners' abilities to take a more detached perspective and personal responsibility for making changes toward a more constructive pattern.

A therapist can begin by pointing out the evidence one has observed regarding the couple's circular pattern and providing psychoeducation about the difference between linear causality and circular causality. It is less important that clients learn those technical terms than that they grasp the concepts and can become adept at spotting the processes as they interact with each other. The therapist initially draws their attention to their circular processes during sessions but increasingly coaches them in taking on that role. These interventions can produce a cognitive shift from adversarial blaming to collaboration.

INTERVENTIONS FOR INHIBITED AND UNREGULATED EMOTIONAL RESPONSES

Intimate relationships often are sources of some of the most emotionally pleasant experiences in individuals' lives (contributing to overall well-being in life), but they also can be sources of some of the greatest emotional distress (contributing to poor psychological functioning). Emotional experiences within a relationship are influenced by the individual's cognitions, capabilities for regulating their emotions, and behavioral interactions with their partner. As we noted in Chapter 1, Greenberg and Goldman (2008) emphasize that partners co-regulate each other's emotions, a process in which they can soothe each other but also one in which mutual emotional distress can escalate.

Interventions for emotions commonly begin with some *psychoeducation* designed to increase partners' awareness and understanding of their emotional responses and factors that influence them. A therapist can emphasize that emotional responses are quite normal, and they can alert individuals to the fact that something important (positive or negative) is occurring in their life, to which they should pay attention. The therapist can explain that people often notice their emotional responses before they become aware of their thoughts about the significance of situations, so emotions can be clues about whether or not one's needs are being met. Using the concept of "clues," the therapist can propose to the couple that the three of them engage in "detective work" to uncover what each partner's emotional responses can reveal about their needs and goals.

Psychoeducation also can focus on how emotions motivate people to take action to try to induce other people to help them fulfill their needs. Thus, a person who becomes angry when a partner repeatedly interrupts her during discussions can be guided in becoming aware that her needs to be respected and have influence on decision making in the relationship seem to be neglected, and she may be motivated to request behavior change from her partner. Thus, the therapist seeks to increase partners' abilities to identify their needs and communicate with each other about them.

Psychoeducation is enriched by referring to relevant examples from the couple's life. Thus, a therapist might comment

> "Walter, you have described often feeling sad when you and Fred first see each other at the end of a work day, and you are aware that at those times you have thoughts that you used to be close but now seem to be leading separate lives. Your sad feelings may be signs that your intimacy needs are not being met as they were in the past. Your emotions are telling you something important."

The therapist should emphasize that being able to learn from and communicate with each other about the meanings of our emotions depends on valuing their significance. Key aspects of effective emotion regulation are being aware that one is experiencing an emotion, identifying what emotion it is, and accepting it as reflecting something important in one's life. Nevertheless, accepting the significance of an emotional response does not necessarily mean concluding that it is realistic or appropriate. The cognitive therapy term *emotional reasoning* refers to interpreting cues of emotion as valid evidence of a condition, as when a depressed individual's low mood leads him to conclude "I cannot accomplish anything." Partners should take their emotional responses to each other seriously and communicate about them, but it is crucial that they develop an ability to take a "detached" perspective for analyzing the conditions (behaviors between partners and each person's subjective cognitions about them) that elicit the emotions.

In addition, the therapist can inform the couple about evidence linking particular emotional responses to cognitive themes (Beck, 1976; Goldman & Greenberg, 2006). For example, sadness and depression tend to be associated with perceived loss, anxiety or fear with perceived danger, and irritation or anger with violation of one's rights and independence. Goals in therapy are to increase partners' awareness of their emotional responses, circumstances that elicited them, and their meanings, as well as to develop the couple's skills for communicating about them to each other. Individual cognitive therapy includes a standard procedure of teaching clients to use "thought records" (which conveniently are available on cell phone apps) to track their automatic thoughts, emotional responses, and behavior. Couple therapists also can use this procedure to help partners enhance their emotional insight: awareness and acceptance of their emotions, and links between the emotions and their cognitions and behavior toward each other.

Another goal the therapist emphasizes in psychoeducation is the partners' *acceptance* not only of their own but also each other's emotional experiences as normal human responses, as well as the importance of expressing emotions constructively, avoiding impulsive venting. This includes developing one's ability to moderate one's reactivity to one's own arousal as well as to a partner's arousal. It involves *being aware* of your internal experiences of your partner's behavior, *understanding* factors that are contributing to your partner's actions toward you, and *communicating* that empathic understanding while also informing the partner about your own experiences. The interventions go beyond psychoeducation to coaching clients in practicing self-monitoring, applying an accepting attitude to the other's emotional experiences, developing self-soothing as needed to regulate strong affect, and using constructive expressive and listening skills to communicate about them.

The therapist also should describe Planalp et al.'s (2018) emphasis on couples having strategies to *enhance shared positive emotional experiences*. Just as reducing negative behavioral interactions must be accompanied by efforts to increase mutually enjoyable behavior, interventions specifically designed to increase positive affect are needed. Pleasure from experiencing less negative emotion is different from pleasure from shared positive emotional experiences. Gottman (1999) describes a CBT-like emphasis on guiding partners to engage in "repair attempts" to counteract damage from negative interactions (e.g., taking responsibility for a problem, expressing affection), which are designed to increase positive emotions. In addition, partners can be encouraged to engage in actions that they know tend to contribute to the other person feeling pleasure; often, simple acts such as preparing them a warm cup of tea on a cold winter night can bring pleasure.

In couple therapy, the therapist is in the midst of the couple's interactions during sessions and intervenes with their emotional responses rather than allowing negative patterns to unfold unchecked. With particular presenting problems such as partner aggression, the therapist interrupts escalation of emotional arousal, draws the couple's attention to the common rapid shift in the emotional state between them, and uses interventions that reduce the risk of aggressive behavior. This involves *targeting partners' cognitions* such as beliefs that fuel anger and justify punitive behavior, as well as teaching members anger management skills, including self-soothing techniques, and use of time-outs to reduce dangerous levels of anger (see Chapter 5). Similar interventions can be used with couples coping with strong anger and anxiety from disclosure of infidelity, fears associated with a partner's serious disease diagnosis and stressful medical treatments, and other major life stressors.

By focusing on links that emotions provide to partners' core needs, the therapist takes an experiential approach that captures each person's subjective life. It is highly individualized rather than a one-size-fits-all approach. A therapist can work with each couple using Handout 4.5 (Strategies for Managing Emotional Experiences in a Couple Relationship; available on the book's web page at *www.guilford.com/epstein-materials*) to select interventions that are most acceptable to them. The therapist coaches the couple in applying the strategies listed in the handout, encouraging them and providing feedback to shape their constructive enactments.

Homework to Enhance Behavioral, Cognitive, and Affective Changes

For all interventions for behavior, cognition, and emotion, it is crucial that new patterns introduced during therapy sessions are generalized to the couple's daily life via structured homework. The therapist guides the couple in devising at-home practice that is feasible, with each person's role specified. It must be a collaborative process of the clients choosing activities they will try at home rather than the therapist assigning tasks. Planned changes should be carried out in gradual steps to avoid having clients attempt large changes that are too difficult. Potential barriers to completing homework and ways to overcome them should be discussed before the couple leaves the therapist's office. The therapist can play a "devil's advocate" role, suggesting factors that might interfere with the homework, stimulating a discussion with the couple about what goals seem realistic. In the next session, the therapist must check on the couple's experiences with the homework in order to reinforce its importance and to troubleshoot any problems.

KEY POINTS

- Partners' behaviors, cognitions, and emotions continuously influence each other.

- Therapists should ensure that their interventions are culturally sensitive by actively learning about their clients' cultural beliefs and traditions.

- Behavior changes are usually introduced early so that partners can change their negative views about the interactions occurring in their relationship.

- Cognitive interventions often are needed early in therapy to identify partners' extreme and inappropriate ways of thinking.

- Interventions addressing partners' inhibited or dysregulated experience and expression of emotion can be prioritized when a therapist identifies that emotional responses are interfering with constructive couple interactions.

- Structured homework allows the new patterns introduced during therapy sessions to be generalized to daily life.

PART II

TREATMENT PLANNER

CHAPTER 5

Partner Aggression

Forms of psychologically and physically aggressive behavior occur commonly in couple relationships around the world, across diverse countries and cultures (Deries et al., 2013; Ellsberg, Jansen, Heise, Watts, & Garcia-Moreno, 2008; Kar & Garcia-Moreno, 2009; Krahé & Abbey, 2013; Krahé, Bieneck, & Möller, 2005; Olayide & Clisdell, 2017). Although there has been much less research on lesbian, gay, and bisexual partner aggression (most of it with North American samples), existing studies have indicated incidence rates and lifetime prevalence rates comparable to or higher than among heterosexual couples (Rollè, Giardina, Caldarera, Gerino, & Brustia, 2018). Spivak et al.'s (2014) review of data in the United States indicated that partner aggression often begins at a young age: 9% of high school students reported physical violence victimization by a boyfriend or girlfriend. Both cross-sectional and longitudinal studies have found that victimization commonly is associated with serious physical health problems (e.g., chronic pain, gastrointestinal problems) and mental health problems (e.g., depression, anxiety, posttraumatic stress symptoms) (Ahmadabadi et al., 2020; Coker et al., 2002; Sugg, 2015). Rollè et al. (2018) note that cross-sectional studies with lesbian, gay, and bisexual couples have found similar associations of victimization with both physical and mental health problems.

In this chapter, we use the term *partner aggression* rather than the common term *intimate partner violence* (IPV), because it is more comprehensive in describing the wide range of aversive and hurtful verbal and physical acts that members of couples exhibit, whereas IPV often automatically brings to mind severe physical violence. It is important that clinicians be on the lookout for all levels of partner aggression.

PHYSICAL PARTNER AGGRESSION

Regarding *physical partner aggression*, behaviors range from relatively mild pushing, grabbing, and slapping to inflicting severe injuries and even death via punching, choking, and use of weapons. This diversity of physical aggression has led writers to attempt to identify possible subtypes of aggression that may have different causes and may require different forms of treatment. Johnson's (1995, 2006) differentiation between the severe violence referred to as *patriarchal terrorism* or *battering* and relatively mild to moderate violence labeled *common couple violence* or *situational violence* has been widely accepted in the field. In heterosexual couple relationships, battering occurs less commonly, primarily involves male-to-female aggression, and has the goal of dominating the victim. Although cases of female-to-male battering also are identified, they are less common. Furthermore, women's violence is likely to involve relatively low-level physical aggression, especially for self-defense. Because professional attention to partner aggression initially developed from concern about severe effects on physically battered women, the focus was primarily on unilateral aggression by male partners. However, when researchers have focused on mildly to moderately severe physical aggression, which occurs more commonly than battering, data have indicated that it often is bilateral within couples, with both members engaging in various aggressive acts (Carney & Barner, 2012; Costa et al., 2016; Johnson, 2006; Stith et al., 2011). This pattern has been labeled situational violence because it tends to arise during specific instances in which a couple is in conflict over particular issues in their relationship, in contrast to the perpetrator's pervasive motivation to control the victim that often underlies battering.

When the full range of physical violence is taken into account, the perpetration rates of heterosexual couples tend to be similar, but men are more likely to exhibit more severe and physically damaging behaviors than women (Afifi et al., 2009; Archer, 2000; Frieze, 2005; Straus, 2009). That gender difference in severity also is found between lesbian and gay couples (Rollè et al., 2018), even though lesbian couples report receiving more partner aggression of any type than gay couples do (Messinger, 2011). Nevertheless, Jose and O'Leary (2009) noted that within samples of heterosexual couples who sought therapy at clinics, the rates of male and female partners who were injured were similar (15% and 12%, respectively). This in no way lessens the importance of clinicians identifying cases of dangerous battering by males. However, even when physical partner aggression by males or females is fairly mild, it tends to have negative effects on the victims' psychological well-being and should be a key target for intervention.

Rollè et al.'s (2018) literature review indicates that the general public and mental health professionals have underestimated the prevalence of partner aggression among lesbian and gay couples considerably. One reason is the myth that relationships between two women are inevitably mutually supportive and nurturing based on females' gender socialization, and that aggression between two men will be limited because they are evenly matched in physical strength (which also ignores psychological aggression). A second reason is silence regarding partner aggression within the lesbian and gay communities, based on fear that publicity about it will add to discrimination and oppression within society. Rollè et al. (2018) also note that feminist writers have tended to downplay same-sex partner aggression because it is inconsistent with the feminist model of male aggression toward females based on misogyny and patriarchy. Nevertheless, research increasingly has identified partner aggression as a significant problem in couples across sexual orientation. At present, there also is a need for research on couples with diverse gender identities.

PSYCHOLOGICAL PARTNER AGGRESSION

Psychological partner aggression consists of forms of verbal and nonverbal behavior that do not involve contact with the victim's body but still cause psychological distress because of their aversive, threatening, and punitive nature. O'Leary and Maiuro (2001) reviewed the variety of forms of psychologically aggressive behaviors described in the literature and included in questionnaire measures, and classified them into four types. (1) *Denigrating* one's partner (e.g., describing the partner in derogatory terms, name-calling, shaming the partner in front of other people) involves direct attacks on self-esteem. (2) *Passive–aggressive withholding of emotional support and nurturance* (e.g., avoiding the partner, sulking, emotionally abandoning the partner) is used to punish the partner for failing to meet the individual's expectations. (3) *Threatening behavior* (e.g., explicit or implicit verbal or nonverbal acts that convey the likelihood of painful consequences, such as making verbal threats of physical violence, engaging in reckless behavior such as fast driving, and threats to take away the couple's children) are used to coerce compliance from the partner with the aggressor's desires. Finally, (4) *restricting the partner's personal territory and freedom* (e.g., isolating the partner from friends and family, monitoring the partner's communication with others, blocking the partner's access to money) controls the partner by blocking access to resources that could allow the partner to function independently.

Recognition of the degree to which psychological partner aggression is harmful to members of couples and to their satisfaction with their relationships has increased. Studies have shown that the negative effects of psychological aggression on well-being and relationship satisfaction tend to be equivalent to, or even stronger than, those of mild to moderate physical aggression (Coker et al., 2002; Khan, Österman, & Björkqvist, 2019; Pico-Alfonso et al., 2006; Yoon & Lawrence, 2013). Furthermore, psychological aggression commonly co-occurs with physical aggression and tends to precede it (O'Leary, Smith Slep, & O'Leary, 2007).

In contrast to physical aggression, where many (but certainly not all) people view even mild forms as inappropriate, standards regarding forms of psychological aggression tend to be less clear. For some couples at least, some actions (e.g., name-calling, the "silent treatment") are relatively normative ways of interacting when in conflict (Jose & O'Leary, 2009). Consequently, therapists who provide couples psychoeducation regarding types and negative consequences of psychological partner aggression need to be prepared to encounter degrees of surprise and defensiveness from some clients (Epstein et al., 2023).

SOCIOCULTURAL FACTORS INFLUENCING PARTNER AGGRESSION

Research identifying the pervasiveness of partner aggression across countries has highlighted the importance of understanding the cultural context within which it occurs (Krahé & Abbey, 2013). Differences in power differentials between men and women, norms for characteristics of masculinity and femininity, concepts of male honor, and religious and ethnic beliefs that men have a right to control their wives and daughters through means including physical force must be taken into account in assessing partner aggression and planning interventions that have potential to be palatable and effective (Kar & Garcia-Moreno, 2009; Krahé & Abbey, 2013). Some other cultural beliefs have less to do with gender and are focused more on individualism, in which one has a right to defend oneself from any form of perceived interference by others by fighting back. Based on their cultural backgrounds, some clients may fail to view their partner aggression as inappropriate and harmful, so therapists need to probe tactfully for information about aggression that clients fail to report or mention but consider normal. When exploring details about a couple's behavioral interactions when in conflict, it is important to exhibit curiosity about their relationship, while avoiding expressions of judgment at that point. Therapists need to identify harmful behavior and intervene promptly to stop it, but they also need to create a therapeutic relationship in which both partners feel valued and safe in sharing information with the clinician about their behavior and cultural factors that influence it. In this chapter, we describe interventions to reduce cultural influences on partner aggression.

RISK FACTORS FOR PARTNER AGGRESSION

Considerable research has been devoted to identifying factors associated with perpetration of partner aggression, which clinicians can keep in mind when assessing couples and designing treatments. As Mackay, Bowen, Walker, and O'Doherty (2018) noted, rather than showing clear evidence that those characteristics cause aggression, many findings show correlations between particular characteristics of individuals and the degree to which they behave aggressively toward partners. However, being aware of those characteristics helps guide therapists in exploring possible risk factors within each couple that may become foci of treatment.

The characteristics listed in Figure 5.1 have been found to be associated with perpetration of partner aggression (Bates, Archer, & Graham-Kevan, 2017; Ehrensaft, 2009; Epstein et al., 2023; Mackay et al., 2018; Schumacher, Feldbau-Kohn, Smith Slep, & Heyman, 2001; Slep, Foran, Heyman, & Snarr, 2010; Stith, Smith, Penn, Ward, & Tritt, 2004). The vast majority of studies have been conducted with heterosexual couples and with North American samples (Rollè et al., 2018). Meyer (2003) described forms of minority stress that increase the risk for partner aggression among lesbian, gay, and bisexual couples. Although external sources of minority stress such as discrimination by people in the community have not been found to be predictors of partner aggression, internalized forms of homophobia and consciousness of stigma associated with one's sexual orientation have been found to be significant predictors.

- Childhood physical/sexual abuse victimization
- Childhood exposure to parental partner aggression
- Personality disorders associated with focus on personal goals and low empathy for others
- Forms of psychological distress (e.g., depression, trauma symptoms)
- Attachment insecurity that elicits anxiety about possibly losing one's partner
- Trait anger/hostility
- Difficulty regulating negative emotions such as anger
- Over-learned aggressive behavior in situations involving interpersonal conflict
- Deficits in relationship skills for communication, problem solving, and seeking intimacy/nurturance/security
- Alcohol and drug abuse
- A high level of life stressors affecting members of the couple (e.g., regarding employment, finances); poor stress-coping skills
- Current couple discord and relationship dissatisfaction
- Ingrained negative couple dyadic interaction patterns involving coercive behavior and reciprocal escalation of negative actions
- In heterosexual relationships, male partners' traditional gender role beliefs that encourage dominance
- Beliefs regarding dominance and acceptability of coercive/punitive behavior in relationships, not necessarily tied to gender
- In lesbian, gay, and bisexual relationships, minority stress from discrimination, especially internalized homophobia and consciousness of stigma associated with one's sexual orientation
- Beliefs about benefits of aggression, versus costs
- Attributing negative intent, selfish motivation, and blame for relationship problems to one's partner

---

FIGURE 5.1. Risk factors for perpetration of physical and psychological partner aggression.

Screening each couple for these characteristics will decrease the possibility of overlooking factors influencing partners' aggressive behavior. In a CBCT approach, although it is important to move quickly toward increasing partners' positive, nonaggressive interactions, it is assumed that ingrained cognitive, affective, and behavioral responses can persist unless therapy explicitly identifies and targets them. Effective treatment planning for each couple depends on identifying factors contributing to their aggression and designing interventions to reduce the impacts of those factors. Each couple comes to therapy with their unique life experiences since childhood, aspects of personal development and psychological functioning, current life stresses, cognitions about each other, attitudes regarding aggressive behavior, and skills for communicating and solving problems together.

PARTNER AGGRESSION FROM A CBCT PERSPECTIVE

The risk factors noted above involve the three domains of cognition, affect, and behavior. Individuals are more likely to behave aggressively toward their partner when they think in particular ways (e.g., holding a belief that a partner who treats you poorly deserves to be punished), have difficulty regulating negative emotions such as anger and anxiety, and rely on aggressive behavior to try to influence others. Some of those factors develop from experiences in their families of origin and other significant relationships (e.g., exposure to parents' partner aggression), as well as through cultural socialization (e.g., learning commonly held beliefs regarding the appropriateness of using aggression to express displeasure or punish another person). Many individuals learn to use aggression to influence others, based on being on the receiving end of coercive behavior, observing other people wielding power by behaving aggressively, or being reinforced for their own aggressive actions that result in compliance from others. Aggressive behavior may serve a function of expressing (venting) an individual's internal cognitive and emotional distress to others; for example, letting one's partner know that their actions hurt one's feelings. It also may be intended to coerce another person to behave in a particular way; for example, using physical force or psychological threats to cut off a partner from the social support of others. The latter type of control is a core aspect of battering and may be carried out without the perpetrator experiencing emotional arousal; that is, it is a calculated control strategy rather than venting.

It is neither necessary nor sufficient to know details about the personal historical roots of an individual's current partner aggression before interventions for positive change are started. However, some knowledge of history can help the therapist and couple anticipate possible barriers to change. For example, it is helpful to be aware that a man's gender role beliefs emphasizing male dominance that were learned in his family of origin may contribute to his aggressive responses to his female partner, even though he espouses egalitarian values.

Even though most people know how to behave aggressively through observing others' aggressive behavior via media or exposure in their own lives, the degree to which they actually behave aggressively varies widely, depending on other factors. Some of these factors involve the extent to which the individual is aware of and skilled in constructive, nonaggressive alternative ways of influencing others. People who lack effective social skills may rely on aggression to influence others. Thus, an individual whose partner has stronger verbal skills and debating ability may attempt to counteract that power imbalance through aggression. Other factors involve the extent to which the individual is adept at self-control, able to monitor and regulate their cognitions, emotions and behavior. Some individuals who engage in partner aggression conceptualize their deficits in self-regulation as "I have a short fuse," which gives a vague sense of poor self-control. Some individuals may use that concept to avoid personal responsibility for their aggression, but even they may have real deficits in self-regulation that require treatment.

Other trait-like personal characteristics that individuals bring to their intimate relationships, likely contributing to partner aggression, involve forms of psychopathology, such as clinical depression, PTSD from traumatic life experiences (e.g., attachment injuries, child abuse, wartime combat trauma), alcohol and substance abuse, and personality disorders. During clinical screening, a crucial distinction must be made to determine whether cognitive, affective, and behavioral aspects of partner aggression can be improved through conjoint treatment, or whether they reflect more severe personal problems that require individual therapy. For example, with milder levels of symptoms such as attachment insecurity and emotion dysregulation, couple therapy can provide the individual with repeated *in vivo* opportunities in sessions and daily life to work toward positive change. In contrast, relatively severe psychopathology can make it difficult for an individual to exercise sufficient self-control when in conflict with a partner.

In addition to the cognitive, affective, and behavioral response patterns that each individual brings to the relationship, the forms and intensity of partner aggression commonly are influenced by *dyadic processes*, as the partners influence each other mutually. As described in Chapter 1, patterns such as one member of a couple pursuing while the other withdraws, or both members escalating negative behavior in a reciprocal manner, can contribute to aggressive behavior that occurs rapidly and seemingly automatically. Couple therapists commonly observe rapid changes during sessions in which a couple that has been discussing a topic calmly quickly shifts to mutual emotional agitation and verbal aggression, triggered by one person's statement, facial expression, or voice tone that the other interprets negatively. Couples often are not aware of the rapid shift until their therapist points it out. When therapists intervene with dyadic patterns, it is crucial that each individual be held responsible for their own negative behavior, without blaming victims for perpetrators' actions.

In addition to focusing on individuals' characteristics and the couple's dyadic processes, a CBCT perspective examines aspects of the couple's environment that can be risk factors and may require intervention. Improving a couple's ability to cope with environmental stressors that affect them individually or jointly is a common aspect of therapy for partner aggression.

Thus, a cognitive-behavioral perspective on partner aggression is multilayered, attending to partners' historical and current life experiences, aspects of psychological functioning that influence their abilities to get their needs met constructively within their relationship, and cognitive, affective, and behavioral aspects of their couple interactions. Clinicians must be attuned to both intrapsychic and interpersonal processes, and they must also be skilled in integrating interventions for the two realms in the treatment plan. Although treatment is not simultaneous individual therapies, interventions are intended to produce positive changes within each person as well as in how they behave as a couple.

TRADITIONAL TREATMENTS FOR PERPETRATORS AND FOR VICTIMS

Based on evidence of severe harm that male batterers inflict on female partners in heterosexual relationships, traditional treatment programs were developed as gender-based, involving separate interventions for male perpetrators and for female victims. Traditional batterer intervention programs (BIPs) have been based primarily on a feminist perspective on the patriarchal structure of heterosexual relationships, providing psychoeducation to batterers who largely were referred by the criminal justice system, mostly in a group intervention format (Eckhardt et al., 2013; Rosenbaum & Kunkel, 2009). These programs are aimed at counteracting perpetrators' beliefs that supported their control of their female partners, as well as increasing their motivation to take responsibility for their coercive actions. Eckhardt et al. (2013) note that treatment programs increasingly have integrated that feminist approach with aspects of cognitive-behavioral therapy designed to reduce aggression-related cognitions, improve anger regulation, increase motivation to change, and build relationship skills for communication and conflict resolution (O'Leary, 2008). Programs for female victims have focused on providing legal advocacy, counseling regarding employment and independent living, safety planning, and cognitive-behavioral interventions to reduce negative symptoms (e.g., PTSD, depression) resulting from partner aggression (Eckhardt et al., 2013). Rollè et al. (2018) emphasize that only limited attention has been given to adapting gender-based treatments for lesbian, gay, and bisexual couples, developments that are greatly needed. Also, interventions for couples with nonbinary and trans members need to take these clients' needs and relationship dynamics into account.

Given the high prevalence and destructive effects of partner aggression on victims, it is unfortunate that research on traditional treatments for perpetrators and victims has shown limited effectiveness. Eckhardt et al. (2013) reviewed studies testing the effects of treatment programs designed for perpetrators and those for victims, primarily with samples involving physical violence. The studies they reviewed examined a variety of BIPs and both brief and extended treatments for victims/survivors. Eckhardt et al. (2013) concluded that many of the limited number of studies had significant design limitations, so it is not possible to draw clear conclusions about the effectiveness of programs in reducing risk factors for future violence. Recidivism rates for perpetrator programs tend to be high (Babcock & LaTaillade, 2000; Murphy & Eckhardt, 2005). Eckhardt et al. (2013) note that studies on the effects of programs for female victims have been few in number and adequacy of research designs, and most examined only one outcome—the incidence of revictimization, with some assessing victims' use of community resources. The findings provided limited evidence that victims obtained lasting benefits regarding revictimization and even less evidence of increased use of resources.

Due to the recognized dangers to physical and psychological well-being that commonly result from aggression victimization, mental health professionals have widely feared that treating couples conjointly would place victims at risk for further harm and should be avoided (Stith & McCollum, 2009). Although such concerns are valid in cases of battering, research in recent years, including Johnson's (1995, 2006) differentiation between battering and common couple violence, has indicated that a population of couples can be treated safely and effectively in a conjoint format (Epstein et al., 2023). Some couples are mutually motivated to stay together, and rather than continuing to interact in ways that leave them at risk for future aggression, therapists have an opportunity to provide them with constructive ways to resolve conflict (Epstein et al., 2023; O'Leary, 2015; Stith & McCollum, 2009).

COUPLE THERAPIES FOR PARTNER AGGRESSION

At present, two conjoint models have been designed specifically to treat couples experiencing psychological and mild to moderate physical partner aggression: CBCT and solution-focused couple therapy. These models have been subjected to research, and the results have been encouraging.

Both approaches have a moderate degree of structure, and both tend to be relatively time-limited (although they can be applied flexibly to meet the needs of individual couples). They are designed to interrupt couples' aggressive interactions quickly and to develop constructive ways of handling conflict.

CBCT programs typically begin with psychoeducation regarding the characteristics and consequences of partner aggression. They include components that focus on reducing individuals' "overlearned" (automatic) aggressive behaviors for expressing frustration with their partner and negative cognitions that contribute to anger and justify aggressive behavior. Interventions also are designed to improve difficulties with regulating negative emotions such as anger, limited skills for constructive communication and problem solving, and the couple's skills for coping with life stresses (Heyman & Neidig, 1997; LaTaillade et al., 2006). In addition, O'Farrell and colleagues' behavioral couple therapy (BCT), which includes cognitive-behavioral components and is used in conjunction with interventions for an individual partner's substance use (e.g., attending self-help meetings, medication), was not designed specifically to reduce partner aggression but has been found to do so (O'Farrell, Murphy, Stephan, Fals-Stewart, & Murphy, 2004; Schumm, O'Farrell, Murphy, & Fals-Stewart, 2009).

Stith and colleagues' solution-focused couple therapy for partner aggression (Stith et al., 2011) is based on the premise that clients not only bring problems to therapy but also personal resources and strengths that often are overlooked when clients and clinicians focus on problems. Therapists strive to uncover strengths that clients can use to resolve presenting problems, including partner aggression. Second, rather than developing conceptualizations of factors contributing to a problem, solution-focused therapists focus much more on engaging clients in generating specific conceptions of the outcomes they desire and outline the steps they can take to achieve those goals. This process overlaps with the problem solving used in cognitive-behavioral therapy, although CBT clinicians tend to spend more time initially gathering information about the characteristics of the presenting problem, in order to identify factors that influence its occurrence (a functional analysis we described in Chapter 3) and may require intervention. Third, solution-focused therapists guide clients in seeing that the problems they view as constant actually vary across time and circumstances, which can encourage pessimistic clients to envision the potential for improvement. This concept is also central to functional analysis in cognitive-behavioral therapy, in which identifying the conditions under which desired couple interactions occur sets the stage for efforts to increase them. Fourth, solution-focused therapists make sure that couple therapy includes goals both partners desire (e.g., enjoying daily life together free of tension and fear) in addition to goals that have been imposed on the couple by professionals and the legal system. This focus on solutions that clients prefer is associated with a fifth premise of solution-focused therapy; namely, that therapists do not impose standard goals on their clients. This potentially differentiates that model from a CBCT approach to partner aggression to some degree, as CBCT does include some common foci, such as practicing expressive and empathic listening skills, intervening with cognitions that fuel anger and aggressive behavior, and enhancing partners' abilities to regulate their emotions.

Research on both cognitive-behavioral and solution-focused approaches to treating mild to moderate partner aggression conjointly has indicated that *active intervention to replace aggressive interactions with constructive and mutually satisfying patterns is feasible and can be conducted safely*. Maintaining safety requires careful screening regarding risk factors for injurious violence, active intervention by therapists to maximize partners' regulation of their emotional and behavioral responses to each other, and constant monitoring of possible increases in volatility. In this chapter, we emphasize a CBCT approach to achieve those goals.

SCREENING AND ASSESSMENT FOR PARTNER AGGRESSION

Because some degree of partner aggression commonly occurs in the general population, and even more often among couples who seek therapy for a variety of relationship issues, it is safe to assume that any therapist who works with couples will encounter some clients experiencing psychological and physical aggression. Given the potential danger of conducting joint therapy that may place victims of battering at increased risk, sensitive screening of all couples is essential. Screening is complicated by the fact that many couples do not disclose partner aggression to therapists spontaneously, or even when the clinician asks about it in general terms (especially using a term such as *abusive behavior*) during the initial intake meeting (Epstein et al., 2023). Failure to disclose aggression may be motivated by a number of concerns, such as embarrassment and concern about disclosing socially undesirable behavior that could be judged negatively by the clinician and other people, lack of comfort and trust in the clinician at the beginning of therapy, a victim's fear of angering a perpetrator, or a view of physical or psychological aggression as normal in couple relationships. Individuals are more likely to report aggression by themselves or their partners when asked to complete, in privacy, questionnaires such as the Conflict Tactics Scale—Revised (CTS2; Straus et al., 1996), with items about the frequency of specific forms of aggressive behavior.

Therapists are faced with an ethical dilemma involving competing concerns for uncovering dangerous victimization while avoiding placing a victim at risk. Screening should not be avoided, given the risks associated with conducting therapy without knowledge of aggression occurring outside sessions. However, screening must be done in a tactful way that minimizes the risk that a perpetrator will punish a victim for disclosing abusive acts.

Because many couples who have experienced partner aggression do not disclose it when asked about their reasons for seeking couple therapy, therapists must screen for it by asking direct questions. However, to reduce potential victims' inhibition about disclosure, it is crucial to conduct screening with the members separately. The following sequence of procedures is designed to uncover types of partner aggression while attempting to maximize safety:

• **During a potential client's initial phone inquiry regarding couple therapy,** when the therapist asks about concerns that led the caller to pursue couple therapy, listen for direct descriptions or hints about partner aggression. In either case, ask, "Do you have complete privacy to talk with me right now, without anyone, including your partner, present? I believe it is very important for each person I speak with to be relaxed and have privacy, so I want that for you now." If the caller indicates a lack of privacy or the therapist senses inhibition in the caller's speech, avoid probing further about aggression at this point. Focus on general goals for therapy, with questions such as "How much have you and your partner discussed seeking couple therapy?"; "How much do you think your partner is interested in having therapy at this time?"; "What goals for therapy have you and your partner discussed?" The therapist should stress that couple therapy works best when both members see value in it and feel comfortable meeting with a third party to talk about their relationship. Offer an opportunity for the caller's partner to speak individually with the therapist so that the partner can ask questions about therapy, the therapist's qualifications, and so on. Given that a caller's partner may be listening, the therapist can convey availability to talk with the caller further when conditions are more private by noting that the therapist is available in the days ahead if either person would like to call and ask more about therapy.

- ○ *With direct descriptions of aggression*, when the caller has indicated privacy for talking, ask:
  - ■ "How much do you think your partner also is concerned about these types of aggressive behavior occurring in your relationship? I can hear that you personally are concerned about it and would like to see improvement. Has your partner directly expressed a desire to address the aggressive behavior during couple therapy? To what extent do you think your partner would be agreeable to the two of you and me talking about it?"
  - ■ "What have the two of you tried so far to try to reduce aggressive behavior in your relationship? To what extent did you seem to work well as a team in your efforts to reduce aggressive actions? How well did the things you tried seem to work? If your success was limited, what seemed to interfere with making progress? If you were successful overall, what positive changes did you notice?"
  - ■ "How comfortable or uncomfortable are you about bringing up, during couple therapy sessions, aggressive behavior occurring in your relationship? If you are concerned about your doing it, please tell me what you are concerned might happen? What do you think your partner's reaction might be if I heard about the issue?"
  - ■ "It is very important for members of a couple to feel safe in their relationship. To what extent do you feel unsafe? If you are concerned about your safety, what plans do you have set up to keep yourself safe? Who else in your life is available to help you stay safe?" The therapist should be prepared to offer the client referral information regarding shelters, legal assistance, among other things.
  - ■ "How comfortable are you with beginning sessions with your partner? Would you prefer to begin individual therapy instead, to sort out your feelings and goals, and maybe to prepare for possible couple therapy?" The therapist should be prepared to offer referrals for individual therapy.
- ○ *With hints about partner aggression*, when the caller has indicated privacy for talking, ask:
  - ■ "What issues in your relationship do you believe the two of you agree could use some attention in couple therapy? What issues, if any, do you think the two of you disagree are problems in your relationship?"
  - ■ "How concerned or fearful are you about bringing up particular issues during couple sessions, especially about your partner's reaction to me as a therapist knowing about those issues in your relationship?"
  - ■ "How safe do you feel beginning couple sessions with your partner? Would you rather begin with individual therapy to sort out your feelings and goals and to prepare for possible couple therapy if you decide that is your goal?" The therapist should be prepared to offer referrals for individual therapy.

• **Once the members of a couple have agreed to pursue couple therapy, the therapist schedules them to attend an initial assessment session.** At this point, the therapist proceeds as if couple therapy could occur, with the crucial caveat that subsequent information about dangerous aggression will preclude conjoint therapy. The therapist informs the couple that the assessment session will involve filling out some brief questionnaires about themselves and their relationship, as well as being interviewed together and individually so that the therapist can get to know them. The therapist should present a brief rationale for those assessment procedures, such as the following:

> "In order to get to know a couple well, I have standard ways I ask partners about themselves and their relationship. It includes brief questionnaires that quickly help me learn about how the two of you interact with each other, communicate, and reach decisions. It also includes my interviewing you together regarding the history of your relationship, and then each of you individually to learn about your background. I need that information in order to work with the two of you to plan treatment that will help you achieve your goals."

• **Use of assessments to decide on an initial treatment plan.** After the therapist provides the couple a rationale for the assessment procedures, the therapist conducts a joint interview and separate interviews with the individual partners, following the guidelines described in Chapter 3. Finally, the therapist gives the couple feedback about overall impressions of their relationship's strengths as well as areas that could be improved through therapy. If the therapist has decided there is no level of physical or psychological partner aggression for which conjoint therapy would be inappropriate, the therapist guides the couple in deciding whether couple therapy is the best approach for them at this point. If the partners decide to pursue therapy, the therapist and couple set goals to begin their work together. Although some couples explicitly identify partner aggression as a problem that they wish to address, many couples present a variety of other goals (e.g., conflict regarding child-rearing practices, strained relations with in-laws, one partner's depression). It is important that the therapist validate those goals as important and emphasize that the therapy will focus on them. However, when the assessment has identified ongoing partner aggression, the therapist also introduces the goal of improving the couple's skills for resolving conflicts constructively and in mutually satisfying ways.

The therapist must consider that some questionnaires and topics covered in the individual interviews make it obvious that the clinician is gathering information about partner aggression and other problems in the couple's relationship. Perpetrators will be aware that their partner may be revealing their aggression and may be upset about the disclosure. Consequently, the therapist must convey that each person's responses will be kept private, so that each person can share their personal views with the therapist comfortably. The therapist emphasizes that after the assessment is complete, the three of them will have a discussion about setting goals for treatment.

• **Completion of questionnaires.** The therapist asks the partners to complete the measures described in Chapter 3 in separate rooms, as part of the standard couple pre-therapy assessment. Most of those forms (Relationship Issues Survey, Couple Satisfaction Inventory, Couple Communication Behavior Questionnaire, Inventory of General Relationship Standards) are relevant for all couples seeking therapy, but the CTS2 (Straus et al., 1996) and our Partner Aggression Scale (Handout 3.3) are especially relevant for screening couples for partner aggression. If the therapist is using telehealth sessions, in order to maintain confidentiality and safety for each individual, we advise that partners agree to complete forms in separate locations, seal them in envelopes, and mail them to the therapist.

• **Joint interview with the couple.** As described in Chapter 3, the joint assessment interview with the couple (Figure 3.1) covers the history of their relationship as well as their current functioning. For the purpose of screening for past and current partner aggression without placing potential victims at risk for retaliation, the therapist asks questions that give partners opportunities to reveal aggression without directly pulling for disclosure; for example, "When the two of you have disagreements about how to do something (e.g., spending money, disciplining children), how do you communicate and behave toward each other?"; "When you are upset with each other, how do you express it?" It is important that the therapist notice any cues that aggressive behavior occurs, but not ask an individual to elaborate to the extent that might result in their partner becoming angry. Because aggressive individuals may show little anger during sessions but vent it toward their partner later, the therapist must be guided by a general principle of protecting victims rather than by the emotional tone in the room at any point.

• **Individual interview with each member of the couple.** The protocol for individual interviews with members of a couple presented in Chapter 3 includes questions that are relevant for identifying partner aggression, as well as risk factors for aggression. Given that these interviews are conducted privately, the therapist has opportunities to ask follow-up questions when a client makes vague statements that lead the therapist to suspect possible aggression, either as victim or perpetrator. The therapist emphasizes that the individual's responses will be kept confidential. Questions that may tap risks for the individual's own perpetration of aggression include:

  ○ Questions about current life stressors
  ○ Follow-up questions when an individual identified areas of conflict in the relationship on the RIS (Handout 3.1) regarding the intensity of conflict and examples of negative or positive behavior on each member's part
  ○ Follow-up questions to the individual's responses to the Partner Aggression Scale (Handout 3.3) screening questionnaire, regarding the frequency and intensity of their own and their partner's particular aggressive behaviors
  ○ Degrees to which the individual and their partner are successful at regulating their emotional responses to upsetting experiences
  ○ Aspects of personal psychological functioning that may be risk factors for aggression perpetration or consequences of being victimized (e.g., substance use, depression, PTSD)

THERAPIST DECISIONS REGARDING THE APPROPRIATENESS OF CONJOINT TREATMENT

A decision to pursue couple therapy to address partner aggression for a particular couple is based on judgments of whether the modality (1) will be safe for the members of this couple and (2) will be effective in reducing current aggression and preventing future aggression.

• **Safety.** The criteria we use to estimate the level of safety in conducting joint sessions, all of which are assessed by the Partner Aggression Scale and questions in the pre-therapy individual assessment interview, include:
  ○ An absence of past and current severe forms of aggression (e.g., punching, choking, use of a weapon)
  ○ An absence of past and current aggression involving infliction of physical injury (e.g., bruises, sprains)
  ○ An absence of untreated alcohol or drug use that is a risk for emotional, cognitive, and behavioral dysregulation
  ○ Positive responses from both members to therapist questions about feeling safe living

with their partner, participating in therapy with their partner, and choosing to participate of their own free will

- o The therapist's perception of a positive therapeutic alliance with both members, with both conveying motivation to work collaboratively with the therapist
- o Both partners' expression of commitment to safety and a realistic appraisal of risk factors
- **Effectiveness.** Although the therapist's ability to predict overall treatment effectiveness from the initial assessment necessarily will be limited, the following criteria can be used to help decide whether conditions for positive changes exist:
  - o As per the safety criteria listed above, the therapist's impressions suggest that the initial therapeutic alliances with both members of the couple are positive.
  - o The therapist appraises the therapeutic alliance between partners as positive; regardless of relationship distress, they both have expressed sincere motivation to improve their relationship and take some personal responsibility for their roles in relationship problems and efforts that are needed.
  - o Neither partner is experiencing a level of individual psychopathology that seems likely to interfere with their ability to engage in and benefit from the couple interventions.

GOAL SETTING AND SOCIALIZATION TO TREATMENT

In Chapter 2, we described ways in which therapists can introduce clients to the concepts, goals, and methods of a CBCT model. As we noted, therapists collaborate with couples to work toward the goals that led them to seek assistance. However, because a notable percentage of couples have not identified their partner aggression as a problem, therapists take responsibility for pointing out ways in which aggressive responses detract from the quality of daily life together and interfere with achieving partners' goals such as resolving specific conflicts. Rather than simply relying on a didactic psychoeducational description of the drawbacks of venting anger and aggression, the therapist looks for compelling examples in the couple's actual interactions.

One approach involves allowing the couple to describe a frustrating argument that occurred at home since the last session. The therapist interrupts them to ask each person what they had hoped would happen when they talked, empathizing with how *disappointing* (shifting the focus from anger) it must have been to have their interaction deteriorate. The therapist then guides the partners in discussing a therapy goal of improving their ability to have satisfying discussions of issues. This technique is consistent with the solution-focused approach of moving couples from problem-focused thinking to envisioning positive goals. It involves harnessing current experiences of frustration, sadness, and other emotions to motivate them to try a new approach.

A second and similar approach involves using the couple's upsetting negative interaction during a therapy session to motivate them to consider new approaches to dealing with the issues that make them upset with each other. The therapist allows the couple to escalate briefly (one might consider this an experiential exercise) and then interrupts them, asking each to describe how they were feeling and empathizing with their disappointment. Because clients with limited self-regulation abilities will have difficulty deescalating at this point, it is important that the therapist provides a mixture of empathy and structure/control.

Thus, the therapist's intent is to guide the couple in generating core goals for therapy that are tailored to their needs and life circumstances (e.g., reducing financial stresses, increasing intimacy, co-parenting their children effectively), ensuring that improving their ability to resolve conflicts without aggression is a high-priority goal. The therapist can emphasize that eliminating aggressive interactions will have the overall benefit of making their relationship more enjoyable, as well as specific benefits of helping them solve particular problems together.

In addition to socializing clients into the CBCT model's concepts and methods in general (see Chapter 2), the therapist introduces clients to the methods used specifically to reduce negative interactions during conflict. Terminology is quite important in establishing a therapeutic alliance in addressing partner aggression. Because the widely used terms *intimate partner violence* and *partner abuse* tend to be pejorative, we have found that members of many couples have negative reactions when therapists use them. They may perceive that the therapist is jumping to conclusions and is insulting them, lacks empathy for their life stresses, and is shaming them. Consequently, we focus on concrete behaviors, referring to them as negative ways of handling conflict, and also examine their effects on the partner and relationship. As we work toward establishing a positive alliance with each person, we do refer to the actions as aggressive, in the sense that they commonly inflict pain on the recipient and undermine the bond between the partners. Perpetrators are more likely to accept input from a therapist, including firm structure, when they perceive the clinician as respecting and caring about them as human beings.

The therapist describes the *components of CBCT treatment for partner aggression* listed in Handout 5.1 (available on the accompanying web page at *www.guilford.com/epstein-materials*).

The therapist also describes *structural aspects of the couple therapy*, which are mostly generic CBCT characteristics:

- *Mostly joint sessions*, with the option of occasional sessions with the individuals if they are experiencing challenges from aspects of the therapy (e.g., difficulty managing anger).
- *Active practice in sessions and during "homework" of positive couple skills* for communication, problem solving, coping with stressors, modification of problematic thinking, anger management, and building of a positive couple bond.
- *The roles of the therapist:* providing educational information; teaching, coaching (with detailed constructive feedback), and supporting the couple as they practice new skills; collaborating with the couple in planning homework they will engage in between sessions to transfer positive changes to daily life.
- *The roles of the couple:* attending sessions consistently, so changes can develop; taking responsibility for making personal changes that will contribute to a better relationship; avoiding competition and win–lose interactions with one's partner; collaborating with the therapist and partner to plan homework, and being consistent in carrying out homework plans between sessions; giving the therapist feedback about aspects of therapy that are helpful, as well as any aspects that feel uncomfortable or unhelpful.
- *Generally time-limited therapy* (often a few months), but each couple and their therapist decide together on when goals have been reached and it is time to end therapy.

PLANNING TREATMENT

When working with couples who have been experiencing partner aggression, the therapist's primary goal is to increase the members' physical and psychological safety by identifying and removing risk factors for aggression. Interventions focus on risk factors involving partners' cognition, emotional responses, and behavior toward each other. A number of interventions are available to modify those cognitive, emotional, and behavioral components of partner aggression. They all draw on interventions detailed in Chapter 4. Due to the damaging effects of aggression on individual and relationship well-being, it is crucial that the therapist's initial interventions quickly reduce current aggressive acts, demonstrating to the couple that they can interact in nonaggressive ways even when discussing sensitive issues. Immediate attention to behavior change is essential, but interventions that reduce poorly regulated emotional responses also are needed to allow the individuals to behave more constructively even when they are upset. Furthermore, when the assessment has indicated that individuals' cognitions (e.g., a belief in retribution) contribute to anger and aggression, interventions for those cognitions should be integrated early in the treatment plan. With partner aggression, the treatment plan should focus on interrupting damaging interactions as quickly as possible, as well as developing individual and dyadic skills for communicating and solving problems.

Interventions to Modify Behavior

Time-Outs

As described in Chapter 4, a time-out is an agreement between partners to interrupt a negative interaction and distance from each other temporarily, in order to prevent it from escalating and to give individuals an opportunity to use strategies to regulate intense emotions and plan a more constructive approach to talking with each other. This intervention might appear simple in structure, but in practice it often is difficult to use. First, couple therapists who suggest time-outs experience resistance from some clients, who complain that their partner already withdraws from them as a means of avoiding dealing with important topics ("He just cuts me off and leaves.") (Stith et al., 2011). Consequently, the therapist must convey that the purpose of a true time-out is to shift the couple away from negative emotional and behavioral interactions, toward relatively calm constructive ones. It is a temporary "cool off and regroup" strategy in which partners are committed to working together to resolve issues. The goal is to avoid negative exchanges, not to avoid each other.

Individuals' withdrawal from their partners may reflect a pattern they learned long ago in their families of origin, either through observing other family members withdraw or through discovering that their own withdrawal was effective in escaping from others' aversive behavior. In discussing the use of time-outs with a couple, a therapist should be on the lookout for evidence that one or both partners have a pattern of avoidance, explore its history, convey empathy for the positive function it has served, but encourage the individual to experiment with time-outs. The therapist emphasizes that successful time-outs require that partners demonstrate to each other that it is safe to return and talk further. When an individual is a pursuer in a pursue–withdraw pattern and is distressed at the prospect that their partner is "getting away" from discussing an important topic during a time-out, the therapist needs to intervene to reduce that person's emotional distress that is fueling the pursuit. This involves a combination of emotion-regulation strategies and commitment from their withdrawing partner that they will return to discuss the issue further (Epstein & Baucom, 2002). We recommend that each person retreat to a private place to use emotion-regulation strategies and write down ideas to discuss when they will reconvene.

Communication Skills Training

Educating and coaching couples in expressive and empathic listening skills (Chapter 4) has a number of benefits for reducing partner aggression. First, psychoeducation regarding communication skills can counteract individuals' prior learning in their families of origin and the broader culture that aggression is an acceptable and effective means of influencing other people. The therapist introduces an alternative model for sharing information about one's needs, making requests (not demands) for change, and conveying understanding and respect for each other. As partners internalize this constructive model, that cognitive shift can contribute to reduced aggression even if the couple does not practice the communication skills on a regular basis. Second, the structure involved in partners carrying out the expressive and listening roles tends to slow the pace of the couple's interaction, reducing emotional and behavioral escalation. In addition, when an individual is able to disclose vulnerable thoughts and feelings rather than primarily anger, their partner is more likely to perceive them as a reasonable human. In turn, when the listener conveys empathy for the expresser's thoughts and emotions, the expresser may develop more positive perceptions of the listener's motives and level of caring. Handouts on communication guidelines (Handout 4.1) are another aspect of structure, serving as reminders to exit escalation patterns as quickly as possible.

Problem-Solving Skills Training

Individuals who lack interpersonal skills for influencing others and tend to feel overwhelmed by their partners' verbal skills are at risk for turning to psychological and physical aggression to "even the playing field." Consequently, improving their skills for resolving problems through collaboration versus competition often helps reduce partner aggression. Problem-solving skills (Chapter 4) have particular benefits for reducing aggressive interactions that are similar to those from expressive and listening skills. Psychoeducation regarding purposes and benefits of working as a team to resolve problems can counteract beliefs individuals learned earlier in life (e.g., that one must always be on guard for others' attempts to exert control; that a strong person is dominant in relationships). For couples who are accustomed to a win–lose approach to conflict, the emphasis on devising solutions that are acceptable to both members initially may be met with skepticism that one's partner can be trusted to cooperate. However, consistent coaching and encouragement from the therapist as the couple experiments with collaborative brainstorming and trials of solutions have potential to build trust.

As with behavioral experiments in general, it is important that the therapist prepare the couple to expect "slips" and that the goal is to catch the slip quickly and shift to a more positive interaction. For example, if one of the members becomes frustrated with the other's proposed solution to a problem and criticizes the partner in a denigrating way, the therapist interrupts, points out the aggressive response, and coaches the perpetrator in acknowledging the slip and substituting a constructive way of disagreeing with the partner. Practicing standard problem-solving steps builds in positive structure to couple interactions that reduces escalation of anger and aggression. Initially, the therapist guides the couple in working through the steps, but gradually partners take responsibility for the process. The handout on problem solving (Handout 4.2) is used in sessions and at home to help couples keep the steps in mind.

Dyadic Coping Skills Training

Given that stressors are risk factors for partner aggression, psychoeducation and practice of positive dyadic coping skills are important interventions. The therapist begins with psychoeducation about the role of stress in emotion dysregulation and use of aggression as a coping response. To build a positive therapeutic alliance and motivate partners to experiment with change, the therapist conveys empathy for the partners' distress but emphasizes the goal of developing nonaggressive coping with the stressors they face in order to strengthen their bond as a couple. Based on information from the assessment interviews and the Dyadic Coping Inventory (DCI; Bodenmann, 2008), the therapist and couple discuss coping strategies they have been using, identifying those that increase tension and the risk of negative interactions, as well as those that have positive effects and that could be increased. The therapist then guides the couple in identifying forms of positive dyadic coping that seem relevant for specific stressors affecting them as individuals or as a couple (see Chapter 4), and the therapist coaches them in role-playing alternative coping strategies, so they can get a sense of how helpful each could be.

As with practice of communication and problem-solving skills, the therapist looks for verbal and nonverbal cues that partners are uncomfortable trying particular coping strategies, and explores their cognitions that may be barriers. For example, an individual may resist a partner engaging in delegated dyadic coping that involves taking over some of the individual's tasks to lighten the load. Exploration of the person's discomfort may reveal a personal standard that a competent person doesn't need help. The therapist can integrate some cognitive interventions to soften the rigidity of the person's standard and open the door to more dyadic coping.

A number of aspects of better dyadic coping can reduce risk factors for partner aggression. Psychoeducation that increases partners' insight into their use of aggression to cope with stress and learning ways to collaborate to reduce each other's stress can contribute to self-regulation. A collaborative bond can be enhanced as they experience the positive effects of working as a team, and the structure involved in repeated practice of dyadic coping can reduce impulsive responses. Focusing on dyadic coping also may reveal vulnerabilities within each individual (such as negative standards about accepting help) that should be addressed in the treatment plan, either as part of the couple interventions or via referrals for concurrent individual therapy.

Increasing Overall Relationship Satisfaction through Positive Behavior Addressing Core Needs

As we have noted, relationship distress is a risk for partner aggression, and increasing partners' satisfaction depends not only on reducing negative behavior but also on increasing positive exchanges (Epstein & Baucom, 2002). Consequently, interventions focused on increasing a couple's experiences of treating each other in pleasing ways are an important component of treatment. As described in Chapter 4, the initial assessment of the couple includes a history of their relationship, including activities they shared that contributed to their attraction to each other and satisfaction with their relationship. Based on that assessment, the therapist uses *guided behavior change* procedures to help the couple develop plans to enact behaviors that create more positive experiences with each other. The therapist emphasizes that the goal is to increase feelings of closeness and satisfaction, so it is important to consider the feasibility of the proposed plans. Some ideas for initiating or increasing particular positive behaviors may be rejected based on the cost/benefit analysis, whereas others are selected for a trial run.

Interventions to Modify Cognition

Increasing Attunement to Automatic Thoughts That Elicit Anger and Aggression

As described in Chapter 4, a core intervention for negative cognitions involves psychoeducation regarding automatic thoughts and building clients' skills for noticing and modifying their thoughts that contribute to negative couple interactions. Handout 1.1 on cognitive distortions can be applied to automatic thoughts that elicit anger and aggression. Skill-building includes guiding individuals in becoming more aware of their stream-of-consciousness thinking (especially during interactions with their partner), helping them track associations between negative thoughts and their anger and aggressive behavior toward the partner, and coaching them in modifying problematic thoughts. During conjoint sessions, the therapist has numerous opportunities to observe a couple reacting negatively to each other, when responding to something their partner said during the session. Those responses give the therapist opportunities to enhance partners' abilities to notice and cope with their negative automatic thoughts and associated aggression.

In addition, individuals can keep logs of their automatic thoughts associated with anger and aggression as homework. Because aggressive behavior often is "over-learned" and occurs in a reflexive manner, the more individuals can catch themselves responding with anger-eliciting thoughts and aggression, the better their chances of weakening the negative response pattern. As described in Chapters 3 and 4, therapists can give couples written thought record forms or links to cell phone apps for recording their experiences *in vivo*. When couples bring their thought records to the next therapy session, the therapist and couple can examine them as a team, learning about each person's internal experiences associated with aggressive responses. This collaboration also allows each individual to introduce information that can challenge the other's negative cognitions. For example, when Tom left the room during a disagreement with Stan, Stan *attributed* it to Tom not respecting him and so he became quite angry. When Stan reported this incident from his thought record during the subsequent couple session, Tom replied that he had always respected Stan. He had felt overwhelmed by Stan's ability to "out-debate me" and had a strong urge to escape the situation. Even so, Stan still was frustrated that Tom cut off their conversation, but the information from Tom changed his negative attribution and reduced his anger.

Many individuals' aggressive responses have been reinforced by producing desired effects, such as motivating a partner to comply with requests or stopping a partner from pressuring the individual to spend more time together. When aggressive behavior has been instrumental in getting what one wants, the individual has developed an *expectancy* that such actions are effective. Weakening that expectancy requires compelling new information that the costs of aggression outweigh the payoffs, and there are alternative ways of behaving that can produce better results. Chapter 4 describes interventions for modifying individuals' expectancies that are relevant for reducing partner aggression. For example, the therapist can engage the couple in thinking about consequences they experienced when one or both behaved aggressively, such as hurt feelings, decreased closeness, and a greater likelihood that both will expect more aggression in the future.

The therapist can guide the couple in setting up experiential behavioral experiments in which they deal with conflicts by using constructive communication and problem solving, and they pay attention to the impacts on their relationship. Repeated positive experiences with nonaggressive behavior may be needed to change ingrained expectancies that favor aggression.

Increasing Relational Circular Thinking about Partner Aggression

It is crucial that the therapist avoid suggesting that a victim of aggression was responsible for the partner's actions. However, the therapist can guide a couple in tracking the process of their ineffective interactions and in identifying actions that each person can take that can contribute to resolving conflicts. Victims of partner aggression still may become caught up in negative couple patterns such as extended debates or a demand–withdraw cycle, so the therapist's goal is to increase their circular thinking; that is, "When my partner does X, I tend to do Y, which increases the chance that my partner will do Z, and so on." Even though couple therapists are accustomed to noticing circular processes, clients often are not. Thus, providing repeated feedback to a couple and enlisting them in noticing patterns that include aggressive responses can produce a key cognitive shift.

Modifying Standards and Assumptions That Justify Partner Aggression

Simply challenging an individual's standard that it is justifiable to use aggression to punish or control a partner is likely to have limited impact. Those beliefs commonly were developed through the individual's life experiences in the family of origin, other significant relationships, and broader cultural context. Consequently, aggression often seems normative to the person, and a therapist's explicit negative value judgments about the person's aggressive acts can be experienced as invalidating. Although it is appropriate for therapists to reveal a personal value that people should not inflict emotional or physical harm on others, their task is to convey positive regard for the perpetrator as a human being simultaneously. The clinician can build the therapeutic alliance by conveying empathy for the individual's experiences that resulted in beliefs about the benefits of aggression. Then, an important distinction can be made between the appropriateness of communicating one's thoughts and emotions to one's partner (e.g., "When you ignore me, it seems like I'm unimportant to you, and I end up feeling both irritated and lonely") and the inappropriateness of punishing the partner with aggression. The therapist can focus on the constructive goal of sharing feelings with one's partner with communication skills to pave the way for positive change *and* the disadvantages of attempting to influence the partner through aggression.

As described in Chapter 1, individuals' diverse personal backgrounds result in differences among their *standards for what constitutes partner aggression* (especially with forms of psychological aggression that do not involve physical contact). Consequently, therapists need to use psychoeducation to broaden many clients' beliefs about actions harmful to recipients and to relationships. Again, it is important to avoid pejorative terms that can increase clients' defensiveness and detract from the therapeutic alliance, while still conveying the negative effects of partner aggression and taking a firm position that the therapist's goal is to help the couple feel safe and satisfied in their relationship. Thus, our handout describing forms of psychological and physical partner aggression (Handout 5.2, available on the book's web page at *www.guilford.com/epstein-materials*) does not include the term *partner abuse,* which is used widely in professional literature and popular media. Rather, it is labeled "Negative Ways of Dealing with Dissatisfaction and Conflict in a Couple Relationship." It does use and define the terms *psychological aggression* and *physical aggression,* focusing on the use of aversive acts to punish or control another person.

Because there are cultural variations in the acceptability of aggression in couple and parent–child relationships, it is important that a therapist inquire about each client's family-of-origin experiences and cultural norms in their background. The therapist must balance respect for cultural diversity with a clear message about the importance of family members treating each other in ways that protect their physical and psychological well-being. Thus, we validate individuals' right to communicate how their partner's actions have affected their thoughts and emotions, and feeling safe to share personal experiences is important for one's mental health. However, we emphasize that the individual needs to communicate in a manner that maximizes that one's partner will understand and take their messages seriously, while also treating the partner respectfully and protecting the partner's well-being. The therapist can give the couple copies of Handout 5.3 (available on the book's web page at *www.guilford.com/epstein-materials*), which summarizes research findings regarding the negative effects of partner aggression on individual well-being, as well as relationship quality and stability. The therapist can explain that routinely sharing this information with clients is based on people often being unaware that even mild to moderate levels of aggressive acts can take a serious toll on recipients' individual self-esteem, depression, anxiety, and overall feeling of well-being, as well as making the couple relationship very uncomfortable. The therapist appeals to clients' common goal of having their partner like them and want to be with them, and the therapeutic focus on eliminating aggressive behavior is described as intended to help them achieve those personal goals.

Challenging Beliefs Supporting Partner Aggression without Shaming Clients

Even though many individuals have developed standards and assumptions that support aggression in relationships, they also may be susceptible to experiencing shame when therapists and other people portray such behavior as damaging and unacceptable. Shame is different from guilt, which involves an individual evaluating their own *actions* negatively (based either on feedback from others or societal standards the individual has internalized) and being motivated to make amends to anyone who suffered from those acts. In contrast, shame involves *condemning oneself* for one's actions and becoming motivated to withdraw (Dearing & Tangney, 2011; Epstein & Falconier, 2017). Shaming is a strategy, which receives some cultural support, used by some parents to socialize children, as well as a method some individuals use to punish and motivate their partners. With its attack on the recipient's self-esteem, shaming falls within the definition of psychological aggression. Epstein and Falconier (2017) note that participating in couple therapy can result in shame experiences, either from partners condemning each other or from therapists defining client behaviors as destructive. Consequently, as therapists provide psychoeducation regarding forms of partner aggression and draw attention to aggressive acts in a couple's interactions, it is important that they convey empathy and respect for the individuals. Differentiating between an individual's negative behavior and the essence of the individual as a person is essential. Allowing an individual to experience guilt and become motivated to behave more constructively can be therapeutic, but eliciting shame that results in defensiveness and withdrawal is counterproductive.

Interventions for Emotion Regulation

Although clients as well as therapists recognize anger as a common precursor of aggressive behavior, anxiety associated with insecure attachment also plays a role for many individuals, as they attempt to control a partner they perceive as withdrawing. Interventions to increase individuals' abilities to notice and moderate strong negative emotional responses toward their partners should be key components of the treatment plan. Because low relationship satisfaction is another risk factor for partner aggression, interventions to assist partners in upregulating positive emotion in their interactions also are important. As described in Chapter 4, emotion regulation includes (1) noticing one's emotional states and tracking their links with particular situations that elicit them, (2) use of self-talk to coach oneself to engage in a time-out if necessary to reduce the intensity of the emotion, (3) use of self-soothing strategies to reduce arousal, and (4) use of constructive communication with one's partner to explain the reason for one's upset feelings and to make requests for change in the relationship as needed. The foundation for these interventions is psychoeducation regarding emotion.

Psychoeducation is used to increase partners' understanding of anger and other emotions, their potential role for alerting both members of the couple about the individuals' needs, and strategies for channeling emotions to motivate positive changes in the relationship. Because many individuals received little education about emotions during childhood, in either their families or school, they often think of their emotions in simplistic terms; for example, "I have a short fuse and just blow up easily." It can be enlightening to them when a therapist introduces information about cognitive, affective, physiological, and behavioral components of an emotion such as anger, as presented in Handout 5.4 (available on the accompanying web page at *www.guilford.com/epstein-materials*). The therapist can emphasize that an emotion such as anger actually is a complicated experience; the more a person understands about it, the greater the chance of using it in a way that improves one's personal life and couple relationship. In contrast to the "short-fuse" concept, this model of the components of emotion offers opportunities for the individual to exercise some control over their emotional responses.

For example, the therapist can describe how awareness of situations that typically trigger one's anger can help one prepare to cope with personal responses in particular situations. This might involve intentionally avoiding certain situations, such as reaching an agreement with one's partner not to initiate conversations about conflict topics late in the evening when one is tired. Furthermore, the therapist can guide clients in noticing when they have experienced a "pile-up" of stressors, in which the accumulation of distressing experiences finally reaches a person's tolerance threshold, and the "last straw" event (e.g., a critical remark from a partner) triggers strong anger and aggression. Reducing the risk of aggression requires decreasing or removing some of the other stressors the individual experienced.

In addition, each individual can learn to pay more attention to their automatic thoughts associated with anger, such as negative attributions about a partner's motives (e.g., "She interrupts me because she doesn't care about my ideas"). The therapist also can probe for each individual's assumptions and standards about the appropriateness of aggressive expression of anger, such as a belief that a partner whose actions lead you to feel angry deserves to be punished. Interventions counteracting cognitions that elicit and support aggressive venting of anger then become part of the treatment plan for emotion regulation. Individuals' "short-fuse" conception of anger and aggressive behavior also can be addressed by psychoeducation about noticing cues of one's physiological arousal that can serve as "early warning" signs and give the individual and couple time for defusing the tension before aggression occurs.

Psychoeducation includes teaching the couple self-soothing techniques that reduce physiological arousal (e.g., progressive muscle relaxation, a relaxing shower, mindfulness exercises). The therapist can use emotion-regulation methods described in Chapter 4, tailored to moderating anger. Finally, psychoeducation focuses on alternative ways of behaving when one is experiencing negative emotion. Some individuals have limited repertoires for responding when they are angry, based on limited prior learning opportunities, but psychoeducation about communication and problem-solving skills can broaden their options. The therapist can present communication and problem-solving guidelines described in Chapter 4 as constructive alternatives to aggression.

As we summarize in Figure 5.2, there are a variety of methods that therapists can use to help couples manage and reduce anger and aggressive behavior. They include increasing awareness of one's personal risk factors for experiencing anger and symptoms of increasing anger, strategies for avoiding or removing such risk factors, modifying one's anger-eliciting cognitions, and replacing aggressive behavior with constructive communication, problem-solving, and dyadic coping skills. These interventions are applications of CBCT interventions for problematic emotional, cognitive, and behavioral responses detailed in Chapter 4.

TROUBLESHOOTING PROBLEMS IN COUPLE THERAPY FOR AGGRESSION

Therapists working with partner aggression must be prepared to intervene with two major types of problems that can arise during treatment:

- Risks for dangerous escalation of psychological or physical aggression that were not identified during intake screening.
- Barriers to effective treatment based on characteristics of the individuals, the couple as a dyad, and the therapeutic alliance.

Risks for Escalation of Partner Aggression

We already have described how therapists use careful screening, clear ground rules for constructive interaction, and interruption of conflict escalation during sessions to minimize the risk that events during couple sessions will increase the likelihood of subsequent partner aggression at home. In spite of these strategies, the discussion of sensitive topics during couple therapy tends to be emotionally challenging, and therapists must monitor the risk level continuously and be prepared to intervene. Useful procedures include:

- "Check-ins" with the couple at the beginning and end of each session, regarding the current level of conflict and tension, identification of events that led to any increase, and problem solving about ways to regulate anger and any aggressive actions.
- Additional "check-ins" during the session when the therapist notices verbal or nonverbal cues that tension is rising, with similar problem solving about ways to regulate anger and aggressive behavior.
- If the therapist becomes concerned that there is significant risk that partner aggression may occur, scheduling separate sessions with the partners as soon as possible to address each person's risk of perpetration or plans to maintain personal safety.

Therapists can use the following descriptions of interventions for reducing anger and partner aggression to provide psychoeducation, then coach the couple in tailoring the interventions to their own aggression difficulties. See Chapter 4 for further details on these interventions.

Increase Personal Awareness of Anger Risks and Symptoms

- Keep track of specific situations that tend to make you angry (who is involved, where it takes place, what time of day or night, what each person is saying and doing).
- Keep track of a possible build-up of stress and tension that occurs before you "blow up"—be aware of a "pile-up" of stressors and an experience of one last stressful event eliciting strong anger and the urge to act aggressively toward one's partner.
- Increase awareness of physical cues or symptoms of becoming angry (e.g., feeling hot; tenseness in face, neck, arms, legs; speaking faster or louder).

Remove or Avoid Situations That Elicit One's Anger

- Plan to avoid situations that have gotten you angry in the past (e.g., do not discuss conflicts with your partner when you are tired or not feeling well). Avoiding situations that have gotten your partner angry in the past also is wise.
- Distance yourself from situations that are beginning to provoke you (e.g., if your partner is criticizing you, say you are getting upset and need to cool off, and take a time-out).
- Take time before responding to another person's actions that are beginning to provoke you (e.g., tell the other person "I need to think that over," and write down your thoughts and feelings about the situation; you then can prepare to respond to the other person in a calm way).
- Shift your attention and thoughts to something else that does *not* make you angry.
- Start doing an activity that distracts you from your angry thoughts and emotions (e.g., listen to music, exercise, talk with friends). This is good temporary avoidance that allows you to stay calm. You then can plan how to respond to the other person.
- Do things that physically relax you (warm shower, cup of tea, walk outside, muscle relaxation exercises, slow deep breathing, visualizing being in a relaxing place).
- Avoid alcohol because it tends to increase the risk of losing control of one's anger, and even the risk of aggressive behavior, rather than relaxing the angry person.

Change Angry Thoughts

- Keep track of "hot" thoughts that increase your anger or keep it alive (e.g., "I'll make her regret it that she treated me that way!"; "What a jerk!").
- Challenge your "should," very high, and possibly unrealistic standards you apply to others, as well as to yourself (e.g., "If I want to talk about our relationship, he should be ready to do it too"; "I should be smart enough to always think of ways to convince my partner to do things my way"). In an ideal world, our partner will think and behave just the way we prefer, but in real life people sometimes respond in ways that are disappointing and frustrating. Similarly, if we expect perfection from ourselves, we are likely to be disappointed in ourselves. If we instead try to give everyone some leeway, and accept their personal limitations, we will be less likely to become angry.
- Notice and challenge your negative <u>attributions</u> (inferences) about the other person's motives (e.g., "He didn't call me when he was going to get home late because he doesn't care about me").
- Catch yourself <u>overgeneralizing</u> (e.g., "She <u>never</u> listens to me") and <u>catastrophizing</u> (e.g., "If she won't talk to me for a while, I won't be able to stand it").
- Challenge your beliefs that anger has positive payoffs (e.g., "Getting angry and venting it at the other person will make sure that she will take me seriously").

(continued)

FIGURE 5.2. Methods to manage and reduce anger and partner aggression.

- Practice positive "self-talk" (instructions to yourself) to keep focused on staying as calm as possible and communicating constructively with others when you are getting upset (e.g., "Keep my body relaxed, breathe slowly, don't get into an argument").
- Remind yourself of the disadvantages of expressing anger through verbally or physically aggressive actions, especially when you are thinking it would feel good to yell, curse, say cruel things about the other person, hit the person, and so on.

Practice Good Communication, Problem-Solving, and Dyadic Coping Skills

- Express your thoughts and emotions about events that led you to feel anger, using brief, specific statements, without blaming or criticizing the other person, using the expressive guidelines in Handout 4.1. Describe what your goals and intentions have been (e.g., "I'm worried that I need to do a really good job on this work project, and I have trouble concentrating when you play music loudly while I'm working. I told you I am stressed about this project, and I'm feeling irritated that you are playing the music loudly. I would like you to keep it low enough that I'll be able to concentrate").
- Practice good listening skills as described in Handout 4.1, focusing on what the other person says they are feeling, not judging whether you think those feelings are right or wrong. This means doing your best to set aside your own feelings temporarily, including anger, to try to understand the other person's view of things, even if it is different from yours. Reflect back to the other person what you heard so that the person can tell you have been listening closely. When it is your turn to express your feelings, you can describe any disagreements and feelings you have.
- When you and the other person face a problem together, instead of focusing on anger you are feeling about it, focus on working as a team to plan a solution that could be satisfying to both of you, using problem-solving skills summarized in Handout 4.2. Discuss a variety of possible solutions with the other person, so that you have a better chance of finding a solution you both can accept. Then discuss advantages and disadvantages of each solution and pick a solution to try. Identify what each person will do. If the solution works, keep doing it; if it does not work well, discuss a new approach to try. Making progress toward solving a problem can help reduce anger.
- When facing stressors that affect you as individuals or as a couple and that produce anger and aggressive responses in your relationship, use the dyadic coping methods described in Handout 4.4 to help each other reduce the negative effects of stress.

FIGURE 5.2. (*continued*)

Barriers to Effective Treatment

In Chapter 2, we discussed characteristics of the partners, couple relationships, and therapeutic alliances that can limit the effectiveness of therapy. When conducting couple therapy for aggression, some factors are especially important: establishing and maintaining a positive therapeutic alliance and reducing partners' self-regulation deficits.

• Establishing and maintaining a positive therapeutic alliance with both members of the couple can be an especially sensitive issue in cases of partner aggression. Although the therapist must convey a strong position that psychological and physical aggression is damaging and inappropriate, that standard must be communicated with respect for both partners as human beings and a goal of helping those who want to improve their relationship. Because confronting an individual's behavior that harms their partner can result in the individual experiencing shame, the therapist should make a clear distinction between the evaluation of the aggressive acts and judgment of the person. This task can be difficult when the victimized partner is trying to shame the individual, based on a desire to change the perpetrator's behavior, and sometimes to retaliate as well. Striving to maintain a perpetrator's self-esteem while supporting a victim's need for safety is essential. Directly stating both of those goals to the couple and intervening in ways to achieve them contribute to a positive therapeutic alliance in which both partners experience care and respect from the therapist.

• This chapter and Chapter 4 describe interventions designed to improve partners' abilities to regulate their negative cognitions, emotional arousal, and over-learned behavioral responses. It is unlikely that "one size fits all," and therapists need to monitor each individual's level of success in using self-regulation skills, being prepared to tailor interventions to provide additional psychoeducation and skill practice as needed. If one or both partners have been unable to demonstrate self-control, referrals for concurrent individual therapy may be needed, and in some cases it may be necessary to put the conjoint therapy on hold temporarily. It is crucial that the couple experience evidence that they can control aggression and interact in pleasing constructive ways.

KEY POINTS

- Clinicians need to be aware of their possible implicit biases about which "types" of couples are at greater risk of partner aggression.

- Clinicians must screen out couples from conjoint sessions who meet risk criteria for revictimization and escalation of violence, intend to stay together, but lack the skills to manage conflict. However, with good screening, monitoring of risks for new incidents, and immediate intervention, couple therapy can be safe and effective in reducing partner aggression. Planning for eliminating aggression involves individualized case conceptualization.

- Therapists must use tact in screening for partner aggression to facilitate disclosure and must maintain a positive therapeutic alliance with both members, balancing empathy and respect for perpetrators while setting firm expectations for nonaggressive behavior within and outside sessions.

- By the time couples seek therapy, their patterns of aggression often involve relatively ingrained patterns of thinking, emotional responses, and behavior that takes time to change.

- When one or both partners have entrenched patterns of aggression-related cognition, emotion dysregulation, and behavior, referrals for individual therapy may be needed.

CHAPTER 6

Infidelity

Broadly defined, infidelity involves a member of a romantic relationship being sexually or emotionally involved with one or more other people in a manner that violates the explicit or implicit understanding between partners that their relationship is exclusive (Hertlein & Weeks, 2007). The professional literature consistently cites data from the United States and other countries indicating a high prevalence of infidelity. For example, about 21% of men and 13% of women in the United States report engaging in sex outside their primary relationship in a manner that violated a partner's assumption regarding monogamy (Gordon, Mitchell, Baucom, & Snyder, 2023), and it is more common in dating and cohabiting relationships than in marriages (Buunk, Dijkstra, & Massar, 2018).

Infidelity is distinguished from forms of consensual nonmonogamy, in which the couple has an explicit agreement that sexual or romantic involvements with others are acceptable (Garner, Person, Goddard, Patridge, & Bixby, 2019; Rubel & Bogaert, 2015; Rubinsky, 2019). Among diverse forms of consensual nonmonogamy, which have similar rates across race (St. Vil, Leblanc, & Giles, 2021), those studied most are open relationships, swinging, and polyamory (Hangen, Crasta, & Rogge, 2020). In open relationships, the partners consider their relationship the primary one and have criteria for acceptable extradyadic sexual activity (EDSA). Swinging involves EDSA that is restricted to social contexts (e.g., a vacation with another couple during which they swap partners) and has clear criteria for acceptable behavior. Polyamory emphasizes mutual consent to engage in concurrent relationships with multiple partners that focus on romantic attachment and also can involve sex. Studies have found a fairly high prevalence of consensual nonmonogamous relationships (e.g., Rubinsky, 2019). There is a common stigma in society involving negative evaluations of consensual nonmonogamous relationships and people who engage in them (Moors, Matsick, Ziegler, Rubin, & Conley, 2013). However, there is research evidence that their members' individual functioning and relationship satisfaction are comparable to those in monogamous relationships and better than those of individuals who participate in nonconsensual nonmonogamy (e.g., one-sided EDSA, partially open relationships lacking mutual consent; Garner et al., 2019; Hangen et al., 2020). Hangen et al.'s (2020) triple-C model of commitment differentiates between consensual nonmonogamy and infidelity in terms of three characteristics: mutual consent, open communication about criteria and actual involvements with other partners, and members' comfort with the structure of their relationship.

Given that a percentage of individuals do not divulge their infidelity to their partner or a couple therapist until the partner discovers evidence of it, and the internet has created easy ways for individuals to become involved with other people, the scope of infidelity may be underestimated by published reports. Surveys indicate that fidelity still is valued highly by a large majority of people across cultures (Buunk et al., 2018; Kröger, Reißner, Vasterling, Schütz, & Kliem, 2012), although there has been a recent modest trend toward greater acceptance of it under some circumstances (Labrecque & Whisman, 2017). The gap between the degree to which fidelity is valued and its actual occurrence creates stress for many couples, and Whisman, Dixon, and Johnson (1997) reported that 30% of clients in couple therapy identified infidelity as a reason for initiating therapy. Because infidelity can undermine the foundational qualities of intimate relationships—safety, security, mutual respect, and caring—for many couples it is a major threat to the stability of their bond, posing a major risk for relationship dissolution (Buunk et al., 2018; Gordon et al., 2023). It also has negative effects on both partners' psychological well-being. Consequently, couple therapists commonly consider it to be among the most challenging problems they treat (Gordon et al., 2023).

Another complication for assessment and treatment planning is that secret infidelity may underlie other relationship problems (e.g., arguments or withdrawal by one member) for which couples sought therapy. If and when the infidelity is revealed, the type of treatment and each partner's goals are likely to change substantially. This chapter discusses strategies for clinical decision making when therapists face such issues, as well as interventions that can help couples cope with stressors and challenges of infidelity as they consider the future of their relationship.

Infidelity poses a challenge for therapists who strive to establish positive therapeutic alliances with both members of a couple. Even though factors that contributed to a member's infidelity often include characteristics of the relationship (e.g., low levels of communication and intimacy) and of the betrayed partner (e.g., clinical depression), the unfaithful individual is personally responsible for responding to those factors by engaging in infidelity rather than pursuing other options such as couple therapy. The couple therapist must convey respect and empathy for the unfaithful partner while focusing on their vulnerabilities that led them to become involved with another person, or else those vulnerabilities will remain risks for future infidelity.

SEXUAL AND EMOTIONAL INFIDELITY

Instances of infidelity can be primarily sexual, primarily emotional, or a blend of the two (Glass, 2003; Hertlein, Wetchler, & Piercy, 2005; Moller & Vossler, 2015). In any case, the violation involves a threat to the couple's attachment bond (Macintosh, Hall, & Johnson, 2007). Sexual infidelity can include a wide range of forms of physical contact, as well as online sexual behavior that often progresses to in-person sexual involvement (Buunk et al., 2018; Rietmeijer, Bull, & McFarlane, 2001). Manifestations of emotional infidelity are even more diverse and can be ambiguous (e.g., the difference between frequent conversations between friends and those that reflect romantic attachment). The diversity of these forms of behavior often contributes to partners' different definitions of what constitutes an affair (e.g., "It was just a kiss"; "I enjoy talking with him because he makes me feel good, but we're not having an affair!"). Whenever a difference exists between partners' definitions of whether a person's involvement constitutes infidelity, that conflict introduces stress beyond the infidelity itself and needs to be resolved.

A common quality of these types of interactions with another person is their potential to detract from the participant's connection with the primary partner. The effort the individual puts into keeping the involvement secret may contribute to the distance. Some individuals who are confronted by their partner for engaging in physical or emotional intimacy with another person, violating the partner's assumption that their relationship was monogamous, realize the significance of the extradyadic relationship but outwardly deny it ("It means nothing to me") in the interest of avoiding conflict with the partner. Other individuals may truly not view their behavior as infidelity, and so the therapist should explore the person's thoughts and emotions regarding the third person. In this way, the therapist will get a sense of whether the individual is denying to themself the significance of the involvement or truly thinks of it as a platonic friendship. If the individual resists reducing or ending involvement with the other person due to the distress it is causing the primary partner, it may be an indication of the depth of their attachment to the third party, and thus is a risk for dissolution of the primary relationship. Without the individual's honest "soul searching" regarding thoughts and emotions about the other person and willingness to disclose them in therapy, accurate assessment of the intensity of the affair is limited. We discuss this issue further in the Screening and Assessment section of this chapter.

EFFECTS OF INFIDELITY ON THE COUPLE AND INDIVIDUALS

An individual who is getting some personal needs met with another person but has no intention of ending the primary relationship may even assume, "I have enough caring and energy to have both relationships." Although individuals engaged in polyamorous relationships commonly state that they are successfully maintaining multiple intimate relationships, that success occurs within consensual nonmonogamy. In contrast, when individuals engage in hidden nonconsensual nonmonogamy and violate an agreement of exclusivity with their primary partner, the risk of disrupting the primary attachment bond seems greater. Furthermore, whenever the primary couple has arguments, the member involved with a third person may temporarily withdraw to the affair partner (with whom life is more positive) rather than making efforts to resolve issues with the primary partner. This coping pattern may produce temporary relief from emotional distress, but it perpetuates the couple's problems and the attachment to the affair partner.

When an individual discloses an affair to the primary partner, either on their own volition or more often under pressure from the other's suspicion, the typical result is severe disruption to their relationship. Many researchers have emphasized the traumatic nature of such disclosure for the betrayed partner (Baucom, Snyder, & Gordon, 2009; Glass, 2003; Gordon et al., 2023; Lusterman, 2005; Macintosh et al., 2007; Spring, 2020; Stefano & Ola, 2008), as the information shatters the individual's core assumptions about their partner and relationship (Janoff-Bulman, 1992). The betrayed person's experience may not meet the full diagnostic criteria for PTSD but nevertheless will involve strong negative cognitions, emotion, and potentially destructive behavioral responses (Roos, O'Connor, Canevello, & Bennett, 2018). The severe disruption of the relationship can also be highly distressing for the partner who participated in the infidelity, as it also poses a major threat to that person's security (stability of the primary relationship, sense of self as a good person, relationships with their social network; Gordon et al., 2023). Factors that may intensify the trauma and shame associated with disclosure of infidelity include the length of the affair, how long it was kept secret, whether the betrayed individual knows the affair partner (who may even be a relative or close friend), who else has known about it, whether the affair partner contacted the betrayed individual, and whether the partner is still in involved with the individual.

COGNITIVE, EMOTIONAL, AND BEHAVIORAL RESPONSES TO A PARTNER'S INFIDELITY

Betrayed partners commonly experience negative cognitions, emotions, and behavior responses to the infidelity, all of which need to be addressed when couples want to work through the infidelity. Using a CBCT approach, the therapist assesses all three realms in planning treatment and, as detailed in Chapter 4, integrates all three during sessions.

Negative Cognitions

The betrayed partner may have extreme negative assumptions (e.g., "I don't know who my partner is any more. I always thought she was a caring person, but she's not!"; "Every nice experience we had together over the years was a sham!";"I can't trust anything she says"; "Everyone thinks I'm a loser because my partner wanted someone else"), extreme standards (e.g., "The only way I can feel at all safe is if my partner stops working on any projects at his job that involve female colleagues"; "I need to monitor him closely, so he needs to FaceTime me wherever he goes"), negative expectancies (e.g., "If my partner pledges in couple therapy to be honest, she'll end up lying to me whenever it's convenient for her"; "If I tell her how her affair made me feel, she won't empathize with my pain at all"), and attributions (e.g., "He told me he had to stay late at the office tonight, but I bet he was spending time with his lover"; "He says he still loves me in order to appease me"; "He had an affair because I was a failure as a partner"). The betrayed partner may also engage in negative selective perception, with hyperalertness to partner actions that might be signs of the partner's continuing infidelity (e.g., "I haven't been able to count on them to follow through on things they agreed to do"; "There's no evidence there was true love between us"). The betrayed partner may also experience negative flashbacks, intrusive memories of discovering a partner's infidelity, or images of the partner engaging in intimacy with a third person (e.g., "I have very upsetting images of her having sex with her lover and enjoying it"). These images tend to have an obsessive quality: they commonly seem uncontrollable to the individual and are associated with emotional distress.

The personal rejection a betrayed individual is likely to experience, and any associated self-blame for failure of the relationship, also may lead to hopelessness and suicidal ideation, with risk of suicidal behavior. Consequently, the therapist should probe for such themes and address them, initiating crisis intervention and referrals for individual therapy as needed.

Negative Emotions

After learning about the infidelity, individuals may experience a variety of negative emotions. They may feel *anxiety*, especially in ambiguous situations such as if the partner is late arriving home, or if the partner received a phone call or text message from a person the individual does not know. Anxiety may also be associated with an assumption that the relationship and the couple's way of life are no longer secure. In addition to anxiety, the betrayed individual may feel depressed, due to the perception of loss of the partner's love and hopelessness about their relationship. *Depression* also may be associated with attributions that one's own shortcomings led the partner to find someone else.

Shame also can be experienced by a betrayed or unfaithful individual who views the infidelity as an indication of their failure as a human being or romantic partner. The experience of shame may be greater if the individual learns that other people know about the infidelity and assumes that others now have negative views of them. In addition, the betrayed person often feels *anger*, which can reach the level of poorly regulated rage, directed predominantly toward one's unfaithful partner for violating one's personal standards for how members of a close relationship should treat each other. Anger also may be directed at oneself for perceived failure to maintain a successful relationship and/or for having missed cues of the partner's unfaithful behavior.

Finally, the betrayed partner commonly experiences *jealousy*, which is a combination of anger, sadness, and fear (Cano & O'Leary, 1997), after learning about the partner's infidelity. This emotion often results from the perception that a third party is a threat for losing one's partner. Some jealousy may be normative, but some people tend to be more jealousy prone than others; severe jealousy may reflect attachment insecurity, which may require individual therapy in addition to couple therapy.

Negative Behavior

A betrayed partner may *attempt to control and monitor the unfaithful partner*. For example, they may make repeated requests that the unfaithful partner reassure them that they will end an ongoing affair or never repeat an affair that has ended. Other attempts at control involve excessive checking behavior (e.g., checking the partner's cell phone for signs of unfaithful behavior) or ingratiating behavior in an attempt to regain the unfaithful partner's interest and affection. A betrayed individual also may attempt to *enact retribution* through psychological and physical aggression (e.g., expressing contempt; disclosing the partner's infidelity to family, friends, and co-workers to shame the partner and destroy the partner's relationships, career, etc.; engaging in infidelity oneself; destroying the partner's possessions).

A betrayed individual's negative behavior may also include *withdrawal and refusal to interact with the partner*, which to some extent may reflect constructive self-preservation but may be carried out to the extent that it blocks potential for addressing issues that could create an opportunity for recovery from the infidelity if both members eventually prefer it. Finally, a betrayed individual may engage in *self-destructive behavior*, such as substance use to cope with emotional distress, physical self-harm, impulsive sexual relationships, and negative health behavior such as poor nutrition, sleep deprivation, and inadequate personal hygiene.

COGNITIVE, EMOTIONAL, AND BEHAVIORAL RESPONSES OF THE UNFAITHFUL PARTNER

It also is important to examine the cognitive, emotional, and behavioral responses of an unfaithful partner. As we will see, they can interfere with the couple's ability to address factors contributing to the infidelity and potentially efforts to improve the relationship if they wish to do so.

Negative Cognitions

An unfaithful partner may make *assumptions that have potentially negative consequences*, such as, "Our relationship is ruined, and it's not worth trying to save it." The consequences of some other assumptions can vary depending on the couple's agreement about acceptable behavior in their relationship. For example, the belief "I can be involved successfully with my new lover and stay with my partner because there are things I like about each person" could be problematic if the couple had agreed on strict monogamy, but not necessarily if they allowed for external relationships with explicit limits. An unfaithful partner also may hold *extreme standards* (e.g., "My involvement with another person is justified because my partner didn't treat me well"; "I'm a horrible person for being unfaithful"), *negative expectancies* (e.g., "Any attempts I might make to improve our relationship will fail"; "The couple therapist will be biased against me for being unfaithful"), and *attributions* (e.g., "My strong feelings for my lover mean that she's a better person for me than my partner is"). They may also engage in *negative selective perception* (e.g., "Whatever characteristics attracted us to each other years ago all seem to be gone now").

If the unfaithful individual's negative appraisal of their life situation escalates to a sense of hopelessness, it may lead to suicidal ideation, with a risk for suicidal behavior. Consequently, therapists need to balance interventions intended to encourage the person to examine the process through which they engaged in infidelity and take responsibility for it, with sensitivity to the vulnerability and hopelessness the person may be experiencing.

Negative Emotions

The unfaithful partner may experience mild to severe *anxiety*, especially when anticipating negative effects that disclosure of one's infidelity may have on one's own life, such as relationships with family and friends, one's job, and financial security. Anxiety also is associated with anticipation (often realistic) of very aversive interactions with one's betrayed partner, including condemnation and pressure to divulge the details of one's behavior with the third person. *Depression* also is common, associated with perception of loss of the betrayed partner's love and hopelessness about the relationship, as well as loss of other positive aspects of life such as relationships with one's children and other family members.

Even though an unfaithful partner may engage in self-enhancing thinking that justifies their infidelity, they simultaneously may experience *shame*, associated with thoughts about being a failure as a human being or romantic partner. This is especially the case if one also assumes that other people have such negative views of one's infidelity. Insulting, degrading accusations from the betrayed individual can elicit or exacerbate shame responses. Finally, the unfaithful partner can experience *anger*, associated with blaming one's partner for treating one in ways that were unsatisfying and led to one's infidelity. The unfaithful partner also may experience anger toward themselves for perceived personal failure to maintain a successful relationship and for violations of moral standards for one's behavior.

Negative Behavior

An unfaithful individual may engage in expressions of criticism, contempt, and punishment toward the betrayed partner, and also may describe the partner in derogatory terms to significant others in order to shame the partner and justify the infidelity. This behavior can include forms of psychological and physical partner aggression, with the individual excusing their behavior by telling others that it is simply an expression of the great unhappiness and frustration that impelled them to engage in infidelity.

Alternatively, an unfaithful individual may *withdraw and refuse to interact with the betrayed partner*, thereby leading the individual to avoid confrontation regarding the infidelity and its harm. The individual may avoid feelings of guilt or shame by denying responsibility for the relationship problems and infidelity. Another way of avoiding negative feedback from the betrayed partner involves repeatedly asking them what actions one can take to move forward quickly to reestablish trust and repair the relationship. In response to this pressure for a "quick fix," the betrayed individual commonly pressures the partner to describe more details of the affair and how the individual decided to engage in it, hid it, and so on. The unfaithful partner may counter those requests with further avoidance (e.g., "Look, I'm very sorry I did those things and hurt you, but let's stop dwelling on it and get back to having a good relationship"). These avoidant patterns by the unfaithful partner block potential for addressing their own characteristics and those within the relationship that contributed to the infidelity and may still pose risks. If both members eventually want to recover from the infidelity, avoidance reduces potential for changes that could produce a more functional relationship.

An unfaithful partner also may engage in *self-destructive behavior*, such as substance use to cope with emotional distress, forms of physical self-harm and other impulsive destructive behavior, and negative health behavior such as poor nutrition, sleep deprivation, and inadequate personal hygiene. Thus, the unfaithful partner's psychological and physical well-being commonly are at risk, and therapists need to screen for signs that individual therapy (at times crisis intervention) may be needed.

DYADIC COUPLE PROCESSES POSING A RISK FOR CRISIS

The major disruption of stable patterns in each person's functioning and in the relationship can reach a crisis level, to the point that constructive individual and dyadic coping deteriorate. A process leading to deterioration of individual and couple functioning occurs when partners reciprocate and exacerbate each other's negative cognitions, emotional responses, and behavior, adding to the stress that was already created when the infidelity was uncovered. As each person observes their negative interactions, the risk increases that they will develop an expectancy that there is little potential for a fulfilling relationship. It is crucial for a therapist to intervene to minimize escalation of negativity, so partners can engage in constructive interactions and see some potential for the future of their relationship.

Alternatively, in some cases both members of a couple decide to stay together without resolving the risk factors that led to infidelity or learning strategies for communicating better about personal needs, managing conflicts, and relinquishing the option of punishing each other for past problems. What initially may appear to the couple and outsiders as a resolution of the traumatic experiences persists as a major risk for relapse.

RISK FACTORS FOR THE DEVELOPMENT OF INFIDELITY

Consistent with our emphasis on treatment planning that identifies and intervenes with risk factors for clients' presenting problems, survey and qualitative research has investigated a variety of characteristics of individuals and relationships that are associated with higher incidence of infidelity (Allen et al., 2005; Buunk et al., 2018; Haseli, Shariati, Nazari, Keramat, & Emamian,

2019; Jeanfreau, Jurich, & Mong, 2014; Vowels, Vowels, & Mark, 2022). Based on those findings, using primarily heterosexual samples, the next section describes the process through which affairs tend to develop and the types of risk factors: characteristics of individuals who are more likely to participate in emotional and sexual infidelity, dyadic patterns in couples at greater risk for infidelity, characteristics of individuals more likely have been betrayed, and contextual factors such as characteristics of a potential affair partner.

The Processes in the Development of an Affair

Allen et al. (2005) described six stages of the process through which an individual becomes involved in an affair, associated with the perpetrator's experiences, the processes between members of the primary relationship, characteristics of the betrayed partner, and contextual factors in the couple's life. The amount of research on the factors contributing to each stage has been limited, with some information coming from reports of clinicians who treat couples presenting with infidelity. Allen et al. emphasize that the stages may overlap:

The first stage, *setting the stage* involves predisposing conditions for infidelity. Studies have identified some characteristics of individuals who are more likely to engage in infidelity, although it is important to be cautious in inferring that characteristics that are correlated with involvement actually caused it, or drawing conclusions about how a demographic characteristic such as gender may influence participation (Allen et al., 2005; Buunk et al., 2018; Jeanfreau et al., 2014). It also is important to note that the strengths of the statistical associations (effect sizes) identified in these studies generally are modest, indicating that for many individuals the association does not exist. Overall, demographic characteristics of perpetrators (e.g., education, religious affiliation) are related inconsistently to infidelity, whereas their subjective feelings about their primary relationship (sexual satisfaction, relationship satisfaction) are more consistently associated with it (Haseli et al., 2019; Vowels et al., 2022). Other personal characteristics that can contribute to engaging in infidelity may include chronic insecurity about one's attractiveness, life stressors such as failure at one's job that reduce self-esteem, desire for excitement and independence, beliefs regarding the acceptability of outside relationships, narcissism, and substance abuse. Serban, Salvati, and Enea (2022) found no difference between same-sex (lesbian and gay) individuals and heterosexual individuals in their engagement in infidelity-related online behavior. Figure 6.1 lists risk factors for perpetration identified in studies.

Vulnerabilities at the couple level can include low emotional and sexual intimacy, differences between partners' needs and life goals, and poor communication and conflict resolution skills. Characteristics of a betrayed individual that may contribute to risk include discomfort with intimacy, life stressors that distract the individual from paying attention to their partner (e.g., caring for a disabled child), and avoidance of dealing with the partner's expression of unhappiness with their relationship. Furthermore, contextual factors such as multiple stressors in the couple's life (e.g., financial problems, needs of ill family members), availability of attractive potential partners, and models of other people engaged in apparently exciting affairs can set the stage for an individual considering involvement. These are all conditions that exist before an individual has begun to consider involvement with a particular person.

Stage 2, the *approach* or *slippery-slope* stage, which can be brief or extended, involves thinking explicitly about whether one would like to get involved in an outside relationship, based on potential costs and benefits. It often consists of a series of decisions, such as whether to meet the

---

Demographic Characteristics

- Men (both heterosexual and gay) tend to be more likely than women (both heterosexual and lesbian) to express approval of infidelity, desire for it, and actual involvement, although this gender difference has decreased in more recent cohorts, and some studies have found no gender difference.
- Greater religiosity is associated with less permissive attitudes about and involvement in infidelity among those with happy marriages, but not among those with low relationship satisfaction.
- A personal history of divorce, as well as previous involvement in nonconsensual extradyadic affairs, is associated to some extent with involvement.

Personal Traits, Attitudes, and Evaluation of Couple Relationship Quality

- A high desire for independence from one's partner
- A desire for variety in relationships
- Having an avoidant or dismissive attachment style in general, or feeling insecure attachment in one's primary relationship
- Low satisfaction with one's primary relationship—for males especially feeling deprived sexually, and for females especially feeling a lack of emotional connection and validation (although cases exist in which individuals who report satisfaction still engage in infidelity)
- For males, substance abuse

FIGURE 6.1. Risk factors for engaging in infidelity.

third person for coffee, spend more time together, increase the intimacy of topics discussed, and reveal one's attraction to the person. Characteristics of the individual's partner also can influence those decisions, as when the partner's failure to respond to one's expressions of unhappiness leads the individual to view an outside relationship as more attractive.

Stage 3, the *precipitation* or *crossing-the-line* stage, can be ambiguous and involves subjective judgment about the significance of one's feelings and behavior toward the other person. This ambiguity tends to be greater in emotional affairs that have not involved any sexual activities. During this process, the individual's growing emotional connection and sexual arousal to the other person can interfere with making logical decisions about one's involvement, and drug and alcohol use may reduce one's inhibitions further.

Stage 4, the *maintenance* stage of the infidelity, after the individual has become emotionally and/or sexually involved with the affair partner, can be influenced by conditions such as the strength of positive feelings for the person, one's attempts to reduce cognitive dissonance by concluding that the primary relationship is not as good as the affair relationship, and increasingly more positive interactions with the affair partner than with the primary partner. Allen et al. (2005) note that this process may interfere with the individual's ability to stop the infidelity even when aware of negative consequences for oneself, the primary partner, and significant others such as children.

Stage 5, *disclosure or discovery* of the infidelity, does not occur in a percentage of distressed couples who seek therapy that is difficult to estimate. As we noted, prior or ongoing infidelity may be an unidentified factor contributing to other problems (e.g., conflict, increased emotional distance) that motivated some couples to seek therapy. Our focus in this chapter is on treatment planning for couples in which an involved partner either initiated disclosure or has been confronted with evidence of infidelity by the betrayed partner, has joined couple therapy to address the major disruption to their relationship, and has committed to ending the affair. Allen et al. (2005) note that literature on infidelity indicates that most involved individuals do not initiate disclosure, although those who have experienced more guilt tend to provide their partner more clues. Whether the involved individual initiates disclosure, or how they respond to being confronted with suspicions and evidence by the partner, can influence the future of the couple's relationship. The potential for restoring trust in the relationship may be greater if the involved individual discloses the infidelity but less if they respond to confrontation with denial and defensiveness.

The final stage, Stage 6, couple *responses to infidelity*, involves interaction patterns that may be constructive or destructive, as well as decisions the partners make individually and jointly regarding the future of their relationship. Overall, infidelity leads to increased conflict, lower relationship satisfaction, major disruption to the couple's emotional bond, and a high risk of dissolution of the relationship, although many couples do not end their relationships and may even use the crisis as a source of motivation to improve their bond (Allen et al., 2005).

Allen et al. (2005) and Buunk et al. (2018) cite research indicating that across cultures infidelity by men in heterosexual relationships traditionally tended to be accepted more and led less to dissolution of the relationship than infidelity by women, who are more likely to feel guilt for their involvement. Frederick and Fales (2016) found that heterosexual men are more likely (54%) to be upset than heterosexual women (35%) by a partner's sexual infidelity, but less likely (46%) than heterosexual women (65%) to be upset by emotional infidelity, whereas bisexual men (30%) and women (27%) do not differ in response to sexual infidelity, nor do gay men (32%) and lesbian women (34%). Leeker and Carlozzi (2014) also found that heterosexual men and women reported emotional and sexual infidelity to be more distressing than lesbian and gay individuals. In response to partner infidelity, women have been found to disengage more from the relationship, whereas men are more likely to respond with aggression. However, with the development of more diverse opportunities via the internet for extradyadic relationships of various forms, as well as increased empowerment of women to seek fulfillment of their needs, one must be cautious about generalizations regarding gender differences in infidelity.

Research reviewed by Allen et al. (2005) indicated that betrayed individuals' emotional distress tends to be greater when they have a personal history of low self-esteem and attachment insecurity. There is a higher risk that the couple's relationship will end when both members have engaged in infidelity. As we noted, the involved person's self-disclosure of infidelity, and acknowledgment of and apology for its negative effects on the partner, can contribute to a more positive outcome for the couple relationship. It is important for couple therapists to remember, and to convey to their clients, that even though certain characteristics and actions of a betrayed individual may have contributed to the couple patterns that their partner found unsatisfying, the involved partner was solely responsible for the decisions leading to the infidelity. Other alternatives to infidelity (e.g., more open communication and empathy between partners, couple therapy, taking steps to end the primary relationship) were available.

INFIDELITY FROM A CBCT PERSPECTIVE

In Epstein and Baucom's (2002) enhanced CBCT model, individuals form couple relationships in order to satisfy core communally oriented and individually oriented human needs, including emotional attachment and intimacy. A variety of cognitive, affective, and behavioral patterns of the partners and their couple interactions influence the degree to which partners experience ful-fillment of those needs in their relationship, and infidelity is one of the possible negative outcomes of limited need fulfillment. A CBCT framework for understanding risk factors that contributed to infidelity in each couple and for setting treatment goals for those struggling with its consequences includes those cognitive, emotional, and behavioral characteristics. A developmental perspective on the processes that led to the infidelity, such as the stage model described by Allen et al. (2005), also is helpful in identifying risk factors that need to be modified in therapy.

A CBCT model also focuses on infidelity as a major stressor that has severely disrupted the couple's relationship and requires effective individual and dyadic coping. For example, at the individual level, attention is needed to a betrayed person's trauma symptoms, shattered assumptions about their partner and relationship, strong jealousy, and impulse to behave vindictively. The involved partner's stress associated with being vilified by the betrayed partner and often by other people, common guilt about hurting their partner, severe disruption of their daily life, and possible use of dysfunctional coping responses that backfire (e.g., blaming the betrayed partner) also require therapeutic intervention. At the dyadic level, interventions are needed to reduce partners' tendencies to inflame each other's emotional distress and to improve their ability to use constructive communication and problem solving. We next describe in more detail the cognitive, emotional, and behavioral factors addressed in treatment of infidelity.

Cognition

Couples vary as to how much they explicitly acknowledge and discuss their personal standards regarding exclusivity (e.g., what types and depth of emotional connection are acceptable with close friends versus what is to be reserved for the couple relationship), and even public statements regarding such boundaries in marriage vows and similar ceremonies generally are vague. Never-theless, surveys have indicated that people across diverse cultures commonly value monogamy and disapprove of individuals who betray their partner's trust. Even when members of a couple have never explicitly stated their commitment to monogamy, individuals may assume such a commit-ment exists and are badly shaken when they discover otherwise. Given the higher frequency of explicit consensual nonmonogamy agreements among gay male couples than same-sex and lesbian couples, it is important to clarify what criteria individuals in such relationships use to identify a partner's behavior as infidelity (Martell & Prince, 2005). In some cases, individuals who choose to be involved in external relationships may have personal standards that include contingencies that never were shared with their partner (e.g., "If your partner doesn't seem willing or capable of meeting your needs for affection and sex, it is normal and understandable to have those needs met by someone else"). Thus, the extradyadic involvement may not have violated the involved individual's personal criteria for consensual nonmonogamy but violated the betrayed partner's standards without explicit discussion. A betrayed individual's standards about appropriate con-sequences for an unfaithful partner also must be considered. Standards that promote retribution (e.g., "Someone who hurts you badly deserves to suffer") are likely to lead to negative actions that further damage the couple's bond. Instead, making a decision to protect one's well-being by assertively requiring future exclusivity by one's partner sets up a standard that creates potential for rebuilding the relationship.

Individuals also enter couple therapy with personal standards about what constitutes *for-giveness* when one member has betrayed and hurt the other, a process that has received a great deal of attention in published treatment models (Gordon et al., 2023; Hertlein & Weeks, 2007; Macintosh et al., 2007; Stefano & Oala, 2008). Defining forgiveness as involving accepting the other person's negative actions and absolving them of responsibility is distasteful to many people and places undue responsibility on the betrayed individual to attend to the involved person's needs. Therapists commonly consider it essential that an involved person take personal responsibility and commit to steps to reduce the risk of future infidelity. An individual's standards that detract from taking personal responsibility (e.g., "If I apologize and promise to never do it again, that should be enough to satisfy my partner") become targets for intervention.

As we have described, a betrayed individual is likely to pay attention selectively to possible cues that their partner is continuing to be untrustworthy and to have negative expectancies about risks of more infidelity. Thus, the individual may become upset about any instance in which the partner has failed to report where they had been and who else was present, while overlooking instances in which the partner made specific efforts to be accountable. Although the unfaithful partner is responsible for consistently behaving in ways that contribute to rebuilding trust, therapists also address challenges facing betrayed partners in catching themselves when engaging in selective perception and untested negative expectancies. Rebuilding trust is a dyadic process involving both individuals' cognitions as well as behavior.

Furthermore, the stages of involvement in infidelity described by Allen et al. (2005) involve a perpetrator's decisions that involve weighing the benefits and costs of an affair, even if the individual argues that the involvement was impulsive. Not surprisingly, betrayed individuals' trust in their partner's decision making has been reduced severely, and the couple must grapple with challenges the unfaithful individual faces in approaching such decisions in the future. Intervention can include improving the executive functions involved in foresight and planning.

A CBCT approach focuses on assisting partners in understanding their own and each other's cognitions associated with an individual's infidelity, modifying cognitions that are detrimental, and making decisions about the future of the relationship. Whether or not individuals explicitly think about it or discuss it with a new partner, they tend to be drawn to and satisfied with relationships that meet their core human needs. Although needs such as attachment have been described as innate to a significant degree, personal experiences beginning early in life shape them in major ways. For example, although all individuals are born with an innate need for attachment to others, their early experiences with caretakers (e.g., as available and nurturing or not) shape their internalized "working model" or schema about their own lovability and the availability of nurturers, as well as their emotional responses (e.g., anxiety) when their needs are not met. Those experiences also shape the individual's ways of behaving toward significant others in attempts to meet their attachment need (Bowlby, 1988). Epstein and Baucom (2002) provide a detailed description of how the cognitive, affective, and behavioral aspects of individuals' needs are highly compatible with a cognitive-behavioral model of individual and interpersonal functioning, as well as treatment.

Extensive research has identified two major types of human needs that involve seeking particular types of outcomes: *communal needs* involving connections with others and *agentic or individually oriented needs* involving one's individual autonomous functioning and ability to influence one's environment (McClelland, 1987). These needs influence many aspects of human functioning, including couple relationships (Epstein & Baucom, 2002). In a CBCT model, we focus on how individuals respond positively to potential partners who have characteristics that can fulfill their core needs and, conversely, respond negatively to partner behavior that fails to meet those needs.

Regarding communally oriented needs, Baumeister and Leary's (1995) review of theoretical and research literature identified a set of needs regarding the formation and maintenance of strong relationships with other people:

- *Affiliation:* the need to share social and other activities with others; it is necessary for intimacy, but it can occur without the deep sharing involved in intimacy. In terms of cognition, the individual is likely to notice and value others' actions that reflect sociability.
- *Intimacy:* the need for close psychological and physical contact, sharing deeply each other's personal experiences. The individual attends to cues that another person wants an in-depth relationship, and will respond positively if another initiates intimate behavior.
- *Altruism:* the need to take care of other people. The individual notices areas in which others appear to need assistance, empathizes with others' distress, and is motivated to reach out to provide support.
- *Succorance:* the need to be nurtured by other people; not necessarily unilateral dependence on a partner, as an individual who can function independently still may enjoy being nurtured at times by their partner. The individual's cognitions include attachment working models, in terms of how worthy of receiving help one is and how emotionally and physically available a potential caretaker is.

Epstein and Baucom (2002) note that these four types of communally oriented needs commonly coexist, but their relative strengths may differ from person to person. For example, the common quality of desiring time together in affiliation and intimacy can lead to a misunderstanding between members of a couple as they develop their relationship. Although both people want to share time and activities, one person's need may be mostly for affiliation, whereas the other is motivated more to move toward a deeper intimate connection. Initially, this difference may not be apparent to them as they both express pleasure at being together, but at some point the individual who has a strong need for intimacy makes efforts to "take the relationship to a deeper level" (e.g., disclosing more personal information and seeking it from the partner) and meets resistance from the partner.

Regarding *agentic* or *individually oriented needs*, Epstein and Baucom describe how theory and research have identified three major types, which we describe here with core cognitions that define them:

- *Autonomy:* the need to make decisions and pursue one's interests and goals independently from others. The individual focuses on opportunities to make individual choices in life and evaluates perceived impediments to freedom negatively.
- *Power:* the need to have observable influence on people and events in one's life. The person notices how much impact their actions have on other people, enjoys experiencing power, and is frustrated by others' actions that seem to block attainment of one's goals.
- *Achievement:* the need to attain mastery in performing well on tasks, as observed by others but especially according to one's own evaluation. The person's self-evaluation is contingent on observing success on valued tasks, and people perceived as interfering with one's achievement may be considered adversaries.

These individually oriented needs potentially could lead to selfish behavior in a couple relationship if the individual fails to take their partner's needs and happiness into account, but they are inherently healthy rather than dysfunctional. In fact, couples can derive mutual satisfaction when they experience each other as supporting fulfillment of their needs for some autonomy, power, and achievement, in balance with meeting their communally oriented needs. Behaviorally, frustration over unmet needs may lead to attempts at coping, such as forms of aggression or withdrawal (Epstein & Baucom, 2002). In couple relationships, coping may include seeking fulfillment of unmet needs in an outside relationship. Thus, assessing partners' needs, how well they are addressed in the relationship, and how they have coped with unmet needs is an important component of assessment for couples experiencing infidelity. Rather than focusing pejoratively on ways in which an individual's infidelity was "a bad idea," this approach emphasizes that much can be learned about the individual's needs and the counterproductive ways in which they have attempted to fulfill them, so changes can be made.

As we have noted, an individual sometimes feels generally satisfied with their primary relationship, so they are not motivated to end it. Yet, they still seek an outside relationship that will satisfy a particular need, such as a boost to self-esteem from being attractive to others when one has been disappointed with one's career achievement. Insight into such an unmet need that may not reflect a shortcoming of the person's primary relationship is important for planning interventions that help the vulnerable person to avoid placing unrealistic demands on their couple relationship to meet their personal needs. Thus, rather than seeking validation of one's value through an affair, the individual could be guided in reviewing their talents, professional interests, and degree of fit with their current job.

Emotion

An individual's negative emotions toward their partner and relationship when their needs have not been fulfilled can contribute to motivation to become involved with another person. Although infidelity can occur when individuals are satisfied overall with their relationship but encounter tempting opportunities for another relationship, gradual erosion over time of the initial positive feelings and sexual attraction due to life circumstances (e.g., child-rearing stresses) and habituation can increase one's vulnerability to forming other relationships. Positive emotions from a third person's attention can add to an individual's motivation to become involved. Individuals' negative cognitions regarding their emotions (e.g., "I haven't had romantic feelings toward my partner in a long time, so our relationship must be dying") can worsen the emotional shift toward another relationship. These processes can be exacerbated if the individual has limited ability to regulate strong emotions and to balance them with rational decision making. The "slippery slope" process described by Allen et al. (2005) includes the effects of emotions on the individual's movement toward an affair partner. In turn, any difficulty a betrayed person has with regulating negative emotional responses (e.g., anger) to disclosure of infidelity can escalate negative behavior toward the unfaithful partner, such as vindictive attempts to ruin the partner's relationships with family, friends, and co-workers.

Behavior

We have emphasized how the subjective quality of the bond between two people, including the emotional "chemistry" they feel, is influenced by the types and amount of behavioral interaction between them. Partners meet each other's needs through daily actions, demonstrating attraction and interest, sharing mutually enjoyable experiences, feeling intimacy from mutual self-disclosure and empathic listening, and so on. If those behaviors diminish over time and the couple lacks skills to communicate with each other, initiate repair efforts (see Chapter 4), and find new ways to stimulate positive feelings, the rewarding power of their relationship likely weakens. By comparison, fantasized or real alternative relationships may become appealing.

COUPLE THERAPIES FOR INFIDELITY

Infidelity has received considerable attention in professional literature, and a few therapy models have been developed: Gordon and colleagues' model that integrates cognitive-behavioral and insight-oriented couple therapies (Baucom, Snyder, & Gordon, 2009; Gordon et al., 2023); Weeks and colleagues' intersystem approach (Weeks, Gambescia, & Jenkins, 2003) that identifies risk factors at the individual and couple relationship levels and intervenes to reduce them; Spring's (2020) primarily cognitive-behavioral model; and Johnson and colleagues' emotionally focused therapy approach to resolving attachment injuries (MacIntosh et al., 2007). To date, little research involving controlled clinical trials has been conducted to test the effects of treatments for this relatively common and distressing problem (Hertlein & Weeks, 2007; Levine, 2014), with notable empirical support for the Gordon and colleagues' integrative model and the Weeks et al. intersystem model. In addition, integrative behavioral couple therapy (IBCT) has been applied to infidelity due to its balance between interventions to improve relationship barriers to intimacy and interventions to increase partners' empathy and acceptance of aspects of each other that are unlikely to change, with some encouraging preliminary results (Atkins, Marin, Lo, Klann, & Hahlweg, 2010). Common factors across models include some crisis intervention to control deteriorated individual and couple functioning, uncovering and reduction of risk factors for infidelity within the partners and their relationship, and strategies to rebuild trust, with some models also focused on achieving some form of forgiveness.

A model applying CBCT concepts and methods is well suited for treating couples experiencing the traumatic effects of infidelity due to violation of the agreement the couple had regarding monogamy or consensual nonmonogamy. In our clinical work, we emphasize the approach developed and tested by Gordon and colleagues (Baucom, Snyder, & Gordon, 2009; Gordon et al., 2023). The model includes three major stages:

1. *Dealing with the impact of the affair(s)* through coping with the major disruption the stressor of infidelity imposes on individual and couple functioning.
2. *Finding meaning* through examining and understanding factors concerning the involved partner, the betrayed partner, the relationship, and external conditions that influenced the individual to decide to become involved.
3. *Moving on* based on a shared couple formulation regarding causes of the infidelity, decisions about staying together or not, with strategies for disengaging as constructively as possible or for strengthening areas of individual or relationship vulnerability in order to avoid future infidelity.

The following sections describe precursors to this treatment model, involving screening and assessment for infidelity; goal setting and socializing couples to the treatment approach; and planning treatment. We then describe procedures used in these three stages of the treatment.

SCREENING AND ASSESSMENT FOR INFIDELITY

Because infidelity occurs commonly in the general population, and even more among couples who seek therapy for a variety of relationship issues, it is safe to assume that any therapist who works with couples will encounter some clients who are experiencing infidelity. Screening is complicated by the fact that many couples do not disclose infidelity to therapists spontaneously, or even when the clinician asks about it in general terms during the initial intake meeting. Individuals are more likely to report their own infidelity, or known or suspected infidelity by their partner, when interviewed individually or asked to complete a questionnaire surveying presenting problems. Failure to disclose infidelity may be motivated by a number of concerns, such as embarrassment, lack of comfort with the clinician at the beginning of therapy, a betrayed individual's fear of pushing away a perpetrator, or a perpetrator's fear of their partner's anger and retaliation. Thus, therapists are faced with an ethical dilemma involving the potential negative effects of uncovering infidelity, and so screening must be done in a tactful way that minimizes the chances of further harm.

Because some couples who have experienced infidelity do not disclose it when asked about their reasons for seeking couple therapy, therapists must screen for it by asking direct questions. The screening and assessment procedures described in Figure 6.2 are designed to uncover infidelity without the therapist pressuring individuals to disclose it when doing so could be harmful, or placing themselves in the position of keeping secrets with an unfaithful partner.

Assessment of Partners' Cognitions, Emotions, and Behavioral Responses Regarding the Infidelity

The previous section focused on procedures to screen for infidelity and facilitate discussions of it in couple therapy, as well as assessment of the partners' cognitions (e.g., concern about a betrayed partner's response to disclosure of infidelity), emotions (e.g., depression), and behavioral responses (e.g., coping with conflict by avoiding discussions with one's partner). It is important to conduct a systematic assessment of those cognitions, emotions, and behaviors in order to plan appropriate interventions.

Assessment of Cognition

Assessment of each person's cognitions regarding the infidelity includes personal standards regarding exclusivity/monogamy, attributions regarding causes of a partner's violation of such standards, how infidelity has altered an individual's assumptions regarding a partner's personality characteristics, selective attention to potential cues that a partner is continuing to violate trust, identification of personal needs that an unfaithful partner attempted to fulfill in an affair, each member's standards about the conditions that would be necessary to rebuild trust in their relationship, and expectancies about the likelihood of future infidelity. As described in Chapter 3, therapists should ask about sociocultural factors (e.g., beliefs about gender roles within a culture) that may influence an individual's cognitions regarding infidelity. Chapter 3 details methods for assessing partners' cognitions, including observation of spontaneously voiced thoughts during sessions, probes when the therapist notices cues that an individual had an internal reaction to a partner's actions, and specific questioning about a type of cognition (e.g., personal standards regarding monogamy).

- **During a potential client's initial phone inquiry regarding couple therapy:**
  - *When the caller describes their own or their partner's infidelity and requests a desire to discuss it privately with the therapist*, the therapist describes their intention to avoid keeping secrets in couple therapy and asks the caller questions to evaluate whether couple therapy will be a safe and productive setting for addressing the infidelity:
    - Whether either member has been keeping their infidelity a secret
    - What concerns a caller has about disclosing their infidelity to the partner
    - Concerns the caller has about confronting a partner with suspected infidelity
    - If the infidelity is out in the open, the extent to which the caller is fearful about bringing it up in couple therapy
    - Strategies the caller has in place to maintain their safety if the infidelity has created risk of partner aggression; offer referral information regarding shelters, legal assistance, etc. (Chapter 5)
    - Degree to which the caller is comfortable beginning joint sessions to address infidelity, or is interested in individual therapy with another therapist, to prepare for possible couple therapy
  - *When the caller has hinted about infidelity as a problem but has not directly identified it, and has requested privacy for this phone conversation with the therapist*, the therapist describes avoiding keeping secrets and asks the caller:
    - The extent to which the individual fears disclosing particular issues during couple sessions and how the caller anticipates the partner may react to the therapist knowing about those issues; the therapist describes how assessment begins with a joint interview, followed by an opportunity for each member to discuss personal concerns individually
    - Strategies the caller has to maintain safety if relationship issues created a risk of partner aggression; be prepared to offer referrals (Chapter 5)
    - Degree to which the caller is comfortable with joint sessions or prefers individual therapy with another therapist to prepare for couple therapy
- **When the caller made no mention of infidelity, the couple agreed on couple therapy, and they have been scheduled for the initial assessment:**
  - *The therapist includes screening for infidelity during the inquiry regarding history of the relationship* (see questions within the joint interview protocol, Figure 3.1)
  - *When one or both members of the couple initiate discussion of infidelity during the joint assessment interview*, the therapist:
    - Asks whether the partners discussed it previously, and if so, how well they were able to discuss it; and how comfortable they are discussing it now
    - Notes that if either partner is uncomfortable discussing it during this interview, the therapist will not pressure them to do so, but it seems to be affecting their relationship and can be addressed in couple therapy
    - Asks whether the partners are willing to discuss the couple's experience with infidelity during the interview, as part of their history as a couple. The therapist stresses that it is essential that the discussion remain safe for both partners, and not lead to negative behavior toward one's partner during the session or afterward
    - Moderates the discussion of infidelity, asking the couple about the events and effects on their relationship. The therapist imposes structure, focusing on constructive interaction and identifying each person's thoughts and emotions as well as goals for addressing it in therapy
    - Observes the couple's behavioral interactions during discussion of infidelity, noting negative patterns (e.g., pursue–withdraw, mutual verbal aggression) as targets for behavioral intervention
  - *When one or both members of the couple identified infidelity as an area of conflict on the RIS (Handout 3.1) but neither brings it up during the couple interview*, the therapist mentions it during their individual interview, and if the person acknowledges it as a concern, the therapist can follow up questions asked above when a caller reveals infidelity and asks for confidentiality

(continued)

FIGURE 6.2. Screening and assessment procedures to identify infidelity.

○ *When infidelity was not identified on a screening questionnaire (e.g., RIS; see Chapter 3) or during the joint interview, but a partner informs the therapist secretly about either person's infidelity during the individual interview:*
- Remind individual about the policy regarding avoidance of secret-keeping and advise that keeping the ongoing infidelity secret results in the therapist colluding in the secret and undermines resolving relationship issues in therapy
- Ask about concern regarding disclosing infidelity to the partner
- Ask about concern regarding confronting the partner with suspected infidelity
- If the infidelity is out in the open, ask about the extent to which the individual is fearful about bringing it up during therapy sessions
- Ask about actions the couple engaged in to cope with infidelity
- Ask what strategies the individual has to maintain their safety if conflict regarding infidelity has created a risk of partner aggression (see Chapter 5)
- Ask about the degree of discomfort dealing with infidelity in sessions, and whether they prefer beginning individual therapy with another therapist
- Ask about sociocultural aspects (e.g., cultural attitudes about infidelity) that should be considered when disclosing and coping with infidelity that may affect individual functioning, the couple, or other relationships
- Ask about aspects of the individual's personal history, sociocultural background, and individual functioning that may have been risk factors for infidelity in the couple's relationship; for example:
  □ trust or infidelity issues in family-of-origin relationships
  □ standards regarding infidelity based on cultural background
  □ infidelity in past romantic relationships
  □ dissatisfaction with the current relationship
  □ current life stressors and losses
  □ styles of coping with life stressors
  □ self-esteem issues, impulsivity, personality disorder characteristics, vindictive beliefs, substance use, depression, attachment insecurity prior infidelity in the relationship, and how they dealt with them

FIGURE 6.2. *(continued)*

Assessment of Emotion

Assessment of emotion involves gathering information from the partners about possible erosion over time of positive feelings and sexual attraction that created a close bond between them earlier in their relationship (and any changes in life circumstances associated with the erosion), difficulties with each person's awareness and expression of their emotions, problems with regulating the experience and expression of strong negative emotions (in general and regarding infidelity in particular), and a tendency for partners to "co-regulate" each other's negative emotions such as anger. As described in Chapter 3, the major methods for assessing these aspects of emotion include observation of individuals' spontaneous descriptions of emotion; probes when the therapist observes cues that one or both members of the couple may be experiencing emotions during a session; and therapist inquiries about partners' personal observations about their own and each other's emotional experiences.

Assessment of Behavior

Behavioral assessment relevant to infidelity includes gathering information about interactions through which partners fulfilled each other's needs initially and any changes over time that were risks for infidelity, the couple's overall communication, problem-solving, and coping skills and how they have used them to address infidelity, and how partners have behaved toward each other in response to the turmoil within their relationship (e.g., interrogation by a betrayed individual, punitive aggression, attempts to "win back" a partner). Behavior assessment methods detailed in Chapter 3 include observation of couple interaction during sessions, individuals' spontaneous descriptions of couple interactions during sessions, and therapist inquiries regarding those types of behavior patterns.

Therapist Decisions Regarding Appropriateness of Conjoint Treatment

A decision to pursue conjoint couple therapy to address infidelity is based on judgments of whether the conjoint modality will be (a) safe for members of this couple and (b) effective in reducing negative ways of coping with the infidelity and relationship issues that contributed to it.

Safety

The criteria that we use to estimate the level of safety for joint sessions include:

- An absence of past and current severe forms of partner aggression (e.g., punching, choking, use of a weapon); see Chapter 5.
- Although it is common for betrayed partners to have thoughts about retribution against an unfaithful partner, no strong intent to act on such thoughts.
- An absence of untreated alcohol or drug use that is a risk for emotional, cognitive, and behavioral dysregulation.
- Depression and suicidal thoughts/behavior associated with the infidelity that could be exacerbated by couple therapy.
- During individual interviews, both members report feeling safe participating in couple therapy with their partner, and choose to participate of their own free will.
- Both partners express commitment to safety and a realistic appraisal of risk factors; for example, when thinking and talking about infidelity elicits strong negative emotions and impulses to behave aggressively, both members commit to learn and use strategies to regulate the emotions and destructive actions.

Potential Effectiveness

Although infidelity places a relationship at risk of dissolution, and the therapist's ability to predict treatment effectiveness from the initial assessment is limited, the following criteria can be used to help decide whether conditions for positive changes exist:

- Regardless of the severity of relationship distress and disruption of partners' individual psychological functioning, both members express motivation to work on understanding and addressing factors that contributed to infidelity, whether that leads to a decision to stay together or to dissolve the relationship, and to minimize further harm. They express willingness to take personal responsibility for their roles in relationship problems and efforts that would be needed if they decide that their goal is to improve the relationship for the future.

- Neither partner is experiencing a level of individual psychopathology that seems likely to interfere with the ability to engage in couple therapy; both are committed to work on regulating negative responses to each other, for their own sake and that of significant others such as any children and extended family and friends.
- Each member of the couple has sufficient personal resources to help them cope with stresses associated with the infidelity, and people who support them do not vilify the other partner and encourage vindictive behavior.

GOAL SETTING AND SOCIALIZATION TO TREATMENT

In spite of partners' initial statements that they are motivated for couple therapy to resolve infidelity issues and stay together, some individuals who engaged in infidelity are secretly ambivalent, continuing their affair, discontinuing it initially but missing the affair partner and thinking about reconnecting, or concluding that they no longer want to be with their primary partner even if they end the affair. Sometimes the individual mulls over this issue for a while and suddenly announces a decision to end the couple therapy and primary relationship, creating a new crisis for their partner and relationship.

At this point, the therapist can point out to the individual that ending the relationship is a major life decision, and can ask whether there are any factors that have led them to conclude that it is hopeless to try to repair the relationship, which they might be willing to address in a time-limited way, to see if progress could be made. If the individual declines further sessions, the therapist can explore how they envision interacting with their partner, any children, extended family, and others in their shared life, so that the therapist and partner will have a sense of what lies ahead.

The therapist also can ask to schedule an individual session with each member of the couple, using a crisis intervention format in which the therapist explores the impact of the person's decision on each individual's functioning. This is important for both partners because the unfaithful individual's life also is likely to be disrupted significantly, and their well-being is of concern. During the crisis intervention session with the betrayed partner, the therapist explores the individual's possible negative cognitions (e.g., "My life is ruined"; "I'm going to make my partner regret they treated me this way!"), emotional responses (e.g., anxiety, depression, anger), and behavioral responses (e.g., vindictively disclosing the partner's actions to family, friends and the partner's boss; withdrawing from social supports; substance abuse). The therapist should evaluate suicidal and homicidal risks, intervene as needed, and guide the client in devising a self-care plan, which will include a referral for individual therapy.

During the crisis intervention session with the unfaithful partner, the therapist explores cognitions, emotions, and behaviors associated with their decision to end the relationship, stating that the therapist's goal is not to try to change the person's mind but to guide them in thinking about how they want to carry out their decision in a manner that will cause the least damage possible to themselves and others in their life. Assessment of suicidal risk also is important.

Often, a betrayed partner also is ambivalent about couple therapy, based on their hurt and angry feelings, as well as their expectancies that they could never trust the unfaithful partner again, in spite of any wish that their relationship could be saved. It is important that the therapist provide the betrayed individual a safe setting in both individual and couple sessions to express feelings and concerns, and to experience some degree of control about goals that would be set for couple therapy focused on understanding the infidelity and making decisions for the future. Because a betrayed individual commonly experienced lack of control over the occurrence of the infidelity, a goal of couple therapy is to build a balance of control between partners. As we note in the description of Stage 1 of the treatment model, betrayed individuals may attempt to regain a sense of control through aggressive actions (e.g., requiring the unfaithful partner to leave their home, revealing the infidelity to other people in a punitive manner). The therapist therefore needs to guide them in devising goals that will achieve a better balance of power and are not destructive.

Sometimes a therapist notices cues that a member of a couple may be ambivalent about couple therapy, but the individual continues to participate and makes no mention of it. The therapist can gently address the individual (e.g., "I noticed that you have been quiet during our sessions and have said little about what you'd like to see improved in your relationship. How are you feeling about what we are doing in our sessions?"). If the individual does not divulge their motives and goals in response to that inquiry, the therapist should not pressure them for more information and can say, "I care about how both of you are doing during this difficult time, so I want you to feel free to share your concerns at any point."

Socializing the couple for treatment involves managing mixed agendas and emotions of both partners and describing the three-stage model, which is focused on managing major disruption to the partners' relationship and individual lives; increasing mutual understanding of factors that contributed to the infidelity (and implications for changes needed for the relationship to improve and survive); and making decisions about the future of the relationship. The therapist can emphasize ways in which couple therapy can benefit both partners, regardless of their final decision about their future, and should state that participating does not obligate them to stay together.

PLANNING TREATMENT

The first stage of treatment planning focuses on setting goals in collaboration with the couple and socializing them to concepts and methods of therapy. Therapists need to be attuned to the common situation in which partners have different goals and may differ in their levels of motivation to engage in the proposed activities that require considerable self-exploration and disclosure. The second stage involves implementing a sequence of interventions focused on managing negative impacts the infidelity had on the partners' behavior, cognitions, and emotions, fostering mutual understanding of factors that led to the infidelity, and guiding the couple in making constructive decisions regarding the future of their relationship.

Coming Together on Goals

In Chapter 2, we described how therapists collaborate with couples to work toward the goals that led them to seek assistance. Infidelity is one of the areas for which members of a couple often have different goals for what will be addressed during sessions and what outcomes are desired. At least initially, their different goals are based on their needs as a betrayed or unfaithful partner. For example, individuals who discover a partner's infidelity commonly feel a need for detailed information from the partner regarding circumstances of an affair (e.g., how the individual met the affair partner and was able to keep the affair a secret) and what forms of emotional and sexual involvement occurred. Because the individual's sense of security has been undermined, the individual also is likely to have a goal of reestablishing some degree of control over their life, both individually and within the relationship. However, the unfaithful partner is likely to perceive requests for more information as either the betrayed person's attempt to gather more incriminating evidence to justify punishing them or as remaining "stuck on the past" rather than moving on to work on the future of their relationship.

An individual who has engaged in infidelity commonly has a goal of self-protection from severe negative consequences of the discovery of the affair and often is highly reluctant to disclose details. The members of the couple also may have different goals regarding the future of their relationship, with one focused on improving and saving it and the other on moving toward dissolving it. The therapist can convey empathy for each person's experiences, motives, and goals, while emphasizing the importance of collaborating as much as possible to minimize harm to the partners and other people when their goals differ. The therapist can coach the betrayed and unfaithful partners in using expressive and empathic listening skills to increase their understanding of each other's needs, so neither member will feel pushed by the partner or therapist to move toward achieving the other's goal.

The therapist's intent is to guide the couple in generating a list of core goals for therapy that are tailored to their needs and life circumstances, such as:

- quick crisis intervention as needed to deescalate severe conflict and disruption of normal functioning as individuals, parents, workers, and so on
- decision making regarding current arrangements for their relationship, such as who will live where, what types of interaction they will have with each other (e.g., family activities), how they can share feelings with each other constructively, co-parenting roles, who should be told about the infidelity, and management of finances
- learning about available community resources such as legal services in case they are needed
- improving their ability to resolve issues without aggression
- identifying individual, relational, and sociocultural factors that contributed to the infidelity and interventions that can help reduce those factors

The therapist introduces the model for addressing infidelity and discusses with the couple whether they would like to apply it to their relationship. The therapist describes the components of CBCT for infidelity that are listed in Handout 6.1 (available on the book's web page at *www. guilford.com/epstein-materials*) some of which are components of couple therapy in general, whereas others are tailored to infidelity.

The therapist also describes *structural aspects of the couple therapy*, which are mostly generic CBCT characteristics:

- *Mostly joint sessions*, with the option of occasional sessions with individuals if they experience challenges from aspects of the therapy (e.g., difficulty managing emotions; a tendency to blame one's partner for all issues in the relationship, defensiveness about self-exploration of personal vulnerabilities/characteristics that affected the relationship and contributed to infidelity)

    • *Active practice in sessions and during "homework" of positive couple skills* for communication, problem solving, coping with stressors, modification of problematic thinking, anger management, and, when relevant, building a positive couple bond

    • *The roles of the therapist:* providing educational information; teaching, coaching (with detailed constructive feedback), and supporting the couple as they practice skills for communication and coping with the stressor of the infidelity

    • *The roles of the couple:* attending sessions consistently; being committed to taking responsibility for personal changes that will contribute to more constructive couple interactions, whether or not they decide to stay together

IMPLEMENTING INTERVENTIONS

The couple treatment for infidelity developed by Gordon, Baucom, and Snyder (Baucom, Porter, et al., 2009; Gordon et al., 2023) that we emphasize involves three stages, each of which applies interventions for problematic cognitions, affect, and behavioral patterns. They all draw on the cognitive-behavioral intervention methods detailed in Chapter 4, as well as insight-oriented couple therapy (Snyder & Mitchell, 2008). We strongly agree with Gordon and colleagues that partners' insight into their own and each other's personal characteristics and life experiences that influenced development of infidelity is very important, and our cognitive-behavioral methods facilitate that insight and mutual empathy.

    The therapist's success in reducing a couple's turmoil will depend in part on the ability to develop a positive alliance with each member. The therapist must be attuned to partners' sensitivity to cues they interpret as indications that the therapist is taking sides, particularly with a betrayed individual who is experiencing trauma symptoms. Infidelity often triggers individuals' personal standards about right and wrong and judgments regarding their own and each other's behavior. The clinician's success at establishing balanced alliances requires communicating respect and support for each person as a human being, even while pointing out an individual's actions toward their partner that were harmful. Given the risk that infidelity tends to elicit partners' adversarial responses, the therapist may need to reiterate that balanced goal repeatedly.

    Due to the damaging effects of infidelity on individual and relationship well-being, it is crucial that initial interventions quickly reduce current negative affect and other trauma symptoms. The interventions can demonstrate to the couple that they can take the negative effects of the infidelity seriously but moderate them and improve their ability to interact constructively to address problems in their relationship and make wise decisions about its future. Immediate attention to behavior change (e.g., eliminating forms of retaliation, setting boundaries on what they discuss and how they do it) is essential. Interventions that reduce poorly regulated emotional responses are needed to allow the individuals to behave more constructively even when upset. Furthermore, when the assessment has indicated that individuals' cognitions (e.g., unrealistic standards for how one's partner should demonstrate caring, a belief in retribution) are contributing to negative emotions and behavior toward one's partner, interventions for those cognitions would be integrated early in the treatment plan. With infidelity, the treatment plan should focus on interrupting damaging interactions as quickly as possible, as well as developing partners' individual and dyadic skills for communicating and solving problems.

TREATMENT STAGE 1: DEALING WITH THE IMPACT OF THE AFFAIR

This initial stage focuses on reducing the negative effects that an affair is having on the functioning of the two individuals and their relationship. The therapist conveys empathy for the distress experienced by the betrayed individual, the stress that the unfaithful partner is experiencing even if that individual had positive experiences within the affair, and the disruption the infidelity caused in their relationship. At this point, it most likely is unclear what decisions the partners ultimately will make regarding their relationship, but the infidelity may be a stark "wake-up call" that there were significant unaddressed problems in the relationship, or that the partners did not adequately think about and discuss possible differences in their views on monogamy. Thus, a couple may never have discussed one member's assumption that even if other people are attractive, one's love and commitment to one's partner will naturally override temptation, and the other member's assumption that humans are not naturally monogamous, and love for one's partner does not preclude satisfying one's sexual needs with others.

A review is conducted with the couple, pointing out the negative effects the infidelity has had on individual and relationship functioning, as well as on significant others such as children. The therapist then engages the couple in setting an immediate goal of behaving in ways that will avoid further harm (e.g., controlling one's impulse to attack each other's self-esteem).

Interventions for Behavior

To counteract negative couple behavioral interactions, the therapist focuses on improving constructive skills for sharing one's feelings, as well as on listening skills for achieving and conveying understanding of each other's feelings. It often is challenging for an individual to convey empathy for a partner's perspective when the listener has been treated negatively by the partner, but at this point the goal is to deescalate intense negative interactions. By listening closely and making sure one understands the other's thoughts and emotions, each person contributes to a calmer atmosphere and understands their partner even if they disagree. For example, a betrayed individual may consider their unfaithful partner's rationale for engaging in an affair unconvincing and selfish, but reflecting back, one's understanding of the partner's experiences will help the couple discuss the pathway through which the affair developed and consider the implications for the future of their relationship.

Because infidelity disrupts the stability of the couple's relationship, the therapist asks about the couple's current living situation and daily interactions, and guides them in discussing possible changes in negative patterns (e.g., a betrayed individual interfering with the partner's opportunities to have time with their children). The therapist provides psychoeducation and coaching in self-care strategies for both members. When an unfaithful individual is motivated to repair the couple's relationship, the therapist can coach the couple in identifying specific actions that person can take to reduce the betrayed individual's distress, such as checking in more often to let the partner know their whereabouts.

If an unfaithful individual has continued to interact with the affair partner, this is likely to be an ongoing source of stress in the couple's relationship, for which the therapist needs to guide the couple in decision making. The therapist should inquire about the unfaithful person's intentions, whether the individual wants to continue the affair relationship and whether that is part of a decision to leave the primary partner. The unfaithful individual may have avoided disclosing such intentions, in a self-protective way, but to the extent possible, the therapist should strive to uncover them in the third stage of this treatment model, which focuses on decisions and directions for the couple relationship. If an unfaithful partner discloses an intention to remain in an affair relationship and to leave the primary partner, the therapist may need to move more quickly to the third stage, although it still is crucial to focus on Stage 1 processes to help the couple cope better with the negative impacts of the affair. Furthermore, evidence that one or both members of the couple have been coping with the infidelity in counterproductive ways (e.g., an unfaithful partner tries to avoid any discussion of possible current contact with the affair partner; a betrayed partner focuses on reducing stress by trying to win the partner back through ingratiating behavior; either partner copes through substance use) must be addressed.

Interventions for Cognition

Cognitive interventions often are needed to counteract partners' extreme negative thinking about the infidelity and provide motivation to increase constructive couple interactions. As we noted previously, learning of a partner's infidelity commonly causes major disruption to an individual's assumptions about the partner and relationship ("I always thought I was safe in our relationship, but I'm not. You are not the person I thought you were."). Such cognitions tend to involve all-or-nothing thinking in which the partner's infidelity is seen as negating all of their prior positive actions within the relationship. The betrayed individual's present negative selective perception, focusing only on negative behavior and ignoring any of the partner's positive efforts to repair the relationship, likely exacerbates the upsetting belief that their relationship has been destroyed. It also can contribute to a negative expectancy that it is hopeless to try to rebuild their bond, which might not be accurate. The therapist can guide the individual in taking a broader view of the partner's behavior over the course of their relationship without negating the seriousness of the infidelity, as well as helping the individual explore how a person who seemed to have many positive qualities could behave in such a hurtful way (see Chapter 4).

Alternatively, a betrayed individual may conclude that they are "stupid" for not knowing their partner well enough to notice signs of involvement with someone else. This may reflect perfectionistic standards for oneself and a downplaying of the unfaithful partner's skills at conducting an affair in secrecy. The therapist can focus on guiding the individual in considering a less critical self-evaluation.

An unfaithful partner who has been attacked verbally by their betrayed partner, and perhaps has been subjected to other forms of retaliation, is likely to view the other's behavior as unfair. This may interfere with expressing remorse for causing hurt and instead may lead to criticizing the betrayed individual, which is likely to escalate conflict. The therapist explains that negative emotions and thoughts about one's partner are common in couples experiencing infidelity but emphasizes that negative consequences often result from acting on them.

Both members of the couple usually experience negative expectancies, in terms of anticipating further negative responses from their partner; the betrayed individual predicts that the unfaithful partner will continue to be deceptive, while the unfaithful individual predicts that the betrayed partner will retaliate and fail to believe anything they say. Although these negative expectancies have some basis in reality, they can be extreme, and they leave no room for good will gestures. The therapist should point out how negative predictions are not surprising at this point, but that the potential for rebuilding trust in their relationship will depend on each person being willing to both make good will gestures and offer their partner opportunities to make them. The therapist can stress that taking some chances probably may make them feel uneasy and anxious, and it will be helpful if they acknowledge it, as well as recognizing each other's willingness to be vulnerable.

Interventions for Emotion

Some betrayed individuals, as well as some unfaithful individuals, are inhibited in their experience and expression of negative emotions about their relationship and about their feelings associated with the infidelity. Avoidance of communication about emotional distress will be a barrier to the couple's ability to reach a deep understanding of this blow to their relationship, make good decisions about its future, and engage in efforts to improve it if they desire to do so. A therapist needs to provide the couple with psychoeducation about the value of noticing and expressing their emotions to each other in a constructive way and engaging in empathic listening.

In contrast to inhibition of emotions, the therapist needs to identify and intervene with emotion dysregulation problems, which often contribute to aversive behavioral interactions regarding the infidelity. The therapist gathers information about each individual's difficulty in moderating emotions such as anger and anxiety, as well as processes in which they "co-regulate" each other's negative emotional states. Interventions described in Chapter 5 for reducing negative emotion in partner aggression are applied as needed. For example, the therapist guides the couple in using "time-outs" to exit negative interactions associated with anger. Cognitions also are addressed that contribute to the co-regulation of negative emotion (e.g., both members view the other's criticisms as unfair, become angry at the perceived injustice, and vent their anger by reciprocating criticism). Observing instances of intense emotions triggered during couple sessions is a major opportunity to assess emotion dysregulation and draw it to the clients' attention. The interventions described in Chapter 4 are used to help moderate the associated cognitions, emotional responses, and behavior both during and between therapy sessions.

Emotion dysregulation in a betrayed individual also is commonly an aspect of flashbacks regarding the partner's infidelity. Gordon and colleagues (Gordon et al., 2023; Baucom, Snyder, et al., 2009) normalize these experiences for the couple through psychoeducation, explaining how flashbacks are common trauma symptoms, regardless of whether the individual would meet the criteria for a PTSD diagnosis. The therapist identifies any negative dyadic coping responses to flashbacks, such as the unfaithful partner suggesting that there is no longer anything to be upset about because the affair has ended. Similarly, it can be harmful to the betrayed partner's self-esteem and well-being if the unfaithful partner engages in superficial, ambivalent, or insincere dyadic coping, in which they hold the betrayed partner responsible for the infidelity (e.g., "I'm sorry I hurt your feelings and you keep thinking about it, but if you had been more attentive to my needs, I never would have had to get them met with someone else"). Gordon and colleagues' interventions include guidelines for strategies the couple can use together to cope with and reduce a betrayed partner's flashbacks (e.g., use of expressive and empathic listening skills).

It can be quite uncomfortable for an unfaithful individual to listen to their partner's expression of emotional pain, but their willingness to do so and to validate that pain has potential to help the healing process. The empathy and willingness to take responsibility for causing pain that is demonstrated by the unfaithful partner may begin to soften the betrayed person's negative view of the partner and build some hope regarding the relationship. Because many unfaithful individuals tend to cope by attempting to avoid listening to their partner's distress, the therapist can coach them to consider the advantages of trying some empathic listening. The therapist also should give the unfaithful partner positive feedback for exhibiting empathy for the betrayed partner's experience and taking responsibility for the infidelity.

We also suggest that the therapist evaluate the degree to which an individual's flashbacks (including significant emotion dysregulation) also reflect the person's broader personal tendency to experience emotional distress (e.g., anxiety and/or depression). There is a limit to which the clinician can address severe individual symptoms such as rage, panic, and suicidality within couple therapy sessions. It is important that therapists assess the severity of individual dysfunction and guide impaired members of couples toward appropriate individual treatment rather than attempting to address the individual issues solely in couple therapy. A referral for concurrent individual therapy, as well as couple interventions for psychopathology symptoms described in Chapter 10, may be appropriate. It is important that the therapist explain to the couple that serving as an advocate for both members' individual well-being is a core aspect of couple therapy and does not reflect condoning the specific ways they have treated each other.

Identification of each partner's positive and negative ways of coping with the stressors they currently are experiencing contributes to interventions designed to reduce counterproductive patterns. For example, an individual who copes with anxiety symptoms through social isolation and alcohol use would be coached by the couple therapist to substitute more constructive coping responses, with a referral for individual therapy if the client fails to demonstrate progress. The therapist also should consider the possibility that an unfaithful individual who has been withdrawing from their partner and exhibits limited empathy for the partner may be considering ending the relationship or has characterological traits that may not respond to couple therapy and may need a referral for individual therapy.

Thus, treatment Stage 1 is intended to control damage that infidelity has produced for the individuals and relationship. It also creates calmer conditions in which the partners can interact in a collaborative rather than an adversarial way to understand the conditions that led to the affair (Stage 2) and make wise decisions about the future of their relationship (Stage 3).

TREATMENT STAGE 2: FINDING MEANING

Given the instability and distress caused by infidelity, it is natural that one or both members of a couple would be motivated to reach some resolution such as dissolving the relationship or reaching a degree of forgiveness that would allow them to put it behind them and move ahead into the future together. They may fear that in-depth exploration of factors that served as risks for the infidelity will "open a can of worms," intensifying negative emotion and behavior between the partners. Therefore, the therapist has a responsibility to provide education and build the couple's motivation to engage in an exploration, not only to reduce confusion about why such upsetting events occurred, but also to help them make appropriate changes to reduce those risk factors in the future. Even if they choose to dissolve their relationship, understanding the risk factors for the infidelity can help them in any future relationships.

Identifying risk factors regarding the couple relationship involves examination of the ways that the partners have interacted as a couple and introspection by the individuals regarding their own needs and motives. Gordon et al. (2023) emphasize use of insight-oriented couple therapy to achieve mutual understanding, an approach with which we concur. However, we focus on achieving insight primarily through cognitive-behavioral methods of identifying themes in each partner's thoughts and emotions (e.g., an unfilled need for emotional intimacy) as well as couple behavioral patterns (e.g., mutual avoidance of open communication) that interfered with mutual need fulfillment. Even with couples who are relatively insightful and have good communication skills, we tend to structure these discussions to a moderate degree, addressing questions to each member of the couple regarding risk factors involving their personal characteristics and sociocultural influences, as well as couple interaction patterns. During this stage, the therapist must emphasize that partners' tendencies to blame each other will lead to emotional upset and defensiveness much more than to useful insight into the causes of the infidelity. The therapist stresses that each person will face the challenge of listening to the other's views of risk factors as calmly as possible and feeling free to present a different view when it is their own turn, but not trying to prove who is right or wrong.

Increasing mutual insight into the process through which infidelity developed involves both individuals being introspective about personal and relationship characteristics that seem to have contributed. Thus, both partners may describe their tendencies to engage in autonomous activities and little shared leisure time over the years, or a pattern of keeping vulnerable thoughts and emotions private. Each person is also encouraged to (and praised for) self-examination of personal factors, such as an unfaithful individual acknowledging that the low level of affection in their relationship made attention from the third person appealing. Similarly, a betrayed individual may disclose that growing up in a family in which members rarely expressed feelings made it difficult to express affection as well as distress to the partner. The individual and relationship history interviews (Chapter 3) provide useful information for this process.

Although making plans for changes for the future of their relationship (staying together with planned changes in ways of relating to each other versus dissolving their relationship) if the partners decide to do so occurs mostly in Stage 3 of this model, identification of risk factors in Stage 2 motivates some couples to begin that process. For example, couples who identified a gradual mutual withdrawal over the years may be motivated to take steps to increase shared time and mutual disclosure of feelings. The therapist can support these efforts while noting to the couple that the more they understand factors that contributed to the infidelity, the more they will be able to plan strategies for strengthening their relationship in the third stage of the therapy.

Interventions for Behavior

We use methods for assessing the couple behavioral interaction described in Chapter 3 to identify risk factors such as inadequate expression and partner empathy regarding personal needs that led to one or both members feeling unfulfilled and frustrated. The therapist guides the couple in using better expressive and listening skills to achieve greater mutual understanding of such unfulfilled needs. The therapist combines the communication skills training with systematic inquiry about the qualities of the relationship that each member had found satisfying and those that were lacking. Identification of partner behaviors that would best communicate caring and respect is emphasized, with the therapist coaching the partner in reflecting an empathic understanding of the other's thoughts and emotions.

At times, partners disagree with each other's portrayal of a couple pattern (e.g., "I did not avoid talking to you about our relationship!") or an individual's characteristics (e.g., "Your sister grew up in the same home you did, and she has no trouble showing her caring"). In such instances, the therapist focuses on expressive and empathic listening skills, so the partners understand each other's perspective even if they have different views. For example, instead of complaining about their partner not demonstrating caring, Partner A might begin by using expresser guidelines, "I know we've been together for a long time, and you say that's because you care a lot about me, but I would appreciate it if you would express your feelings for me more openly, telling me what you value about me and giving me some hugs from time to time." Partner B could then respond empathically, "I hear that you believe me when I say my long commitment to being with you reflects caring, but I don't express my feelings for you in visible ways much, and it would feel good to you if I did that." Partner A could confirm Partner B's empathic reflection, "Yes, that is how I feel about it." Then they could switch roles, with Partner B expressing their thoughts and feelings about the issue: "I do experience warm feelings for you often, and at times I try approaching you to express them, but you are so busy and preoccupied with things like your job and the daily disasters in the news that you don't notice my efforts. I've gotten to giving up quickly." Partner A might disagree with Partner B's portrayal of A as being too preoccupied to notice B's expressions of caring, but A's job is to reflect back B's thoughts and feelings, "So, your experience is that you try to express caring for me, but I seem so preoccupied with work and news stories that I don't notice it. You'd like me to stop what I'm doing more and notice you." Although this couple has different perceptions of who has been responsible for their disconnect regarding expressions of caring, they have begun the process of identifying aspects of their interaction pattern that each member could help change. Those can be targets for treatment if they decide to try to improve their relationship.

Unfulfilled needs also may be associated with joint stressors the couple has faced that limit attention to their relationship (e.g., loss of sleep from having a newborn; a child with a serious disability; caring for an ill parent; financial strain; discrimination) or individual stressors that affect both partners (e.g., job loss, a medical condition). The assessment of couple functioning described in Chapter 3 commonly uncovers such stressors, but in exploring risk factors for infidelity, it is helpful to inquire specifically about factors related to unmet needs. The therapist emphasizes that if the couple desires to strengthen their relationship, the treatment plan should include interventions focused on improving dyadic coping with stressors.

When an individual partner's behavioral deficits or excesses are identified, such as a general tendency to withdraw from conflict or compulsive attention to job tasks that limits time with one's partner, the therapist can evaluate with the couple how much that pattern can be addressed in couple therapy. For example, behavioral experiments can be set up in which an avoidant person tries graded exposure experiences that involve remaining in discussions of conflict topics with their partner for increasing lengths of time. When it appears that an individual's pattern is too severe to be treated solely in couple sessions, the therapist can provide referrals for individual therapy that often can be pursued concurrently.

The therapist must guide an unfaithful partner in tracing the development of increased interaction and attraction to the third party in a sensitive manner, as this leaves the individual vulnerable to negative responses from the betrayed partner, as well as personal shame and defensiveness. The therapist can note that relative levels of satisfaction with one's primary partner and an outside person typically depend on how much enjoyable time is spent with each person, and planning changes in both relationships can help shift the balance away from the affair relationship. This approach would involve minimizing or ending interactions with the affair partner, while planning opportunities for enjoyable shared time with the primary partner.

Interventions for Cognition

During the practice of communication skills for expressing and understanding each other's unmet needs, the therapist also is probing for each member's cognitions regarding satisfying and unsatisfying aspects of the couple relationship, such as unmet personal standards for ways their partner should demonstrate caring. Similarly, the therapist explores each individual's attributions about the causes of a partner's unsatisfying behavior, such as attributing a partner's repeated failure to ask about one's daily experiences to a lack of interest. Furthermore, the therapist guides the couple in noticing selective attention to instances when the other person failed to meet one's needs, while overlooking instances of attentive partner behavior. Cognitive interventions described in Chapter 4 are introduced and practiced.

The Role of Forgiveness

As addressed in Stage 1, when an individual learns that their partner has been unfaithful, it often results in very negative beliefs about the partner (e.g., "My partner is not the good person I assumed them to be"). Although the unfaithful partner indeed engaged in very hurtful behavior, an exclusively negative view of them is a barrier to considering possible ways to strengthen the relationship and perhaps move ahead together. In turn, the unfaithful partner may shift to a more negative conception of the betrayed individual to justify the infidelity (e.g., "My partner continues to show how we were never right for each other"). Therefore, a goal of Stage 2 of the treatment model is to help the members achieve a more balanced conception of each other, as people with mixtures of characteristics, including positive ones that attracted them to each other. Furthermore, through learning more about each other's developmental struggles and current vulnerabilities, partners can increase their compassion for each other's ways of behaving within their relationship.

Gordon et al. (2023) describe the process of achieving empathy and compassion for someone who has behaved in a hurtful way as fostering forgiveness. The empathy is not equivalent to finding the other's behavior acceptable, but it can soften intense negative emotions and harsh behavior toward the person. For example, an unfaithful individual may describe how repeatedly being passed over for promotions at work exacerbated chronic low self-esteem developed in childhood and how attention from an affair partner provided a temporary ego boost. The betrayed individual still may consider the affair to be an unacceptable way of coping with self-esteem problems, but they may experience some level of compassion for the unfaithful partner. The compassion may lead the betrayed person to take a strong stand declaring that in order to continue their relationship the individual must develop better ways of coping with blows to self-esteem. Therapists need to identify any negative beliefs partners hold regarding extending forgiveness for hurtful behavior, such as considering forgiveness a form of weakness (Baucom, Snyder, et al., 2009; Gordon et al., 2023). This involves clarifying the idea that forgiveness involves extending compassion for one's partner and willingness to try to continue the relationship, while not forgetting or accepting past negative behavior, requiring the other's remorse for hurtful behavior and a commitment to achieving a mutually satisfying relationship.

Interventions for Emotion

When one or both partners' deficits in identifying and expressing their emotions have created a distance between them and increased the risk for infidelity, the therapist can use interventions to increase awareness of feelings and to express them to one's partner, described in Chapter 4. Likewise, when one or both members demonstrate poor regulation of negative emotions that detracted from the quality of their relationship, the therapist can use the interventions covered in Chapters 4 and 5 to help them moderate negative affect.

Infatuation with an affair partner can present a stark contrast to any dissatisfaction an individual feels with their primary relationship, and it may fuel decisions toward forming a deeper bond with the affair partner. Because it could be painful for a betrayed individual to hear about their partner's infatuation with the other person, it is wise to discuss it during an individual session with the unfaithful partner. During that session, the therapist can express understanding of how powerful those feelings could be, but for that reason special attention may be needed to manage them if the individual wants to repair the primary relationship. Plans can be made to avoid reminders of the affair partner (e.g., deleting photos, avoiding locations where the person might be encountered). Because memories of the affair partner can trigger strong emotions, the therapist can coach the individual in methods for moderating them (e.g., distraction techniques).

As described in Stage 1, a betrayed individual's emotions such as anxiety and anger often occur in response to current partner behavior (e.g., arriving home late, mentioning a personal leisure interest that the partner had shared with the affair partner) or flashback memories (e.g., daydreams focused on the affair). In addition to addressing these responses during Stage 1, the therapist commonly needs to continue to intervene with them during exploration of risk factors in Stage 2. The therapist can focus on roles both partners can play in helping the betrayed person cope with negative emotions. For example, the betrayed individual can disclose upset feelings to the partner, who can respond empathically. As needed, the therapist can hold an individual session with the betrayed individual, focused on strategies for coping with distress, with the option of suggesting adjunctive individual therapy.

TREATMENT STAGE 3: MOVING ON

Based on the understanding the couple and therapist achieved during Stage 2 regarding factors that contributed to the infidelity and the current functioning of the relationship, the therapist shifts to the goal of guiding the couple in making decisions about directions for their future. Constructive decision making will be based on Stage 1 success in reducing disruption of individual and relationship functioning, plus Stage 2 understanding of factors that require change to strengthen the relationship and prevent future infidelity. During Stage 2, some couples have identified changes they would like to make and may already have begun working on them. Other couples may not have reached the point where they decided whether to commit to making changes rather than dissolving the relationship. A therapist can note that it need not be an all-or-nothing decision at this point, as a couple could decide to experiment with some changes for a while before they conclude whether they prefer to end their relationship rather than work on risk factors further. A trial period of therapy can be a relief to some couples who are unhappy with their relationship but are concerned about negative consequences of ending it.

Interventions for Behavior

We concur with Gordon and colleagues about the importance of creating with the couple a concrete record of a narrative that describes the factors contributing to the infidelity. Such a record aids in treatment planning, whether their goal is to strengthen their relationship for the future or to disengage with the least damage possible. The procedure is either for each partner to write a separate narrative of the contributing factors based on information identified during Stage 2, or for them to collaborate in writing a joint narrative. In either case, the therapist serves as a consultant to maximize the degree to which the narratives reflect the range of risk factors identified in Stage 2. At this point, partners may still blame each other for the infidelity in their versions of the narrative, and the therapist must provide structure in reducing adversarial communication. The therapist coaches the couple in using constructive expressive and listening skills to identify risk factors they agree were present and could be addressed in future therapy.

The therapist then coaches the couple, as needed, in defining each risk factor (e.g., avoiding discussions of areas of conflict; a deficit in shared enjoyable activities; a member's chronic depression) and in using problem-solving skills and dyadic coping strategies to generate interventions to reduce each type of risk. We recommend that the therapist emphasize the value of spending time on problem solving and coping strategies even when one or both members are ambivalent or even strongly leaning toward ending the relationship. The therapist can note that sometimes couples identify interventions that decrease their hopelessness about improving their relationship, which can be tested during a trial period. Even when a couple is headed toward dissolving their relationship, they may not disengage fully (e.g., if they have children together), and addressing behavioral patterns that contributed to the infidelity (e.g., avoidance of open communication) could improve their ability to collaborate in other roles such as co-parenting.

At this point, the problem solving shifts toward decisions about whether the couple will work toward staying together and implementing mutually satisfying changes. At this point, the partners may have different goals for the relationship, as one partner may be committed to the relationship and the other may be ambivalent or even determined to end it. The therapist may be able to bridge the partners' discrepant goals by emphasizing the difference between short-term and long-term goals. Thus, in the short term, the couple might agree to use a trial period to examine whether mutually satisfying changes (e.g., in communication, emotion regulation) can be achieved, with each person delaying making a final decision during that period. Progress on those goals will benefit them whether or not they stay together.

Decisions also should be made about practical arrangements, such as whether the couple will live together, types of interactions they will have, and how they will manage finances and their relationships with relatives and joint friends. These decisions may differ from those in Stage 1 to decrease disruption and emotional stress associated with the initial impact of the infidelity.

Interventions for Cognition

Although the therapist intervenes to reduce partners' negative cognitions about each other during the first two stages of this therapy model, facilitating problem solving to address risk factors for infidelity in the narrative also often includes attention to negative cognitions. Ideally, the narrative a couple constructs includes some *relational circular thinking* about mutual contributions to unsatisfying couple interactions, but some individuals still may mostly blame their partners.

Pointing out instances of mutual contributions to a negative behavior pattern is not equivalent to relieving an individual of personal responsibility. In Stage 3, some individuals also may still cling to *unrealistic standards* for their relationship (e.g., narrow standards for the "correct" way to demonstrate love for one's partner) that make it difficult to collaborate on new solutions. In order for partners to devise potential solutions to a problem, they need to be open to new ideas. If they do not view themselves as having shared goals in life, it will be difficult for them to collaborate on behavior changes that may improve their relationship. When members of a couple have different cultural backgrounds that involve different conceptions of intimacy, the therapist can guide them in seeking ways to incorporate diverse ways of connecting. This may extend to addressing the possibility that partners still hold different standards for what behaviors and feelings about a third person constitute infidelity, but reaching a joint decision regarding future boundaries.

Interventions for Emotion

Even though therapists intervene with negative emotions such as anger, anxiety, depression, and shame in Stages 1 and 2, the focus in Stage 3 on constructing a narrative regarding the infidelity and identifying changes at the individual and couple levels to reduce risk factors can trigger further negative emotions. For example, attention to an unfaithful partner's vulnerabilities that led to infidelity can elicit shame within that person in the presence of the therapist and betrayed individual. In turn, reminders of how the individual decided to be involved in an affair may trigger flashbacks and anxiety for the betrayed individual. Furthermore, daily life events that remind members of the couple of the affair (e.g., a movie that involves an affair, comments from other people who know about the infidelity) may elicit emotional distress, even when the couple decides to continue their relationship and "live with" the affair. The therapist can coach them in counteracting a negative attribution that feeling upset in such situations indicates trouble in moving on. It is important that the therapist prepare the couple for such reactions, including plans to use dyadic coping to help each other get through them. For example, the couple and therapist can agree that whenever a member experiences shame, anxiety, or another negative emotion, that member will disclose it, and the other partner will coach the distressed individual in using self-soothing methods.

The therapist also can prepare the couple for instances in which they are susceptible to co-regulating each other's negative emotions. Thus, when discussing the narrative regarding development of the infidelity, a betrayed individual may express residual anger toward the unfaithful partner, triggering the unfaithful partner's defensive anger and criticism. The therapist should prepare them for such negative scenarios and help them plan how to manage them.

TROUBLESHOOTING PROBLEMS IN COUPLE THERAPY FOR INFIDELITY

Couple therapy for infidelity requires that a therapist maintain a balanced alliance with members of the couple while holding each partner responsible for their own actions and protecting the well-being of each individual. In addition, infidelity commonly produces a crisis state of disequilibrium in each member's functioning, as well as in the couple's relationship. It is essential that the therapist monitor signs of disturbed functioning and risks to well-being that may arise. The following are brief descriptions of problems that may occur in therapy and strategies therapists can use to address them.

Difficulty Maintaining a Balanced Therapeutic Alliance

The therapist needs to convey caring and respect for each person's well-being, as well as fairness in evaluating sources of responsibility for relationship problems.

- In cases with unilateral infidelity, it is crucial to communicate that the unfaithful partner was responsible for pursuing another relationship, but that both members' physical and emotional well-being are important. However, the therapist's goal of protecting both members' well-being regardless of how they behaved within the relationship may conflict with the partners' own goals. For example, during Stage 2, identifying factors that contributed to the infidelity associated with the betrayed individual or the couple's patterns might lead the betrayed person to feel blamed for the partner's actions. Similarly, focusing on the unfaithful individual's characteristics may elicit that person's defensiveness when they believe their partner also contributed to problems in their relationship. One way to reduce such reactions is to suggest beforehand that an exploration of all factors influencing the infidelity might make them feel "on the hot seat" at times, but the goal is for the therapist and couple to understand this distressing period in their relationship as well as possible, so that the couple can make wise decisions about how they can move ahead. The therapist's empathic feedback regarding each partner's concerns about being a focus of the assessment can reduce defensiveness.

- Potential for a therapist to become caught up in a couple's mutual blaming and to take sides can be strong with infidelity, whether or not the therapist had similar experiences in their own or significant others' lives. The therapist must monitor self-of-the-therapist responses and address any biases one notices in reactions to members of the couple. For example, a therapist might become aware of disliking an unfaithful individual who shows little empathy for a betrayed partner's pain and might blame the unfaithful partner for failure of the relationship. It is crucial to reduce the risk that negative feelings for the unfaithful partner will result in the therapist demonstrating little respect and empathy for that individual. If one or both partners perceive the therapist's bias, this can cause a rupture of the therapeutic alliance and loss of focus on the goals of the therapy. Chapter 2 describes strategies for dealing with personal responses to such biases, such as obtaining supervision from a professional peer and focusing more on the vulnerabilities of an unfaithful partner.

Difficulty Fostering Partners' Mutual Empathy and Defining Forgiveness

During all stages of the intervention, both members may have difficulty engaging in empathic listening to the other's thoughts and emotions regarding their relationship, especially if they interpret doing so as agreeing with the other's perspective and forgiving the other person for their painful actions.

- It may be difficult for a betrayed individual to empathize with an unfaithful partner's disclosure that low self-esteem contributed to being attracted to another person who made the partner feel special. This is a general issue in coaching couples who have experienced conflict in using communication skills (see Chapter 4). The therapist must introduce the rationale for empathic listening—in this case, helping the couple and therapist understand factors that contributed to the infidelity as well as possible so that they can identify changes the couple could focus on if they decide to continue their relationship.

• The emphasis on empathic listening raises the issue (especially for betrayed individuals) of the role forgiveness is supposed to play in recovery from infidelity. Although conceptions of forgiveness are a greater focus in Stage 3, they also likely arise in Stage 2 when individuals are asked to adopt an empathic perspective regarding the experiences of a partner with whom they are very upset. When an individual is having difficulty understanding the other's thoughts and emotions associated with behavior they consider unacceptable, the therapist can emphasize that one can understand what influenced a partner's actions while evaluating those actions as unacceptable. The therapist can model an appropriate way that a betrayed individual might speak to their unfaithful partner; for example:

> "I understand you were at a low point in your life, and you gave into the good feelings you got from the other person's attention. However, I consider it unacceptable that you sacrificed our relationship in order to make yourself feel better. Any similar behavior in the future would be unacceptable to me if we are to continue our relationship."

• When a therapist notices that an unfaithful individual exhibits little or no empathy with their partner's thoughts and emotions regarding extradyadic involvements, it is important to assess whether this attitude may be due to a characterological barrier. An additional individual interview may be needed in order to identify a significant psychopathology that may indicate the need for some individual therapy. Similarly, if the therapist learns that a member of the couple copes with stress through substance abuse, discussion of this pattern with that individual and a referral for individual treatment would be appropriate.

Discrepant Partner Definitions of Infidelity

Sometimes partners disagree about whether infidelity has occurred. In some cases an individual who has become involved emotionally and/or sexually with one or more other people may claim that they believe their behavior fell within the limits of the couple's agreed-upon standards for monogamy or consensual nonmonogamy, but their partner disagrees. The partner may argue that the individual is "rewriting history" to avoid taking responsibility for a betrayal.

This type of exchange is similar to other situations in which members of a couple report different memories of past events, and the therapist has no way of definitively deducing what they said and did in the past. One possible approach the therapist can take is to state:

> "I was not present to hear how you discussed your preferences in the past regarding monogamy and any negotiations you engaged in to reach an agreement that you both were willing to live with. I can see at present you have different beliefs about whether Sabrina's involvement with someone else was acceptable. Whether or not you had clear agreement in the past, you do not agree now. If you want to leave open the option of staying together and both being satisfied, it seems crucial for each of you to look within yourself and decide what kind of boundaries you want in your relationship, and begin new decision-making discussions about what types of relationships with other people, if any, are acceptable from this day forward. If there has been some ambiguity, it will be important to remove it. If on the other hand your discussion reveals your standards are incompatible, further discussion will be needed about future commitment to your relationship on each of your parts."

The Risk of Destructive Behavior

Given the intense emotions that commonly occur with revelations of infidelity, therapists must be attuned to risks of destructive behavior, including psychological and physical partner aggression. Although the therapist should be empathic with each individual's emotional distress, it is important to monitor signs that it is fueling aggressive actions and intervene promptly to maintain safety (see Chapter 5).

Experiences of shame on the part of either an unfaithful or a betrayed partner creates some risk for suicidal ideation and behavior. It is important to monitor the cognitions and emotions of partners throughout treatment and be attuned to symptoms of suicidal risk. The therapist also should be prepared to intervene if a member is engaging in shaming behavior to punish their partner, as it may pose a risk to the recipient's well-being.

KEY POINTS

- Infidelity shakes the foundations of intimate bonds—safety, security, and emotional support.

- Therapists are likely to encounter clients experiencing severe symptoms associated with infidelity and must be prepared to devise treatment plans to ameliorate damaging effects.

- A useful approach to working with couples focuses on (1) controlling and reducing the negative effects of the infidelity on the couple's well-being, (2) increasing the couple's understanding of the factors that contributed to the infidelity, and (3) guiding the couple in making constructive decisions regarding the future of their relationship.

- The therapist's maintenance of a strong balanced alliance with both members of the couple is essential to facilitating the partners' empathy for each other, potential forgiveness, and collaboration to move forward, together or separately.

CHAPTER 7

Sexual Relationship Problems

Similar to other presenting problems we address in this book, sexual difficulties and dysfunctions commonly occur in the general population, and more commonly among couples who seek therapy for the overall quality of their relationship. Because many members of the lay public are unaware that some professionals have specialized expertise in the treatment of sexual issues, the first professional approached may be an individual's physician or psychotherapist rather than a clinician who focuses on relational processes. Even though a couple may be aware that sexual issues contribute to distress in their overall relationship, they may attribute sexual problems primarily to characteristics of a symptomatic individual (e.g., viewing a partner with low desire for sex as having physical or psychological problems).

A couple therapist also may be the first professional to learn about sexual difficulties when conducting an intake interview to understand factors contributing to a couple's relationship distress. Because many people are uncomfortable discussing sexual issues with outsiders, especially if they experience shame from these issues, they might be less forthcoming about them than about other problems such as arguments about aspects of daily life. If a couple therapist also is uncomfortable broaching the subject of sexuality, mutual avoidance by the couple and clinician can significantly contribute to overlooking partners' distress in the treatment plan.

Therefore, our goals in this chapter are to describe roles a couple therapist can play in assisting clients who are experiencing sexual difficulties and dysfunctions in their relationships and to provide guidelines for assessment and intervention. By no means does the material in this chapter prepare a clinician to practice as a competent sex therapist, and couple therapists must make decisions about appropriate referrals as needed. Nevertheless, relationship dynamics have significant effects on sexual functioning, and in turn sexual dysfunctions and dissatisfaction commonly influence overall relationship quality. Thus, couple therapists can make major contributions to addressing the concerns of couples experiencing sexual issues.

Even though sex therapy traditionally has focused on treatment of individuals with particular sexual dysfunctions, clients have been assessed and treated within a couple context in which those dysfunctions play out. From historical roots such as Masters and Johnson's (1966, 1970) pioneering work, sexual desire, arousal, and orgasm have been viewed as significantly biologically based but also influenced by individuals' psychological experiences and relationship patterns. However, dysfunction diagnoses in those three aspects of what has been assumed to be normal human sexual response—sexual desire, arousal, and orgasm—predominantly have differentiated between those of males and females, without consideration of diversity in individuals' gender identities and sexual orientations (Nichols, 2014). This binary approach to assessment and treatment, reflected in DSM-5-TR, the most recent edition of the American Psychiatric Association's (2022) *Diagnostic and Statistical Manual of Mental Disorders*, has limitations for assisting nonbinary and transgender clients who present with distress regarding sexuality in their couple relationships. Increasingly, professional literature has addressed ways in which traditional sex therapy models and methods are relevant in many ways to both cisgender clients and those with diverse gender identities but they must be adapted to needs of the latter population (Holmberg, Arver, & Dhejne, 2020).

In addition, mainstream approaches to human sexuality and sex therapy have been developed primarily in Western countries and reflect Western beliefs and values (Hall & Graham, 2020). However, there are significant variations in cultural models of sexuality (e.g., models that place different levels of constraint on female experience and expression of sexual pleasure) that have been found to be associated with prevalence of sexual dysfunctions. This chapter cites literature on the needs of diverse couples who seek help for sexual issues and describes culturally sensitive adaptations to established concepts and methods of sex therapy, with an emphasis on applications from our cognitive-behavioral couple therapy framework. Consistent with our emphasis on cultural sensitivity (especially Chapter 11, on intercultural couples), we concur with Hall and Graham (2020) that treatment is more likely to be effective when cultural beliefs underlying a therapist's approach to sex therapy are discussed in ways that do not clash with clients' own cultural assumptions and patterns. Examples of such common Western cultural beliefs are that sex education regarding normal functioning is important, mutual sexual pleasure is a goal, partners need to communicate openly about their relationship, and consent from each individual is important in a sexual relationship. Therapists cannot assume that all clients from diverse cultures share those common sex therapy beliefs. Consequently, therapists should not be surprised if clients do not describe sexual aspects of their relationship spontaneously when they present their reasons for seeking therapy. When the therapist's assessment suggests that sexual issues are affecting problems for which the couple sought help, the therapist should not automatically prioritize improvements in the clients' sexual relationship. Those whose beliefs and traditions regarding sex differ from the clinician's may not be comfortable pursuing sex as an explicit treatment goal. This does not mean that sexual issues must be avoided, but the therapist needs to strive to create a shared understanding with the clients regarding their presenting problems and should set goals based on that shared understanding. In this chapter, we describe how integration of the clinician's culture regarding therapy with the couple's cultural background occurs through developing a strong therapeutic alliance and empathic inquiry into their cultures.

TYPES AND PREVALENCE
OF COUPLE SEXUAL RELATIONSHIP PROBLEMS

When couples who seek help for relationship distress include issues regarding sexual functioning, they commonly focus on concerns about a discrepancy between partners' levels of interest in sex, as well as about aspects of physical response (such as a member's limited arousal during sexual interactions), difficulties with orgasm (such as premature ejaculation or inability to reach orgasm), or genital pain. Typically, they conceptualize those problems as being primarily due to characteristics of the symptomatic person. Even when the presenting problem is a difference between partners' levels of desire, partners commonly blame the discrepancy on one person, or both individuals view the other person as having abnormally low or high desire. The sex therapy field is based on a medical model, which is still reflected in the set of sexual dysfunction diagnoses described in the DSM up through the most recent edition (American Psychiatric Association, 2022). Diagnoses focus on intrapersonal causes, whether biological or psychological. Although advances in understanding individual psychological factors such as anxiety disorders, depression, and obsessive thinking have contributed to more comprehensive assessment and treatment planning, a more refined understanding of relationship factors influencing sexual dysfunction has lagged behind. Traditional sex therapy methods, beginning with the work of Masters and Johnson (1966, 1970), did include symptomatic individuals' partners, but primarily in the service of alleviating problems within the individual. For example, the frequently used sensate focus intervention we describe in detail later in this chapter involves partners taking turns touching each other in increasingly sensual and then sexual ways, which does change a couple's dyadic interactions. However, the traditional goal has been to reduce the pressure and anxiety experienced by an individual with sexual dysfunction symptoms.

More recent models of sexual response that integrate intrapersonal and interpersonal processes (e.g., Metz, Epstein, & McCarthy, 2018; Johnson, Simakhodskaya, & Moran, 2018; Weeks & Gambescia, 2015) have enhanced clinicians' abilities to treat couples with sexual presenting problems. Those models capture ways in which each partner's internal experiences shape the couple's dyadic interactions in general (e.g., managing conflicts) and specifically regarding sex (e.g., the degree to which partners create a sexually inviting atmosphere between them). We begin our discussion with a brief overview of traditional models of sexual response and types of sexual dysfunction, the importance of attending to sexual experiences of clients with diverse sexual orientations, gender identities, and cultural backgrounds when assessing forms of dysfunction, and then we describe developments in sexual dysfunction concepts that more fully capture systemic couple patterns.

TRADITIONAL MODELS OF SEXUAL RESPONSE AND DYSFUNCTIONS

Masters and Johnson's (1966) physiological model of normal human sexual response included stages of the level of sexual arousal (excitement, plateau, orgasm, and resolution). Kaplan (1974) subsequently modified the model to include an initial stage of desire, which has a major psychological aspect. The model has evolved into the three major stages of *desire, arousal* (the original excitement through plateau), and *orgasm* (the original orgasm through resolution). Basson (2001) further differentiated female and male sexual desire, emphasizing female desire as more responsive to situational conditions such as level of intimacy and other relationship factors, whereas male desire (at least among younger males) as based more on physiological drive. Dysfunctions in sexual response have been conceptualized in the DSM diagnostic system as occurring in the desire phase (male and female hypoactive sexual interest/desire disorder), arousal phase (erectile disorder, female arousal disorder, genitopelvic pain/penetration disorder), and orgasm phase (delayed ejaculation, premature ejaculation, female orgasmic disorder). In DSM-5-TR (American Psychiatric Association, 2022), low female interest and arousal have been merged as a single disorder. Three components of sexual dysfunctions are (1) a chronic condition (rather than occasional difficulties with desire, arousal, or orgasm), (2) resulting personal distress, and (3) contributions to relationship problems (Levine, Risen, & Althof, 2016; Metz et al., 2018). A couple may occasionally experience various sexual difficulties but may not be distressed by them, so the subjective meanings people attach to such difficulties play a major role in a difficulty becoming a dysfunction. Sexual dysfunctions typically include cognition (e.g., thoughts of personal inadequacy, worry about displeasing a partner), emotion (e.g., anxiety in anticipation of sexual activities), behavior (e.g., avoidance of sex), and physiological responses (e.g., limited sexual physiological arousal). A CBCT approach that we emphasize is highly relevant for providing clients with multifaceted assessment and treatment of sexual dysfunction. In this chapter, we also note aspects of other couple therapy models, such as emotion-focused therapy (EFT; Girard & Wooley, 2017; Johnson et al., 2018), and the intersystem model (Gambescia, Weeks, & Hertlein, 2021; Weeks & Gambescia, 2015), which can be used in the treatment of couples with sexual presenting concerns, as well as collaboration with physicians in addressing possible biological processes influencing sexual response.

Although these models of normal sexual response and types of problems that may occur in each stage can be relevant to sexual concerns regardless of an individual's sexual orientation or gender identity, they have potential limitations due to their focus on binary female–male responses and disorders. For example, stressors in the lives of same-sex couples (e.g., discrimination experiences, internalized homophobia, differences between partners' degrees of coming out) may contribute to low sexual desire and need to be addressed in psychoeducation and therapeutic interventions (Pepping, Halford, Cronin, & Lyons, 2020; Rutter, 2012). In addition, although sexual nonmonogamy tends to be more acceptable among gay male couples than lesbian and heterosexual couples within the context of an emotionally close and committed relationship, relationship satisfaction depends on partners' ability to agree on the parameters of any outside sexual relationships, such as a lack of secrecy and the range of acceptable sexual behaviors (Bettinger, 2004).

A transgender male or transgender female individual's low desire, arousal, or orgasm response may be influenced by gender dysphoria that is not addressed in traditional sex therapy concepts and procedures (e.g., distress during sexual interaction with a partner that focuses attention on one's genitals that are inconsistent with one's gender identity). It also is important to differentiate between gender dysphoria resulting from the effects of gender-affirming medical treatments (hormone treatments that alter sexual responses, surgeries that modify sexual anatomy) and gender dysphoria experienced by individuals who choose not to have such medical treatments and continue to live with bodies inconsistent with their identities (Holmberg et al., 2020). Anzani, Lindley, Prunas, and Galupo (2021) note that some transgender individuals experience gender dysphoria and low desire, whereas others do not. In qualitative reports of their sexual experiences many describe enjoyment of a variety of sexual activities, especially when their partners support their comfort and gender affirmation. Their sexual orientation is independent of their gender identity—they may feel attracted to males, females, both males and females, transgender individuals, or nonbinary people, or they may experience low desire, as do some cisgender individuals. Again, we concur with writers such as Hall and Graham (2020) that traditional concepts and methods of sex therapy can be useful for clients with diverse sexual orientations and those with diverse gender identities, but competent clinical practice requires attunement to the needs and experiences of each client and couple.

PREVALENCE OF SEXUAL DYSFUNCTIONS

Research that has surveyed the prevalence of particular cisgender female and male sexual dysfunctions has found considerable variation from one study to another, which can be attributed to methodological limitations such as diverse samples and imprecise use of diagnostic criteria

(Simons & Carey, 2001). Although caution must be used in interpreting inconsistent findings across studies, surveys with heterosexual samples show that sexual dysfunctions are common among women and men (Frühauf, Gerger, Schmidt, Munder, & Barth, 2013; Laumann, Gagnon, Michael, & Michaels, 1994; Laumann, Paik, & Rosen, 1999; Simons & Carey, 2001). For example, the National Health and Social Life Survey conducted in the United States (Laumann et al., 1994, 1999) found that among women prevalence rates were 33.4% for low desire, 24.1% for orgasm disorder, 14.4% for painful intercourse, and 10.4% for lubrication problems, whereas among males the prevalence rates were 28.5% for premature ejaculation, 15.8% for low desire, 10.4% for erectile dysfunction, and 8.3% for delayed ejaculation. Hall and Graham (2020) review research findings indicating that the prevalence of female and male dysfunctions is high overall around the world. For example, an average of 40% of women reported experiencing one or more sexual problems, with the most common types varying from one culture to another (e.g., low desire most common among women in North American, and arousal and orgasm problems most common in countries such as India, Iran, Nigeria, and China). However, considerably fewer women reported feeling distress about those problems, underscoring the importance of subjective evaluations of one's sexual issues. Furthermore, cultural differences in norms and values regarding females' experience and expression of sexual pleasure, including the degree to which it is appropriate for a woman to take an active role in sex, influence women's sexual responses (Hall & Graham, 2020). For example, McCool-Myers, Theurich, Zuelke, Knuettel, and Apfelbacher (2018) reviewed 135 studies on the prevalence of female dysfunctions across 41 countries and found that dysfunction was higher in countries with male-centered versus gender-equal cultures.

Among cisgender men, erectile dysfunction (15–40%) and premature ejaculation (8–30%) are the most prevalent concerns reported worldwide (Hall & Graham, 2020). Even though a problem such as premature ejaculation is common across cultures, individuals' concerns about it may be greater if their cultural beliefs include an assumption that semen loss can produce physical ailments such as weakness. Thus, clients' cognitive evaluations of their sexual problems that are influenced by cultural beliefs are important considerations in understanding sexual presenting problems and devising appropriate treatment plans.

The sensitivity that clinicians must use in identifying diverse cultural factors influencing various sexual problems and the degree of subjective distress that members of couples experience from them is equally essential when treating clients with diverse sexual orientations and gender identities. Findings from heterosexual samples regarding the prevalence rates of types of dysfunctions and the intrapersonal, relational, and environmental factors influencing them likely have limited applicability to gender-diverse clients. Clinicians therefore need to explore nonbinary and transgender individuals' presenting concerns regarding sexual relationships with partners without imposing conceptions of cisgender experiences. As discussed in Chapter 2, examination of areas of one's potential implicit bias is a critical part of cisgender heterosexual therapists' sociocultural sensitivity and humility when they work with gender and sexual minorities.

RISK FACTORS FOR COUPLE SEXUAL DYSFUNCTION

A CBCT model is highly relevant for assessing and treating couples' sexual concerns. The common sexual dysfunctions identified in DSM-5-TR (American Psychiatric Association, 2022) and treated with sex therapy methods involve not only physical responses of arousal and orgasm and biological factors contributing to them, but also partners' associated cognitions, emotional responses, and behavioral interaction patterns. Dysfunctions also are influenced by environmental conditions such as work demands, family and other relationship stresses, and discrimination on the basis of one's sexual orientation, gender identity, race, and other characteristics. The following are descriptions of biophysiological factors, cognitions, emotional responses, behavioral patterns, and environmental stressors that should be elements of assessment and treatment planning.

Biophysiological Factors in Sexual Dysfunction

Because individuals' physical health influences their sexual function, it is important for couple therapists to take biophysiological factors into account and collaborate with clients' physicians in identifying medical issues that may be contributing to presenting problems (Bergeron, Rosen, Pukall, & Corsini-Munt, 2020; Metz et al., 2018). These issues include chronic and acute physical illnesses (e.g., hormone deficiencies, cardiovascular disease, sleep apnea, prostatitis, cancer, stroke, diabetes, arthritis) as well as physical problems such as pelvic floor muscle dysfunction, which either directly affect sexual response or have symptoms (e.g., fatigue, pain) that can distract an individual from enjoying sexual experiences. Furthermore, some medications used to treat physical conditions such as hypertension, as well as psychological disorders such as depression, some over-the-counter medications such as antihistamines, and substances such as alcohol have sexual side effects (Wincze & Weisberg, 2015). Physical injuries involving trauma to the nervous system (including traumatic brain injuries), skeletal-muscular system, genitalia, and any surgeries used to treat them also can impair sexual function. In addition, an individual's negative cognitions (e.g., hopelessness), emotions (e.g., depression, anxiety), and behavioral responses (e.g., avoiding a partner's efforts to initiate sex) to injuries and associated disabilities may detract from sexual desire and function. Some clients may need support in adjusting to normal physical changes associated with aging (e.g., an older male's need for more physical stimulation in order to have an erection). Finally, a transgender individual who chose gender-affirming medical treatments may experience physical side effects that interfere with sexual response. For example, a transgender female who chose hormone therapy to alter secondary sexual characteristics may experience a decrease in sexual desire, arousal, and orgasm that may be disconcerting. More detail regarding biophysiological factors can be found in sex therapy texts such as Hall and Binik (2020), Metz et al. (2018), and Wincze and Weisberg (2015).

Cognition in Sexual Dysfunction

All the types of cognition we focus on throughout this book may contribute to sexual problems and dysfunctions in couple relationships. Members of a couple are likely to have personal *standards* about the characteristics that normal and desirable sexuality should have. Some standards involve beliefs about their own sexual responses (e.g., "I should become physically aroused when I'm close to an attractive partner") or about a good sexual relationship (e.g., "Our levels of desire should be 'in sync' with each other"). Often those standards have been influenced by media depictions of exciting sexual relationships, such as those portrayed in movies or in pornography on the internet. Many children and adolescents, for example, obtain beliefs about intimate relationships and sex through their extensive use of social media. In addition, some clients grow up in cultural contexts that portray sex (or particular forms of sex) as inappropriate, and as adults they have persistent negative thoughts and emotions associated with their sexuality. Individuals who grow up in a societal context in which normal sex is considered to be restricted to relations between two cisgender heterosexual people may experience internalized conflict and distress over their sexual orientation or gender identity.

Because people rarely compare their sexual experiences in discussions with friends, they are unlikely to collect a realistic sample of information about normal human sexual function, and they compare themselves and their relationships with unrealistic standards.

In addition to distress that can result from each individual's own sexual standards, conflict may develop when two partners have different standards and lack adequate problem-solving skills for resolving their differences. For example, partners may have different beliefs about the appropriate way to initiate sex with each other. One individual may focus on trying to seduce the other with suggestive talk and physical touch, whereas the other may emphasize creating a relaxed romantic atmosphere, providing an emotional "oasis" from the couple's usual hectic life.

Couples' *assumptions* about normal sexual function also can influence the ways they interact sexually. For example, a partner or a couple may assume that "[c]hanges in older couples' bodies inevitably result in their inability to have an enjoyable sexual relationship." Or they may think, "People who are sexually interested in each other get aroused even if they have been upset with each other." As with unrealistic standards, inappropriate assumptions about what constitutes "normal" or appropriate sexual function may be developed through exposure to media portrayals, social stereotypes such as those regarding aging and sex, and inadequate sex education. In addition, the diversity of sexual behaviors that exist among individuals with various gender identities make it complicated to define what constitutes normal sexuality, rather than healthy functioning. Adults seeking good information regarding sex may not know where to look for reliable sources or may be embarrassed to ask friends or professionals for leads.

Members of a couple are likely to make *attributions* about causes of problems with sexual functioning, which can vary in their accuracy and potential to produce upset feelings and problematic behavioral responses. Some negative attributions involve inferences about one's own sexual symptoms (e.g., "I'm defective because I rarely have orgasms"), about a partner's reactions to one's symptoms (e.g., "My partner doesn't think I'm sexually interesting anymore because of my erection problem"), or about a partner's symptoms (e.g., "My partner's decreased interest in sex means she doesn't love me anymore"). An individual who has such thoughts commonly believes them without investigating their validity.

With regard to *expectancies*, individuals commonly make negative predictions about the future associated with sexual problems. For example, they may think, "If we try to make love, I won't perform well, and we'll both be upset," and "If I keep disappointing my partner sexually, my partner will find someone else and leave me." The fear of inadequate performance has been a core concept in the field, beginning with Masters and Johnson's (1970) work. Once a couple has experienced an upsetting instance of a sexual problem, one or both partners may develop an expectancy of future occurrences. The negative impact of those distracting thoughts on sexual response the next time they try to be sexual can result in a self-fulfilling prophecy.

Selective perception, in which an individual notices some aspects of a situation but overlooks others, can produce a negative bias when sexual problems occur. Examples include, "When I'm trying to please my partner sexually, he *never* shows *any* signs that he's enjoying it," and "*Nothing* seems to get me in the mood for sex these days." As with many life problems, concern about an issue can focus one's attention on it, restricting one's attention to other information. The selective focus on the adequacy of one's sexual responses has been labeled "spectatoring" by sex therapists (Kaplan, 1974). Thus, individuals who are worried about their own or a partner's lack of pleasure and arousal during sexual touching commonly tune out cues of positive responses. Consequently, the sex therapy procedure of *sensate focus* that we describe in this chapter is designed to shift clients' attention from negative cues, such as lack of an erection, to positive cues such as pleasurable sensations from touching a partner's skin or from being touched. The opposite of negative self-consciousness in spectatoring is *self-entrancement* (Metz et al., 2018) in which an individual focuses on erotic sensations and emotional arousal.

Linear thinking rather than circular thinking also can contribute to individual and couple distress regarding sexual problems. The medical model that has dominated sex therapy and is reflected in the DSM diagnoses focuses on desire, arousal, and orgasm symptoms of an individual, and of course physical and psychological factors are involved in many sexual presenting problems. Nevertheless, interpersonal and environmental factors also play major roles in many cases, and a tendency for helping professionals or clients to focus on deficits in a symptomatic individual can result in one or both partners blaming that person. We strongly recommend a relational approach to assessment and treatment that emphasizes contributions both members can make to create an environment that nurtures mutual sexual interest and enjoyment (see Metz et al., 2018, for a detailed discussion of this framework).

Finally, variation in individuals' awareness of their internal experiences, including their momentary automatic thoughts and underlying schemas, must be taken into account in understanding sexual dysfunctions and treating them. The more obvious symptoms of lack of interest in a partner's initiation of sex, cues of limited physical arousal, and anorgasmia easily can draw both partners' attention, precluding introspection regarding internal cognitions and emotions, as well as subtle behavioral interactions (e.g., fleeting facial expressions). Consistent with our CBCT model, it is important to assess partners' awareness and enhance it as needed.

Emotion in Sexual Dysfunction

Although Masters and Johnson (1970) emphasized the cognitive component of anticipation of failure in sexual performance (i.e., a negative expectancy), emotional anxiety symptoms are likely to be associated with the negative predictions. Kaplan (1974) also described anticipatory anxiety involving a prediction that one will perform inadequately and cause a negative response from one's partner. She identified interventions (e.g., sensate focus exercises) designed to reduce the negative expectancies and anxiety. Furthermore, individuals who experience anxiety commonly attempt to cope with it by avoiding situations that elicit it. Avoidance can be behavioral (e.g., staying busy until one's partner has gone to sleep) or cognitive (e.g., ignoring cues of sexual interest from one's partner). Therapists also need to differentiate between anxiety that is restricted to a particular aspect of sex (e.g., anticipation of erectile dysfunction) and more pervasive anxiety disorders that meet criteria for a DSM diagnosis (e.g., generalized anxiety disorder) and may require concurrent individual therapy.

Anger, either at one's partner regarding specific sexual issues or conflicts in the broader relationship, is another common emotion that can interfere with sexual desire, arousal, and orgasm (Metz & Epstein, 2002; Metz et al., 2018). Even though some couples have arousing "make-up sex" after an argument, on the whole accumulated frustration and anger tend to counteract a positive atmosphere that facilitates sexual intimacy. Furthermore, if an individual's anger toward a partner is expressed through aggressive, vindictive actions, the damage to a sense of safety and connection in the relationship will detract from the sexual relationship.

Transitory sadness and more pervasive depression, which often are tied to perceived losses in one's life, also can detract from sexual experiences, and loss of sexual desire is a common symptom of clinical depression (American Psychiatric Association, 2022). Because depression also is associated with self-criticism, low self-esteem, and a sense of hopelessness regarding one's life, it is important to evaluate symptoms for a potential clinical disorder.

Shame (a blend of anxiety, sadness, and anger toward oneself) also arises commonly with sexual dysfunction, as the individual judges themself harshly. In contrast to feeling guilty for actions one judges to be unacceptable and is motivated to improve, experiencing shame involves attacking one's core self ("I'm defective. I'm a worthless human being"). As we described in Chapter 1, shame tends to be dysfunctional because it typically immobilizes the person and blocks opportunities to solve problems. Many people experience some shame when sexual dysfunctions occur, or even from communicating with a partner or therapist about intimate sexual responses. Consequently, therapists must use tact in exploring sexual topics with clients, creating privacy for each partner for describing their sexual history and current functioning.

Another issue that involves a mixture of behavior, emotion, and physical arousal that can affect couple sex is a partner's reliance on pornography for sexual pleasure. During an individual assessment interview, some individuals may reveal secret use of pornography, or during a couple interview, an individual may report discovering their partner's use. Individuals for whom pornography is one of their sexual outlets may disclose that they are attracted to their partner but rely on pornography for additional excitement, to experience types of sexual behavior vicariously in which the partner will not engage, or to cope with the partner's lower level of desire or their own insecurity about being a good lover. This may become a relationship problem if the individual sexual behavior begins to replace couple sex.

Individual and Dyadic Behavioral Patterns in Sexual Dysfunction

Individuals' behavior patterns associated with couple sexual interaction, as well as in response to signs of sexual problems, can influence whether normal transitory problems develop into a pattern of dysfunction. For example, a male who quickly tries to stimulate a partner, rushing toward a performance goal, may be ignoring his own need for a build-up of relaxed pleasurable sensations, resulting in erectile dysfunction. Furthermore, his focus on stimulating his partner may backfire as the partner feels pressured to respond and has an urge to withdraw. In addition, individuals who have developed negative expectancies of sexual failure commonly avoid sexual interactions with a partner, which may develop into a pursue–withdraw pattern (with the pursuing partner criticizing the individual for the lack of sex) or mutual avoidance. Because avoidance commonly has some positive consequences, as the individual is temporarily spared the emotional distress of dealing with an upset partner, clinicians must consider treatment strategies that engage the individual in reducing the avoidance. Often both partners have limited awareness of these patterns until a clinician conducts a detailed inquiry about how they interact sexually.

It also is important for therapists to avoid assuming that adult clients have good knowledge about sexual function and effective ways to share erotic arousal with a partner. Those whose sexual skills are limited often fail to ask what a partner enjoys or finds unpleasant, and partners who are wary of upsetting each other may avoid giving each other constructive feedback. They also may be unaware that conflict may have lingering effects on a positive atmosphere in their relationship that would encourage mutual interest in sex. A couple's deficits in communication and problem solving may be specific to a topic such as sex. Furthermore, a couple may use good expressive and listening skills when discussing some topics (e.g., finances ways to spend leisure time) but may avoid direct communication about sex. One or both members of a couple may avoid talking about their sexual relationship because they have an expectancy that "analyzing your sexual relationship will take the spontaneity and fun out of it." However, a couple's problematic communication and problem solving may be a broader pattern across many areas of their relationship. In either case, those skills should be targets of the treatment plan.

Relational and Environmental Stressors Contributing to Sexual Dysfunction

Stressors that change the dynamics of a couple's relationship can affect the quality of their sexual relationship. Some of those stressors originate within the couple, whereas others have sources in their interpersonal and physical environment. Clinicians need to identify those stressors and resources a couple has for coping with them.

Stressors Internal to the Couple's Relationship

A couple's experiences with a member's physical illness (e.g., heart disease, cancer), disability (e.g., arthritis, stroke), or other conditions that may change the partners' roles and patterns (e.g., couple treatment for infertility) can affect their sexual relationship. Partners' self-consciousness about the individual's physical pain, shared grief regarding the loss of prior health and concerns about mortality, shifts from a long-term partnership to a caretaker–patient relationship, and distracting intrusive medical treatments all can affect intimacy and mutual sexual enjoyment. A couple who previously had a smooth and mutually satisfying sexual relationship may feel helpless in the face of these factors that result in sex being far from smooth and natural. The less knowledge they have about ways to adjust to illnesses, disabilities, and so forth, the more helpless and hopeless they may feel. If they also hold a standard that "sex should be spontaneous and natural," the idea of making plans to interact sexually in specific new ways may seem to them like accepting failure.

Stressors in the Couple's Environment

Common sources of stress in a couple's environment include job demands, financial problems, child-rearing stressors (e.g., child health and educational problems, management of problematic child behavior), caregiving responsibilities with extended family, threats of neighborhood violence, and discrimination and violence based on social location characteristics such as race, ethnicity, religion, gender identity, sexual orientation, disability, or socioeconomic status. One major pathway through which these stressors can affect a sexual relationship is through primary effects on a member's individual functioning, as when job stresses dominate the individual's daily experiences, taking priority over intimacy with a partner. The effect on that person spills over, influencing the other partner. Another pathway is through a stressor's interference with a couple's typical ways of interacting sexually. For example, attending to children's needs may dominate a couple's time that earlier in their relationship was available for shared relaxation and sex. Similarly, if both members work long hours at low wages in order to support their family, they may be too tired chronically for sex. Couples may not think to describe environmental stressors during an intake assessment.

COUPLE THERAPIES FOR SEXUAL RELATIONSHIP PROBLEMS AND EMPIRICAL SUPPORT

Although sexual dysfunctions have been identified as disorders of individuals, to a large extent treatments have involved an individual's partner whenever possible, based on an assumption that benefits from exercises performed on one's own have limited generalization to couple interactions. Nevertheless, the role of an identified patient's partner in traditional sex therapy has been largely supportive, encouraging the individual and engaging in couple exercises designed to reduce that person's anxiety and increase focus on pleasurable sensations. Those interventions have been based primarily on cognitive-behavioral principles for counteracting anxiety and associated counterproductive behavior such as avoidance of sex (Guttman, 2020; Metz et al., 2018). The therapist would intervene when appropriate to modify the other partner's behavior (e.g., reducing their pressure on the individual to respond sexually), but dyadic patterns were less a focus than is typical in couple therapy. Conversely, couple therapists commonly receive limited education and training in treating sexual dysfunction and often depend on referrals to certified sex therapists. However, mutual influences between overall relationship issues and sexual problems are significant, and couple therapists are likely to hear about sexual concerns from clients who sought therapy for a variety of other issues. Because sex therapy is a specialized field of knowledge and skills, it is crucial that couple therapists not venture beyond their areas of expertise. However, Binik and Meana (2009) argue that exaggerating the specialized expertise necessary to provide *any* sex therapy runs a risk of marginalizing the field and inhibiting competent clinicians from treating sexual problems. We concur with that position and believe the key is taking responsibility for accumulating depth of knowledge about sexual dysfunctions, their determinants, and interventions with empirical support.

Thus, we believe there is much that a couple therapist can do to assist clients with sexual problems, as long as they develop sufficient knowledge and skills and know their limits of expertise. A number of publications have described applications of various couple therapy models to sexual dysfunction, focusing on an integration of interventions for dyadic couple processes and intrapsychic processes within a symptomatic individual. Nelson's (2020) edited volume includes chapters on the theory and methods of several diverse treatments, such as EFT, Imago Relationship Therapy, Internal Family Systems, nutrition-focused intervention, art therapy, and mindfulness treatment. Overall, limited research has been done on the effectiveness of the approaches that are covered, but the trend toward integrating work on sexual problems into diverse popular couple therapies is valuable. We previously noted the application of EFT to sexual presenting problems (Johnson et al., 2018), which focuses on empirically supported interventions that address attachment and emotional bonding problems that are relevant to assisting couples whose sexual issues include partners' attachment problems. The highly integrative intersystem approach (Weeks & Gambescia, 2015; Weeks, Gambescia, & Hertlein, 2020) assesses and intervenes with multilayered factors contributing to sexual dysfunction, such as individual attachment problems, couple relationship conflicts, family-of-origin influences, environmental stressors, cultural values, and religious beliefs. Metz et al. (2018) detail a biopsychosocial model of sexual function that integrates the influences of physiological, individual psychological, and couple dyadic interaction processes and emphasizes cognitive-behavioral interventions at both the individual and couple levels. That approach is the primary focus of this chapter.

RESEARCH ON SEX THERAPY EFFECTIVENESS

There is consensus in the professional literature that empirical research on sex therapy interventions has been limited (Binik & Meana, 2009; Metz et al., 2018; Hall & Binik, 2020). The vast majority of studies have used individual or group therapy formats and have been based on case studies and pilot studies without control groups rather than randomized clinical trials. The lack of rigorous research may be due to the lasting enthusiasm from the original findings from Masters and Johnson's institute indicating high success rates and the very limited external funding available for research on sex therapy (with more funds for tests of pharmacological treatments; Metz et al., 2018). Nevertheless, the published studies show a pattern of encouraging results, with greater success found for female low sexual desire and inorgasmia (Frühauf et al., 2013) and male erectile disorder (Bilal & Abbasi, 2020). Most research has focused on cognitive-behavioral protocols, which are the most common interventions for various sexual dysfunctions (see Hall & Binik, 2020). Encouraging results from cognitive-behaviorally based group mindfulness interventions for females and males, primarily case studies and uncontrolled outcome studies, are a recent development (Brossio, Basson, Driscoll, Correia, & Brotto, 2018; Brotto, Chivers, Millman, & Albert, 2016; Patterson, Handy, & Brotto, 2017). Outcome studies are needed on couple sex therapy models, including the CBCT approach that we use. Furthermore, given that sex researchers and therapists have only recently focused on the needs of clients with diverse sexual orientations and gender identities, it is not surprising that there is a dearth of outcome research on any modality of sex therapy for those populations.

THERAPIST DECISIONS REGARDING APPROPRIATENESS OF COUPLE SEXUAL THERAPY

Because interventions pioneered by Masters and Johnson (1966, 1970) and Kaplan (1974) and sex therapy methods that have grown from those foundations include significant attention to diagnosed individuals' couple relationships, the key question that arises revolves around when it would *not* be appropriate and preferential to use couple therapy. Some important considerations include individuals with sexual trauma histories for whom partner involvement may trigger intense levels of distress (and partner inclusion may be appropriate at a later stage of treatment), individuals with severe shame responses regarding sex, and those whose partners pose a risk for psychological and physical aggression. Even without partner aggression, a couple's severe conflict and relationship distress may have created an aversive environment in their relationship, and couple therapy addressing those relationship problems may be needed before treatment of sexual problems. Aspects of an individual's sexuality, such as compulsive sexual behavior and high reliance on specific paraphilias for arousal, also can interfere with partner sex and should be part of intake assessment procedures.

DECISIONS REGARDING REFERRALS TO OTHER PROFESSIONALS

Regardless of a clinician's expertise for assessing and intervening with sexual dysfunctions, unless they have an appropriate medical specialty degree, it is important that they have the capacity to make referrals to gynecologists, urologists, and other physicians for adequate evaluation of biological factors in clients' dysfunctions. In addition, some clients may prefer a clinician who shares their gender identity or sexual orientation, so it is advantageous to know colleagues who may be options. Finally, assessment may indicate that a symptomatic individual (and/or their partner) experiences clinically significant psychological symptoms such as depression and anxiety, as well as problematic patterns such as compulsive sexual behavior, and referral for concurrent individual therapy is advisable.

SCREENING AND ASSESSMENT FOR SEXUAL PROBLEMS

Initial Couple Assessment Interview

Some clients mention sexual issues in their initial contact with a couple therapist, but many do not. In either case, it is important to at least briefly inquire about the quality of the couple's sexual relationship during the first couple assessment session (see Chapter 3). We routinely ask about the sexual relationship in a matter-of-fact manner, embedded among questions about a variety of topics, such as opportunities the partners have to spend leisure time together, how they express caring for each other, and how they communicate when faced with a problem. If the therapist has administered the Relationship Issues Survey and one or both members have indicated that their sexual relationship is a source of some conflict, the therapist can inquire about it during the individual interview with that person.

When one or both members of a couple spontaneously mention sexual issues or respond affirmatively to the therapist's general inquiry, we begin by asking an open-ended question, "How would the two of you describe the concern you have about your sexual relationship?" We notice not only how they describe the problem, but also their apparent emotional responses and behavior toward each other (e.g., one person expressing dissatisfaction while the other says little). Without going into additional detail, we try to get a sense of the extent to which partners agree on whether sexual issues concern desire/frequency, arousal, or orgasm. Because at this point we have not established a comfortable therapeutic alliance, we do not push for more information, but we ask whether the sexual concerns are one of the topics they would like to spend time on in our sessions. If one or both partners decline, we take note of it and say, "Okay. Let's begin with concerns you both have about topics you have mentioned, such as. . . ."

If both partners have discussed a sexual concern relatively comfortably in this session, the therapist can ask for more information, including whether there was an earlier time when they did not experience the problem, when they first noticed the problem, and what they have tried to improve it. At this point, questions about the type of problem (e.g., a difference in partners' levels of sexual desire or types of sexual behavior they most enjoy, difficulties with desire, arousal or orgasm, how they behave toward each other whenever the problem occurs) are reasonable. However, the therapist should preface them with a statement that although a clinician needs to understand what occurs with a problem, it is important that the couple feel comfortable with the questions and free to request that they go more slowly, as they and the clinician hardly know each other. It also is important to state that the clinician's only goal in asking personal questions about the history of their sexual concerns is to design a treatment plan to help them, and the clients are in control of what they choose to disclose.

Information about the timeline of a sexual problem can be integrated into the relationship history component of the joint assessment interview, perhaps identifying links between occurrence of the sexual problem and particular stressors the couple experienced together. This exploration can include both partners' beliefs about how the stressors influenced their sexual relationship and their memories of how they communicated about their experiences. Information about the timeline of the occurrence of the problem is helpful in distinguishing between a chronic issue that may have predated the couple's relationship and a situational one. The therapist explains how it is helpful to explore possible factors that have contributed to a sexual problem and to take them into account when setting therapy goals and planning treatment.

With regard to inquiry into the couple interaction patterns associated with their sexual relationship, at this point the therapist notes any details the clients describe but lets them know that during treatment further assessment will focus on the sequence of actions and responses between them during sexual interaction (who does what; how each person responds to the other).

Individual Interview with Each Partner

The individual interview with each member of the couple is another opportunity to gather information about a sexual problem and factors contributing to it. Again, the therapist should describe reasons for asking about details of the problem and related experiences in the person's life and couple relationship and reemphasize the client's control over what is discussed. It is crucial to monitor evidence of an individual's discomfort regarding their sexual problem, including cognitions (e.g., "I'm a failure sexually"), emotions (e.g., anxiety), and behavior (e.g., defensively criticizing their partner; avoiding sex).

Actions a therapist can take to reduce a client's distress about discussing sexual problems include describing one's training and experience in working with similar problems; demonstrating warmth, empathy, and validation when clients disclose personal material; demonstrating comfort with discussing sexual topics; and emphasizing details of client–therapist confidentiality (Metz et al., 2018). These qualities not only help individuals feel more comfortable sharing information; they also can help counteract prior experiences a person may have had in which sexual topics were taboo. The therapist states that goals include not only improving any sexual difficulties the couple is experiencing, but also helping them feel better about themselves. This process results not only from developing one's self concept as a "good lover" (focused on the other person's pleasure) but also from understanding one's own body and sexuality (what produces one's own physical and emotional pleasure).

It is important that a therapist not take for granted a couple's description of a sexual problem as being due to a dysfunction within one partner. Often, a more detailed inquiry uncovers factors within the other partner (e.g., a sexual dysfunction, psychopathology symptoms), as well as couple dynamics, that influence the individual's sexual issues. For example, a heterosexual couple may present with a female's low sexual arousal, but the therapist may uncover erectile dysfunction on the male's part. Past experiences of the male becoming defensive about his erectile dysfunction may have led to the female being distracted from her own pleasure. Patterns such as this require the therapist to use tact if neither partner has been comfortable discussing the other's problems or willing to set goals that include help for both partners' difficulties.

The therapist includes questions about the individual's sexual history within the broader personal history interview (see Chapter 3). The sexual history covers the topics listed in Figure 7.1, and the clinician should follow up with further questions to clarify each person's experiences.

Use of Questionnaires

Researchers have developed a number of questionnaires to assess aspects of sexual response, including desire, arousal, orgasm, and individuals' patterns of sexual behavior with a partner. An example of a fairly brief scale that is readily accessible in a published journal article and can be used for initial screening is Spector, Carey, and Steinberg's (1996) Sexual Desire Inventory (SDI). This questionnaire includes items such as "How strong is your desire to engage in sexual activity with a partner?" (rated from 0 = no desire to 8 = strong desire), and it has subsets of items regarding sex with a partner and sex by oneself. However, instruments such as the SDI tend to focus on cisgender individuals and forms of sexual behavior. Using such questionnaires to ask transgender individuals (both those who have chosen medical treatments to modify their bodies and those who have not) to report on sexual attraction, desire, arousal, and orgasm provides the clinician little information regarding the impact of being transgender (including gender dysphoria) and the impact of treatments on the ability to enjoy one's body and have mutually pleasurable interactions with a partner (Holmberg et al., 2020; Spencer, Iantaffi, & Bockting, 2017).

Due to the limitations of standardized questionnaires, we primarily use interviews to assess the types, frequency, and intensity of clients' sexual presenting problems, although an individual's responses to questionnaire items can be useful cues for more in-depth assessment. Through interviews, the clinician can inquire about sensitive material in a socioculturally attuned manner that is tailored to clients' gender identity and sexual orientation, as well as their ethnicities, races, and religions, etc. that may influence their ways of thinking and behaving sexually. This attention to diversity contributes to a positive therapeutic relationship. Interviews also allow the clinician to assess areas such as partners' levels of sex education regarding diversity in human sexual responses, their knowledge about ways to please a partner while also seeking pleasure for oneself, the impact of prior sexual trauma, and each person's comfort with setting limits with a partner on sexual consent. Figure 7.1 includes questions regarding sex education, sexual knowledge, comfort with and interest in various sexual behaviors, and the sexual relationship with one's current partner.

Assessment of Cognitions during Assessment Interviews and Treatment Sessions

We rely on cognitive therapy assessment methods (Chapter 3) to identify partners' cognitions related to their sexual concerns. Because some couples reveal a lot about their sexual relationship during joint and individual assessment interviews, whereas others choose not to discuss sex, the methods we describe here are used either during initial assessments or are delayed until a couple decides to address sex later during treatment sessions.

One approach to identifying individuals' cognitions regarding their own sexuality and the couple relationship is to listen for spontaneously voiced thoughts. An individual may voice an automatic thought that describes potential selective perception (e.g., "My partner never responds positively when I hint that I'm interested in sex"), an attribution (e.g., "My partner doesn't get aroused from my touching because she's not attracted to me"), or an expectancy (e.g., "I'll prob-

Introductory statement by the interviewer: Because you told me you have concerns about your sexual relationship with your partner, it will be very helpful to me to learn some things about your personal background regarding sexuality and how you feel about sex as part of your life now. I am accustomed to talking with people about sex, but I realize that many people may have some discomfort talking about it. I want you to know you have control about the topics we will discuss regarding sex. Please feel free to tell me at any point that you prefer not to talk about a particular topic, and we will move to another topic. I also want you to know that anything we discuss is confidential between you and me, and I will not share any information you tell me with your partner or anyone else. [If the interviewer is a mandated reporter regarding child sexual abuse and is required to report instances in which the client was abused at any point in the past, the client should be informed about that before the interviewer asks any questions.] Some of my questions will include experiences you had as you grew up, and then other questions will be about your sexual relationship with your current partner.

- Who did you learn about sex from (e.g., parents, siblings, friends, school, TV and movies, books and magazines, internet, social media, religious organizations, sexual partners)? Who taught you what? From what you know now, how accurate was the information that you learned from them?
- To what extent were you taught that sex is a positive aspect of life or negative?
- Children often are curious about bodies and sex, and do some exploring of themselves and with other children. What exploration do you remember doing as a child? To what extent do you remember the exploration being comfortable or uncomfortable?
- What sexual experiences do you remember having during adolescence, and how comfortable or uncomfortable were they?
- What sexual experiences did you have as a young adult and after that, that you think influenced your feelings and comfort about sex?
- If you had any stressful or disturbing sexual experiences, what, if any, help did you receive in dealing with them (from friends, family, helping professionals)?
- Describe any other types of stress in your life (e.g., job demands, raising children, health problems) that seem to affect your experiences with sex.
- Please describe any ways in which your cultural background, religious beliefs and traditions, gender identity, sexual orientation, or any other aspect of who you are influence how you think about sex and the role that sex has in your personal life.
- Overall, how would you describe the quality of your relationship with your partner?
- What aspects of it seem fine to you? Describe any ways you wish it was different.
- How often do you and your partner tend to engage in sexual activity together? Who tends to initiate it? If one of you is interested in being sexual but the other is not, how do the two of you deal with it?
- What, if any, types of sexual behavior with your partner do you experience as pleasant? Unpleasant?
- If there is a difficulty in your sexual relationship with your partner, please describe it.
- How long has this been a difficulty? When did you first notice it? How mild or severe is it? [If the individual vaguely acknowledges some difficulty, follow up with specific questions about lack of sexual desire, a desire discrepancy between partners, lack of or limited arousal, lack of or limited experience of orgasm, sexual pain.]
- How often does this difficulty seem to occur? Describe particular situations when it seems most likely to occur. What do you think causes it?
- What is your sense of how your partner thinks and feels about this difficulty?

(continued)

FIGURE 7.1. Topics for individual sexual history and current functioning interview.

- When this difficulty occurs, how does it affect the relationship with your partner?
- How much and how well do the two of you communicate about your sexual relationship?
- What have you and your partner done so far to try to improve this difficulty? How helpful have your attempts to solve it been?
- To what extent would you like an aspect of your sexual relationship with your partner to be part of what we discuss and work on during our couple therapy?

FIGURE 7.1. *(continued)*

ably fail to get an erection, which will deeply disappoint my partner"). Because people commonly believe their attributions, accurate or not, those that involve negative inferences about oneself or one's partner likely result in emotional upset. Similarly, Metz et al. (2018) note that negative expectancies often become self-fulfilling prophecies, as when an individual who expects to experience erectile dysfunction is distracted from noticing pleasurable sensations and fails to become aroused. Individuals also may spontaneously describe an underlying belief, such as an assumption about sex (e.g., "Losing interest in sex is an inevitable part of getting older"), a standard (e.g., "Now that I've had [gender-affirming] genital surgery, my body is too unattractive to let anyone see and touch it"), or an expectancy (e.g., "Now that I had top surgery and no longer want to get sexual pleasure from my former breasts, my partner is still going to want to touch me there and will be frustrated with me about it").

A second but related approach is to notice that an individual is exhibiting cues of an internal reaction to a partner's actions or an inquiry from the therapist during a session and to probe for the person's cognitions. For example, when the therapist says, "As I understand it, there's a difference between you in how often you are interested in some sexual activity," one partner may nod in agreement but the other partner looks downward, exhibits a slumped posture, and says nothing. The therapist then addresses the latter individual: "I noticed you had a reaction to my comment about an apparent difference in sexual interest between the two of you. Please tell me what thoughts you had when I said that, as well as any emotions you experienced." The client responds, "I was thinking, 'I'm such a loser for not showing interest in my partner. No one is going to want to be in a relationship with me,' and I was feeling sad." The therapist can use this inquiry to track the interaction between the partners. Thus, when the therapist notices the partner's negative facial expression in response to the individual's comment about being a loser, the therapist can ask about the partner's thoughts and emotions at that moment. The partner may reply, "I feel like I have to walk on eggshells or else my partner sinks into depression. I'm frustrated." This tracking of the couple's moment-to-moment reactions to each other contributes to treatment planning by identifying points for interventions with their interaction sequences.

Finally, the therapist can ask partners directly about particular types of cognition. For example, one can ask about their assumptions regarding normal human sexual response and factors that can interfere with a person's desire, arousal, or orgasm. This may uncover inaccurate beliefs and suggest topics for psychoeducation. Clients can be asked about their standards for personal sexuality (e.g., how automatically one should respond sexually to an attractive partner), characteristics of one's partner (e.g., how important it is for one's partner to remain as physically attractive as possible as the couple ages), and the sexual relationship (e.g., how much sexual "chemistry" should exist regardless of circumstances such as life stressors). Similarly, the therapist can tap individuals' attributions by asking questions such as "What do you think contributed to your recent decrease in sexual desire?" and uncover expectancies with questions such as, "If one of you expresses interest in sexual activity but the other politely says they are not in the mood presently, what do you think will happen next between you?" Finally, the therapist can probe for selective perception by asking members of a couple what they notice through their senses (e.g., sights, sounds, physical sensations) during joint sexual activity. Members of couples who experience sexual dysfunctions often selectively notice cues associated with the sexual problem (e.g., a partner's negative reactions to one's touch, signs of one's own limited physical arousal) and overlook pleasant sensations (e.g., how it feels to touch a partner's skin, a partner's vocalization that conveys enjoyment of one's touching). Educating clients that "there's a lot going on at any moment when a couple are interacting physically" and increasing their attention to overlooked positive cues are important components of a treatment plan.

Assessment of Emotion during Assessment Interviews and Treatment Sessions

Consistent with CBCT procedures for assessing emotional responses (see Chapter 3), the options are similar to those for assessing cognition. First, the therapist can inquire about cues to emotion expressed by each member spontaneously either verbally (e.g., "Seeing my partner giving me hints about wanting sex immediately makes me very anxious.") or nonverbally (e.g., an individual exhibits possible signs of shame such as lowered head, sighing, and holding their head after their partner criticized them for having low desire). Because emotional contagion occurs very quickly between partners, the therapist can point out that process as it occurs during a session. For example, the therapist can interrupt the interaction and ask, "Did the two of you notice how a few minutes ago you were having a calm discussion but very quickly you both seemed to become very tense, talking faster and speaking with greater emotional intensity? Let's look at how that emotional build-up happened."

The tracking of emotional responses often reveals situational triggers that need to be addressed with the individual and couple. For example, it may become evident that a member of a couple becomes anxious most often as a result of expectancies that their partner's actions signify a risk that the partner will withdraw love. This insecure attachment response may be the result of a lifelong attachment issue but may also have developed from an attachment injury within the couple's relationship, such as infidelity. Information about the origins of emotional responses helps the therapist and couple plan interventions at the individual and couple levels.

In addition to tracking moment-to-moment emotional responses, the therapist can inquire about particular emotional responses. A sample question is "When you are talking about sex or showing sexual interest in each other, what helps both of you feel relaxed? What makes you feel anxiety?" Another question that captures a dyadic process is "When one of you would like to have a positive sexual response but it doesn't go as you wish, what emotions do you tend to experience?" To the other partner: "When you notice your partner is having negative emotions about their sexual response, how do you feel? How do you tend to respond to your partner?"

It also is important to ask about partners' beliefs about emotion itself, because their assumptions about emotional processes can influence their expectancies about the potential for change. For example, when an individual assumes that anger is a powerful force that takes control over a person's actions ("I have a short fuse, so my strong anger comes on quickly, and I can't stop myself from yelling and cursing"), interventions to reduce partner aggression resulting from sexual frustration must address that rigid belief (see Chapter 5). Many individuals experiencing sexual dysfunction have similar assumptions about anxiety, interpreting it as a powerful and seemingly unchangeable force that interferes with sexual response. That belief about anxiety must be identified and addressed in the treatment plan.

Sometimes individuals are confused about the strong emotions they experience during interactions with their partner and how to process them in a constructive way rather than responding impulsively. An example is when an individual's partner discloses dissatisfaction with an aspect of the couple's sexual relationship (e.g., "I've been getting bored by how routine our sex has become") and the individual suddenly experiences a mix of strong negative emotions (e.g., anger, anxiety, shame) and reacts defensively (e.g., with criticism of the partner). This pattern can escalate conflict between the partners and interfere with their understanding of each other's needs and feelings. A therapist can interrupt the negative exchange, help the upset person explore the emotions the partner's comments about their relationship triggered, and identify what it was about the partner's comments that was so upsetting.

Assessment of Behavior during Assessment Interviews and Treatment Sessions

Although direct observation of couples' sexual interactions is not possible, therapists do have opportunities to watch partners discuss their relationship during sessions and obtain samples of how they communicate about sex, express dissatisfaction with each other, and attempt to solve sexual problems. The therapist can assume that the clients may not be demonstrating their typical behavior in the therapy room. However, therapists commonly experience partners becoming emotionally involved while discussing a topic and exhibiting behavior that seems minimally censored.

When the therapist asks a couple to describe their typical behavioral patterns associated with sex, at times there is a high degree of agreement, but at other times notable disagreement, especially when they hold each other responsible for a sexual presenting problem. Therapists can deal with this challenge by asking the couple why they think their memories are so different. The therapist can emphasize that each person has a unique perspective about events, and it will be helpful for them and the therapist to keep each viewpoint in mind when trying to devise a plan for improvement in their sexual issues. By using input from both partners, the therapist can work toward achieving a reasonable approximation to the couple's moment-to-moment behavioral interactions (e.g., who initiates sex and how, who avoids or responds favorably and how).

In addition to assessing a couple's sexual behavioral pattern, it is helpful to gather information about partners' sexual behavioral skills (e.g., for exhibiting enticing behavior, touching a partner in ways that the recipient finds pleasurable, increasing erotic touch when the partner wants it). Individuals with couple sexual problems often develop unrealistic ideas about sexual relationship skills from watching idealized portrayals of intense lovemaking in movies and other media (Metz et al., 2018). Depending on each couple's comfort level with discussing their sexual behavior, the therapist has the option of asking about skills initially during individual rather than joint sessions. The therapist may be able to piece together from the separate reports a reasonable view of each member's sexual skills and how satisfying the recipient experiences them. However, for purposes of treatment planning, it will be important for the therapist to engage the couple eventually in discussion of these behavioral patterns and desired changes. When one or both members exhibit discomfort with expressing dissatisfaction with specific aspects of their sexual interactions, it is important to explore associated barriers, such as a desire to avoid hurting the other person's feelings or inciting the partner to withdraw sexually.

Identification of Individuals' Characteristics That May Require Individual Treatment

The cognitive, emotional, and behavioral responses regarding sexuality exhibited by each member of a couple may reflect individual psychological characteristics or disorders and may require individual therapy in addition to couple interventions. Examples are posttraumatic stress disorder (especially from prior sexual trauma), clinical depression, anxiety disorders, substance use disorders, and sexual addictions and compulsions (Metz et al., 2018). An individual's stressful life experiences regarding sex that do not qualify for a DSM diagnosis also should be explored. These life experiences include humiliation by a sexual partner, resulting in a poor sexual self-concept; a tendency to be perfectionistic that one applies to sexuality; an insecure attachment style that interferes with intimacy; and a tendency to be overwhelmed by life stressors such as job demands. Therapists should inquire about such characteristics during the individual assessment interviews. However, some clients may fail to reveal some of their individual challenges before they have developed a good alliance with the therapist, so therapists should continue to be alert for symptoms of individual disorders throughout therapy sessions with the couple as well.

GOAL SETTING AND SOCIALIZATION TO TREATMENT

Based on assessment of the partners and their relationship, goal setting for the treatment plan is based on information regarding physical, cognitive, emotional, couple behavioral, and environmental factors influencing the sexual presenting problems. Although the primary sex therapy interventions are delivered in the couple context, one or both partners may have historical or current personal issues that conjoint sessions may be insufficient to address. Some individual characteristics may be specific to sexuality (e.g., past sexual trauma, gender dysphoria involving discomfort with one's genitals), whereas others may have broader negative influences on the person's life (e.g., chronic depression, substance abuse). The latter category of personal issues likely is affecting the couple's overall relationship as well as their sexual relationship. As we describe in Chapter 10, individual psychopathology in one or both partners can be addressed through a combination of individual and conjoint interventions, with the individual therapy component being essential for severe disorders.

Thus, a couple may present with both members viewing one person's low sexual desire as a significant problem, and they both may hypothesize that the low desire is due to the individual's chronic clinical depression, a factor that may be supported by the therapist's assessment. However, the therapist also may have learned that the other partner has persistently engaged in psychological aggression toward the symptomatic individual, a likely risk factor for both depression and low desire. The bottom line is that sexual presenting problems often have multiple determinants, and goal setting must incorporate changes in those factors. Because many clients enter therapy conceptualizing a sexual problem in a simpler way, the therapist faces the challenge of helping the couple understand the reasons for setting subgoals to the overall goal of improving the specific sexual problem. This process is similar to educating couples regarding multiple determinants of an individual's psychopathology symptoms and engaging both partners in changing patterns that influence the problem (see Chapter 10). It involves shifting the sole focus from an individual with a diagnosable disorder to one in which members of the couple collaborate to create conditions that are more conducive to a mutually satisfying sexual relationship. That means striking a balance between improving physical, cognitive, emotional, and behavioral factors within a symptomatic individual and improving couple interactions.

Engaging both members of a couple with collaborative treatment goals necessitates avoiding blame toward either person. The therapist can emphasize that the symptoms of the individual with the sexual dysfunction are stressful for both people, and improvement is likely to increase satisfaction for both. The therapist socializes the couple to a dyadic approach that, among other things, involves practicing good communication and problem-solving skills, showing mutual emotional support, and taking personal responsibility for regulating one's emotions, which results in both partners feeling understood and respected. As we stress throughout this book, discussions with a couple regarding the rationale for working on open communication must involve sensitivity to the clients' cultural beliefs and traditions regarding communication, especially discussions about sexuality. The therapist emphasizes that the foundation for a good sexual relationship is a strong overall couple relationship. The treatment will therefore focus on how they relate to each other in general as well as specifically regarding sex. There will be no pressure to talk about sensitive topics regarding sex, but because a couple has mentioned a sexual difficulty, the couple will benefit if they and the therapist can identify ways to reduce the difficulty.

Socializing the couple into the CBCT approach to sexual dysfunction also involves providing a strong rationale for any goals that involve improvement of an individual partner's functioning. The rationale must avoid blame but emphasize taking personal responsibility for one's behavior and making good faith efforts to improve the couple relationship. For example, a therapist may explain to a couple:

> "As I've gotten to know you through our assessment sessions, I noticed that when the two of you disagree about something, it gets tense between you fairly quickly. The tension includes some negative forms of communication, such as criticism, name-calling, refusing to talk, etc. Negative interactions are likely to take a toll in the moment and also over time on both your overall relationship happiness and the quality of your sexual relationship. It seems to me that setting a goal of reducing conflict and improving communication could help a lot toward achieving your goal of a better sexual relationship."

If the therapist views the nonsymptomatic partner as more responsible for the aversive interactions, this wording is intended to engage that person in change efforts, and during treatment sessions the partner's negative behavior would be addressed clearly. In cases in which a partner engages in abusive behavior, the therapist would take a strong stand to protect the victim.

Subgoals would target physical, cognitive, emotional, behavioral, and environmental factors identified in the assessment. Both members' cognitive, emotional, and behavioral responses to an individual's sexual symptoms are addressed. For example, a couple may present with a transgender female who received hormone therapy to modify secondary sexual characteristics and is experiencing low sexual desire. A goal may involve reducing the individual's own negative reactions, including cognitions such as "I used to look forward to sex, but now I'm a sexual mess because my desire is gone"; emotions such as anxiety associated with concern about losing her partner; and behavior such as avoiding talking with her partner about the problem. In turn, therapy goals may focus on the partner's negative reactions, including cognitions such as "My partner's lack of interest in sex with me means she doesn't really love me"; emotions such as deep sadness; and behavior such as criticizing the partner ("What's the matter with you!"). Therapy goals also target any environmental factors that affect the sexual relationship. For example, an individual's desire and arousal may be diminished by distractions such as chronic work demands, exhausting caretaking of an ill family member, or discrimination on the basis of sexual orientation, gender identity, race, and so on. An example of a dyadic stressor directly interfering with couple sex is a newborn in the family. Treatment goals for any of those stressors would include enhancing dyadic coping skills for collaborative problem solving.

Goal setting and treatment methods for sexual dysfunctions apply principles of partner-assisted, disorder-specific, and couple therapy interventions that we also use with psychopathology presenting problems (Chapter 10). An example of a partner-assisted goal would be both members of the couple receiving psychoeducation about a dysfunction and a nonsymptomatic individual providing encouragement and coaching as a symptomatic partner practices sex therapy exercises such as challenging anti-erotic negative automatic thoughts or engaging in mindfulness tasks. In contrast, an example of a disorder-specific goal would be modifying dyadic patterns that maintain sexual dysfunction symptoms. The therapist would give the couple feedback about their pattern (e.g., when they begin sexual touching and an individual exhibits no signs of arousal, they mutually back off and avoid each other for a while) and focus on changes that both members can work toward. Finally, traditional couple therapy for the overall relationship would include improving communication skills, reducing escalation of mutual negative emotion during conflict, and expanding the couple's shared behavior that contributes to emotional intimacy.

PLANNING TREATMENT

Our approach to treating sexual dysfunctions within the couple context integrates traditional sex therapy interventions derived from Masters and Johnson's original methods and later developments that mostly have been cognitive-behavioral. For the sake of clarity, we present interventions regarding physical factors, cognitions, behavior, and emotion in separate sections, but therapists commonly combine them.

Interventions for Physical Factors

Because the foundation of sexual responses is biological processes, it is essential that treatment plans include attention to medical conditions and medical treatments that may be influencing individuals' functioning. Sometimes a physical factor is quite obvious, as when an individual describes chronic pain associated with arthritis that interferes with sexual behavior and distracts the person from pleasurable sensations. In other cases, the role of physical factors may be less obvious at first. Thus, an individual may state, "My body works fine once I'm in the mood and we start sexual touching; it's just that I rarely feel any desire." Although this problem may reflect the psychological processes we described earlier or a relationship issue such as a lack of emotional intimacy, it is wise for the therapist to explore possible physical factors and rule them out or identify the need for adjunctive medical treatment. As we have explained, low desire can result from chronic health conditions, the side effects of medications, and use of recreational substances. When the assessment identifies any of these potential physical factors, it is prudent for the therapist to provide the couple psychoeducation about physical health factors that commonly influence sexual response and to request written permission from them to consult with their physicians. Changes such as reducing alcohol intake or switching to a medication with fewer sexual side effects can contribute to progress. Furthermore, the therapist can enlist an individual's physician to provide additional psychoeducation to the couple regarding physical conditions, medications, and health behaviors that may be contributing to a sexual problem.

Individuals' sexual functioning also can be influenced by their partner's physical health. For example, a partner of an individual with painful arthritis may become preoccupied with efforts to minimize the individual's suffering. This focus can restrain the partner from engaging in sexual behavior that the partner finds exciting, and continuously monitoring the other person for signs of pain (selective perception) can result in overlooking one's own physical and emotional pleasure. A partner's tendency to avoid communicating openly with an individual regarding physical health problems may be based on the partner's standard that a caring partner protects their loved one and negative expectancies that direct communication will upset the individual further. When a couple therapist uncovers such counterproductive partner cognitions and behavior that interfere with finding solutions to health problems and ultimately ignore the partner's own needs, the treatment plan can include interventions to modify those cognitions, as well as to improve open communication between partners. Thus, the therapist can intervene with the cognitions and behavioral responses of both partners that may be eliciting or maintaining an individual's sexual symptoms.

Interventions for Cognition

In the preceding description of interventions for physical factors affecting sexual function, we noted that interventions for unrealistic and inaccurate cognitions often are needed. Psychoeducation is a valuable intervention for changing partners' assumptions about their own and each other's sexual responses and for broadening their knowledge about factors that can detract from or enhance pleasure from sex. Many adults have limited knowledge about sexuality and have been exposed to unrealistic idealized portrayals of sex in movies and pornographic materials. Most people have few, if any, opportunities to "compare notes" with other people regarding their sexual experiences and develop realistic assumptions and standards. A therapist can provide psychoeducation during sessions, focused on topics that are relevant at the moment (e.g., the sexual side effects of particular medications, the rationale for using sensate focus to reduce performance anxiety and attune partners to pleasurable physical sensations).

In addition to presenting information, the therapist can engage the couple in discussing how the information may apply to them. In addition, the therapist can recommend books about sex written for lay audiences. Excellent examples are Zilbergeld's (1999) *The New Male Sexuality*, Barbach's (2000) *For Yourself: The Fulfillment of Female Sexuality*, Barker and Iantaffi's (2019) *Life Isn't Binary: On Being Both, Beyond, and In-Between*, and Metz and McCarthy's (2011) *Enduring Desire: Your Guide to Lifelong Intimacy*. Some clients enthusiastically read these books, but others may not follow through due to the time involved. In some cases, members of a couple differ in their motivation to read, and the therapist may need to take a more active role in summarizing material from a book for them. We tend to break up the material into relatively small portions on particular topics that the couple agrees to read as homework for discussion with the therapist during the next session.

Modifying Unrealistic and Inappropriate Assumptions and Standards about Sex

The psychoeducation readings we have described address unrealistic and inappropriate assumptions and standards individuals hold regarding individual sexuality and couple sex. They counteract misinformation and unrealistic models of sex portrayed in movies and other sources. Discussion with the couple can explore beliefs they hold, how they developed them, and the disadvantages of trying to live according to them. In contrast, the therapist presents information from professionals who work with vast numbers of sexually normal and imperfect people. Metz and McCarthy (2011) espouse a "Good Enough Sex" (GES) model in which partners experience periodic difficulties and limitations but still share a very satisfying sexual relationship, accepting imperfections in themselves and each other. A couple therapist can promote the GES model and encourage assumptions and standards that involve acceptance of the qualities of their existing relationship. However, the therapy combines the focus on acceptance with interventions to produce behavior changes that can enhance the quality of the couple's relationship.

A particular standard that often merits special attention is the belief that one's partner is the person primarily responsible for one's enjoyment of sex. This belief places pressure on a partner to sense what a person needs to enjoy sexual activity. Although learning about each other's sexuality and developing good sexual skills are important contributions each person can make to a mutually satisfying relationship, the concept of "self-entrancement" emphasizes that each individual can contribute to their own desire, arousal, and orgasm by focusing on erotic thoughts, images, and physical sensations (Metz et al., 2018). If a client's cultural background includes a belief that it is inappropriate to have sexually arousing thoughts or to pursue activities that produce sexual pleasure, the therapist can explore how the individual developed those views, as well as what consequences would occur if they allowed themself to seek sexual pleasure with their partner. The therapist also can include sex education about natural and normal pleasure that results from voluntary stimulation of people's bodies—that people are born with the natural capacity to experience sexual pleasure, and as an adult one can make choices about what, when, and with whom one would like to have those experiences. Thus, it is important for a therapist to explore partners' beliefs about roles and responsibility for sexual enjoyment, and empower them to take greater charge of their own sexual experiences.

Modifying Inaccurate and Inappropriate Negative Attributions about Sex

Because individuals commonly make upsetting, inaccurate attributions about the causes of difficulties with sexual desire, arousal, and orgasm, therapists need to catch those as soon as possible and guide the client in checking their validity. For example, many factors might contribute to an individual's lower than usual sexual arousal during the past week or so. Therefore, either partner's attribution that the individual is losing interest in their partner can be discussed as a possibility, but alternative causes (e.g., increased fatigue and distraction from recent stressors, unresolved upset regarding a recent couple argument) should be identified and considered. Psychoeducation about multiple determinants of sexual arousal can broaden the partners' thinking of alternative causes. The therapist often initially takes an active role in guiding clients in considering alternative causes of observed sexual issues, but increasingly the therapist shifts the responsibility to the clients for actively examining the validity of their attributions.

Modifying Inaccurate and Inappropriate Negative Expectancies about Sex

A combination of interventions also can be used to counteract negative expectancies about sexual experiences, such as one or both partners predicting that an individual will repeatedly experience erectile dysfunction (ED) or the inability to experience an orgasm. Because performance concerns (fear of failure) often become self-fulfilling prophecies, the clients already have evidence that the sexual problem can recur. The therapist should acknowledge that but emphasize that negative expectancies need to be considered in the therapy treatment plan, using psychoeducation to explain how such negative cognitions and associated negative emotions can contribute to sexual problems but are treatable. The couple is also asked about memories of any times when the sexual problem did not occur (exceptions), both as evidence that the individual is capable of a more positive sexual response and as an opportunity to explore the conditions that seemed to facilitate the positive response. The next step is collaboration between the couple and therapist in devising a plan to create the favorable conditions in the future and set up behavioral experiments to observe how those changes in conditions affect the sexual experience. Sensate focus exercises are designed to create positive conditions (e.g., a focus on pleasurable sensations rather than distressing negative expectancies, no demand for performance, a positive expectancy of mutual pleasure from touching). Handout 7.1 (available on the book's web page at *www.guilford.com/epstein-materials*) describes the steps of the sensate focus procedures and their rationale, which the therapist discusses with a couple in preparation for their trying them as homework.

Often an individual's negative expectancies occur as a cascade of negative predictions, with the person imagining one negative outcome leading to another. The downward-arrow technique can be used to track such a cascade of negative expectancies, in which the "bottom line" final outcome is the greatest source of the individual's distress. For example, an individual initially might report an expectancy, "If my partner begins to touch me in a suggestive way, I will become tense and withdraw." When the therapist asks, "What do you think may happen if you become tense and withdraw?" the client may respond, "My partner will be irritated and ask, 'What's the matter? Don't you like my touching you?'" The therapist then asks, "What would happen if your partner responded that way?" and the client responds, "I'd have trouble getting my words out and so I might say, 'I'm just not comfortable.'" Further downward-arrow questioning might lead to a catastrophic prediction, "My partner's frustration with our sexual relationship and difficulty communicating with me will result in them finding someone else and leaving me."

An advantage of working through this process in a couple session is the opportunity for a person's partner to get a close view of the intimidating expectancies that inhibit the individual. Because the partner may have difficulty empathizing with the negative thinking, it is important that the therapist normalizes it through psychoeducation. The therapist can emphasize how common it is for people to jump to negative conclusions, especially when the stakes are high, as when the relationship is important to this individual and the thought of losing the partner is painful. The therapist can guide the partner in expressing understanding of the individual's concerns and in giving feedback that they are not headed toward a breakup. The therapist can propose that the couple consider it an opportunity to use good expressive and listening skills to discuss each other's feelings about sex and possible ways to increase the anxious individual's comfort, beginning with low-level affectionate touch. If there are complicating circumstances, such as a transgender individual who has not had gender-affirming surgery feeling uncomfortable about using their genitals during sexual activity, the therapist can use psychoeducation to normalize the person's experience and engage the couple in problem solving to devise a strategy to address it. Another common presenting problem involves a difference between partners' preferred frequencies of having sex. The clients may experience negative cognitions about this difference (e.g., that there is something abnormal about one of them; that their incompatibility will doom their relationship). The therapist can use psychoeducation to normalize this issue, intervene to reduce the negative attributions and expectancies, and focus the couple on using communication and problem-solving skills to find a mutually satisfying way of interacting sexually. The therapist encourages partners to express curiosity and willingness to empathize with each other's cognitions, while providing each other with feedback that may help reduce the other person's negative thinking.

Modifying Negative Selective Perception Regarding Sexual Activities

The counterproductive tendency for individuals with sexual problems to engage in self-conscious "spectatoring" (closely monitoring their own or a partner's sexual responses) easily becomes automatic and routine. In sex therapy, sensate focus exercises and other forms of mindfulness techniques are methods for shifting partners' attention away from distressing stimuli and toward sensual and erotic stimuli (e.g., attractive aspects of a partner's body, pleasant sensations from touching one's partner and from being touched). Sensate focus instructions emphasize shifting one's attention to pleasurable aspects of sensual and sexual touch. The therapist facilitates that shift by instructing the couple to refrain from their usual performance-oriented sexual behavior, and to engage instead in graduated levels of sensual and eventually sexual touch, paying attention in a mindful way to pleasant sensory experiences and altering negative expectancies about the outcomes of physical touch (see sources such as Metz et al. 2018 for detailed descriptions). The other goal of sensate focus—reducing pressure and anxiety that many people feel regarding sexual activity—is achieved as the therapist takes control of the couple's sexual behavior, restricting actions that typically are focused on excellent performance as a lover.

Common CBCT interventions for selective perception also are used when individuals reveal skewed attention to unpleasant aspects of sexual experiences (e.g., "My partner never lets me know that the ways I touch her feel good"). On the one hand, the therapist can ask the individual about any memories of times when the partner did exhibit signs of pleasure, verbally or nonverbally. On the other hand, the person's partner is available to provide disconfirming information (e.g., "I know I don't say much, but I know that when you caress my face, arms, and other parts of my body I smile at you and sometimes make sounds like 'Mmmm!'"). If the individual replies, "I don't remember you doing any of that," the therapist can suggest that perhaps the person was busy trying to please the partner and didn't notice those cues, and perhaps the partner's cues may have been a bit too subtle. The therapist could ask whether the partner would be willing to be more direct in the future, perhaps saying, "That feels nice." This intervention targets potential selective perception, but it also can initiate a small behavior change that reduces the likelihood of partners missing each other's messages.

Another approach to reducing selective perception is identifying a few behaviors by each member of the couple that may be overlooked, asking each person to intentionally enact those behaviors during the next week, and having the other person keep a log of instances when those actions occurred. This approach has potential to increase the likelihood that each person will behave in ways that their partner desires, and that recipients will notice it.

Interventions for Behavior

From its earliest roots, sex therapy has included behavioral interventions designed to alter counterproductive interactions of individuals who experience symptoms of dysfunction and their intimate partners. The goals of the interventions have been to reduce avoidance of sex by individuals who have developed negative expectancies regarding sexual activities, increase knowledge and comfort with one's own and one's partner's body (including genitals), increase individuals' skills for increasing their own physical and emotional relaxation, gradually expose individuals to increasing levels of pleasant sensual and sexual behavior, improve clients' repertoire of knowledge and skills for sensual and erotic ways of interacting as a couple, and improve couple communication about sex. Because most sex therapy literature describes use of sensate focus with cisgender couples with various sexual orientations, there has been relatively little information about ways to adapt the exercise for couples with nonbinary (e.g., transgender, gender fluid, gender queer) members, including some transgender individuals who experience discomfort with their bodies as sexual beings (Anzani et al., 2021; Holmberg et al., 2020). Although many transgender participants in Anzani et al.'s (2021) qualitative study reported a variety of sexual behavior and used their bodies for sexual pleasure, some who struggled with their current bodily characteristics relied on avoidance of sex or behaved as asexual and performed sex for their partner's pleasure. Therefore, therapists' use of exercises such as standard sensate focus that emphasize mutual sexual enjoyment would seem applicable for the former group of transgender individuals but could be problematic for the latter group. When it is the latter group's turn to receive touch, it could be restricted to pleasurable, affectionate touch excluding breasts and genitals. However, in some cases the partners may have conflict about such an unbalanced sexual relationship, whereas other couples are mutually comfortable with it. For those in conflict, other procedures to facilitate constructive communication and problem solving would be needed. Overall, therapists must be prepared to tailor sex therapy exercises for clients with diverse gender identities.

Generic skills training for communication and problem solving are highly relevant for treating couples presenting with sexual dysfunctions. Many individuals take sexual issues very personally in terms of self-esteem and degree of attachment security with their partner. It is important that partners are able to express their thoughts, sexual preferences, and emotions clearly and constructively and that they receive empathic, validating feedback from each other. In addition, we have described many characteristics of individual partners, their relationship and environmental conditions that can influence their sexual relationship, and their ability to collaborate on devising solutions to these challenges is essential. Therefore, the treatment plan should include building the couple's communication and problem-solving skills, with an emphasis on sexual topics. It is helpful to include psychoeducation regarding accurate terms for sexual body parts and sexual acts, so everyone is using the same concepts during discussions.

Metz et al. (2018) describe phases of psychosexual skill development exercises used in a cognitive-behavioral couple sex therapy model, which each include homework to modify the behavioral patterns of the couple and each individual. These exercises have a cisgender bias and need some modification with other clients, such as those transgender individuals who feel uncomfortable with the sexual parts of their bodies. Furthermore, cisgender clients also can vary in their comfort about a partner seeing and touching them, and the therapist must monitor both members' comfort levels and adjust interventions accordingly. The length constraint of the present chapter does not allow us to describe all these interventions in detail, and how clinicians can modify them for couples with various characteristics. Consequently, the reader is advised to consult sex therapy texts such as Hall and Binik (2020), Metz et al. (2018), and Weeks et al. (2020). The therapist introduces all behavioral exercises with brief psychoeducation regarding their goals and procedures, and we recommend giving the couple handouts with guidelines for each exercise to use in sessions or at home, as appropriate.

The first phase described by Metz et al. (2018) (developing couple comfort, relaxation, and cooperation) includes couple exercises in which the couple talk about sexual feelings and partner spooning (with or without clothing, depending on comfort levels) to create nondemand low-pressure physical contact. Interventions that can be practiced individually or as a couple are deep breathing and physical relaxation exercises, and for individuals, pelvic muscle training that can address sexual issues such as orgasmic disorder. The second phase (promoting desire, pleasure, and arousal) includes behavioral interventions of couple-relaxed pleasuring (related to sensate focus) that involves psychoeducation and practice of affectionate touch, sensual touch, playful touch, erotic nonintercourse touch, and intercourse, as well as an exercise focused on partner genital exploration. The third phase (enhancing arousal and eroticism) involves couple erotic pleasuring in which one partner uses "intentional teasing" touch to stimulate the other person in ways that are increasingly erotic and arousing, but backs off (with feedback from the partner) before the person experiences an orgasm. The couple then switches roles. This procedure gradually focuses the recipient on enjoying erotic touch without pressure to perform or reach orgasm. It also increases partners' sexual attunement to each other.

The fourth phase (enjoying eroticism and flexible types of highly arousing sexual behavior) includes couple practice of initiating intercourse and/or other forms of highly arousing behavior, experimenting with a variety of sexual behaviors to discover their preferences and options to avoid routine. Some individuals experience difficulty as they engage in sexual behavior that focuses them on performance (e.g., ED when they attempt intercourse or do not reach orgasm, even though they had done so during the prior phase of enhanced arousal). In such cases, the therapist returns to a discussion of cognitions that create sexual pressure, such as standards for adequate performance, and has the couple shift to relaxation techniques and nondemand erotic touch before eventually trying the high-intensity sexual behavior again. This phase also includes exercises for the couple to devise and use forms of playful sexual interaction, which fosters relaxation and intimacy. The final phase (couple relapse prevention) focuses the couple on making an explicit agreement to continue exercises that have contributed to an improved sexual relationship. The therapist emphasizes that maintaining a mutually satisfying sexual relationship involves nurturing it. One exercise asks each of the partners to list the positive features of their sexual relationship that they have experienced through therapy. Their lists may include factors such as physical relaxation, mutual pleasuring, realistic standards, low-pressure interactions, and good communication about forms of pleasing touch. The therapist also can review with the couple the exercises they used to improve their sexual relationship and highly recommend that they keep their handouts with guidelines available for easy access at home. Clients may have favorite exercises, but the therapist reviews the value of using all of them in the future.

For the common presenting problem of low desire, a number of behavioral interventions can be helpful. Because memories of past pleasurable experiences and anticipation of future ones facilitate desire, it is important for the therapist to guide clients in developing new cognitions of that type even though they have a history of feeling neutral about sex and lacking positive experiences. Therapists need to distinguish between neutral feelings about sex and sexual aversion, which often is associated with a trauma history and calls for a treatment plan to address it. Interventions for low desire begin with a focus on cognition and then introduce behavioral exercises. Cognitive interventions include altering cognitions associated with low-desire: negative attributions such as "I'm defective"; negative expectancies such as "No matter what my partner does to get me interested, I won't feel any interest in it"; and unrealistic assumptions such as "Sexual desire is an automatic instinct that I should feel because I love my partner." Psychoeducation focuses on the influence of past experiences that influenced one's anticipation of pleasure or lack thereof, and ways in which new experiences can form more positive anticipation. Behavioral interventions then are essential to develop those new pleasurable experiences. A number of interventions can be helpful, and the therapist should collaborate with each couple to devise the treatment plan. For example, the exercise on relaxed couple pleasuring that we have already described begins with affectionate touch, with no pressure to feel desire or arousal, gradually moving to mindful sensual touch (again with no performance goal), and eventually to erotic touch. The participation of a partner who is sensitive to barriers influencing the individual's low desire can be reassuring and reduce distracting thoughts about performance or failure. Exercises in which the couple mindfully shares other experiences through their senses of sight, small, touch, and taste, such as having a meal together, taking nature walks, listening to music, or visiting an art gallery can be used to increase joint mindfulness and a concept of "Stop and smell the roses—together," which can be extended to mutual physical touch. All these exercises emphasize Basson's (2001) responsive sexual desire model, which was developed regarding low desire in women but is relevant for anyone who experiences it.

In planning relapse prevention, the therapist includes interventions for partners' cognitions, emotions, and behavior. The negative thoughts and emotions they may experience if any symptoms that brought them to therapy recur are discussed. A distinction is made between a temporary lapse and a relapse in which the couple consistently returns to a problematic level of sexual functioning. This involves counteracting negative attributions (e.g., "Our improvements were just superficial, and we aren't sexually compatible") and negative expectancies (e.g., "We are in a free fall sexually, and if we try more it will be awful"). In contrast, the therapist emphasizes the importance of partners reviewing evidence of progress they had made and making a plan to return to the exercises that helped them improve. The therapist can let the couple know that a tune-up refresher session is available if they feel a need for guidance in implementing their relapse prevention plan. Interventions described in the next section to moderate negative emotions such as anxiety and anger also are used. Behavioral interventions to counteract a lapse further emphasize use of exercises the couple used successfully during therapy.

Interventions for Emotional Responses

Interventions for emotion in sexual problems involve both decreasing negative emotions (e.g., anxiety, sadness/depression, shame, anger) and increasing positive emotions associated with sexual satisfaction. As we noted previously, it is important to distinguish between transitory emotional states that are responses to current experiences such as difficulty becoming aroused and couple interactions such as arguments and criticism from one's partner, and characterological emotions such as chronic depression or anxiety. The latter may require referrals for concurrent individual therapy, but the former typically are addressed within couple therapy sessions.

We already have described interventions for cognitions (e.g., unrealistic sexual standards, negative expectancies) and interventions for behavior (e.g., desensitization to anxiety-eliciting sexual activities via the hierarchy of exposure exercises in sensate focus and related procedures) for decreasing negative emotions associated with sex. In addition, behavioral interventions that increase individuals' sense of safety and security with their partner can help reduce negative emotional responses. Those include expressive and empathic listening skills, as well as joint problem solving and nondemand pleasuring exercises in which sexual pressure from one's partner is removed. Finally, each individual learns to use breathing, relaxation, and mindfulness procedures to reduce their emotional distress. In couple therapy sessions, the therapist can observe and intervene with the actions of a person's partner that contribute to the person's negative emotions about sex. Both members can be guided in contributing to an atmosphere that is conducive to overall and sexual intimacy.

Many couple exercises within the Metz et al. (2018) model and other sex therapy models are designed to increase positive emotional experiences. Those include nondemand physical intimacy exercises such as partner spooning and taking turns as giver or receiver of sensual and erotic touch, as well as exercises for sexual playfulness. Positive emotions also are common when individuals experience empathic responses from a partner during communication skill sessions. The therapist emphasizes that removal of negative interactions does not guarantee a significant increase in positive feelings. Consequently, the treatment plan includes interventions to enhance positive emotions, and evaluation of progress will examine those changes too.

TROUBLESHOOTING PROBLEMS IN COUPLE THERAPY FOR SEXUAL CONCERNS

Because sex is commonly a source of anxiety for couples and a topic that many find difficult to discuss, there are many points in couple therapy where the assessment and treatment procedures may elicit partners' emotional distress and avoidance. The following factors that can interfere with progress in therapy, and strategies therapists can use to address them.

Ambiguous Cues of Client Discomfort with Therapy

Sometimes clients are transparent about their distress, so the therapist can address it and discuss ways to make the therapy more comfortable for them. However, other clients keep their distress and concerns about steps in sex therapy to themselves, exhibiting ambiguous cues of discomfort at most. In some cases, the first clear sign of such a problem is the client's cancellation of a session or dropping out of treatment.

• One approach to forestall such responses is to include in one's introduction to therapy a statement that sex is one of the more challenging topics for people to discuss with an outsider and to work on with one's partner, so that the therapist wants to collaborate with the couple to create a safe and relaxed atmosphere. We ask partners to let us know whenever they are concerned about the methods we are suggesting because no one should feel pressured to do anything. We note that therapy for sexual concerns does ease people into going "out of their comfort zone" at times, but it always is up to the individual what they will try and when. It is important to repeat this message throughout treatment.

• Therapists are accustomed to monitoring clients' moods during sessions, and this is very important when working on sexual issues. If an individual's behavior changes in a noticeable way (e.g., becoming less talkative than usual), the therapist can briefly interrupt the session, tell the person what behavior was noticed, ask how the person is feeling, and inquire whether there is any discomfort regarding the session's topic or activities. Remind clients that it is normal to feel uncomfortable at times and talking about it will allow the therapist and couple to make adjustments when needed.

• Sometimes the evidence that one or both partners is experiencing an issue with an aspect of therapy is their failure to complete homework. Because many sex therapy exercises require the couple's private activities at home, the therapist is not able to monitor their reactions to assignments at those times. One approach to forestalling homework noncompliance involves asking a couple to think about any factors that might get in the way of them completing homework that the therapist is proposing. The therapist can open this discussion with comments such as "Sometimes an exercise sounds like a good idea to a couple when I propose it, but once they get home they realize they have mixed feelings about it. If you will imagine yourselves at home thinking or talking about trying the exercise I just described, do you have any thoughts and emotions that might decrease your motivation to do the exercise at home? That can include personal discomfort with it, but it also might involve situations at home, such as a heavy workload from your job, child-rearing responsibilities, or a lack of privacy." Troubleshooting about homework noncompliance also can occur afterward, during the following therapy session. This involves the therapist asking partners about any ideas they have regarding factors that interfered with their completing the planned exercises. This discussion should cover personal issues such as negative expectancies of an exercise creating couple conflict, as well as situational factors such as job demands.

Partners' Continued Blaming of Each Other or Themselves for Sexual Problems

Although the therapist emphasizes couple collaboration and avoidance of blaming, some couples still engage in blaming by one or both partners, which must be reduced. Because sexual dysfunctions have been labeled as disorders within an individual by professionals (see DSM) and also can appear to laypeople as originating within one partner, the therapist needs to be alert to cues of symptomatic clients blaming themselves or being blamed by their partner. Prompt intervention is needed to block blaming messages and engage both members in developing a mutually safe and pleasurable sexual relationship.

• The therapist can reiterate messages that tension and conflict in a couple's relationship interfere with positive sexual responses, whereas an atmosphere of calm, safety, and enjoying activities in life together contributes to positive emotional and sexual responses.

• When the therapist has knowledge about an earlier time when the couple had mutually enjoyable sexual experiences without the current problems, the therapist can conduct a review with the couple of what each of them contributed to such pleasant experiences. The therapist can emphasize that they were capable of having a satisfying sexual relationship and can focus them on contributions each person can make to restoring it.

• The therapist can engage the couple in identifying contextual factors that have contributed to sexual problems, such as stressors from jobs, child rearing, financial problems, and caring for ill family members. This can lead to identification of dyadic coping strategies they can use to manage those stressors and protect their relationship.

KEY POINTS

- Sex therapy includes interventions for both individual partners and couple patterns.

- Therapist sensitivity to diversity (gender identity, sexual orientation, race, cultural background) is essential when working with sexual concerns.

- Transitory sexual difficulties in relationships are common but can develop into pervasive dysfunctions when partners' understanding of them is inadequate, and their ways of coping with them are counterproductive and distressing.

- Multiple factors commonly combine to create a sexual presenting problem, so the clinical assessment and treatment plan must be multidimensional.

- Because many sex therapy exercises are conducted in the privacy of the clients' homes, the therapist must collaborate with the couple to set up favorable conditions for their homework and troubleshoot instances of noncompliance.

CHAPTER 8

Financial Issues

The American Psychological Association (2017) has found consistently in their annual surveys of stressors experienced by American adults that money is at or near the top of the most frequently reported stressors. Stress and conflict regarding finances is one of the main reasons why couples seek therapy (Whisman et al., 1997). Papp, Cummings, and Goeke-Morey (2009) found that couples argue about money more intensely and longer than other topics. Furthermore, longitudinal data from the National Survey of Families and Households have shown that financial disagreements are the strongest predictors of divorce compared with any other area of conflict (Dew, Britt, & Huston, 2012).

Researchers and clinicians have made an important distinction between *objective* financial or economic situations in people's lives (e.g., low income, insufficient funds to pay one's bills; loss of a job that suddenly interrupts income) and the subjective concerns individuals experience about current and future financial demands, which have been labeled *financial strain* (Voydanoff & Donnelly, 1988). Thus, two individuals who have similar financial conditions may differ in their levels of subjective financial strain. Differences in financial strain depend foremost on objective economic circumstances, but also on individuals' financial history (e.g., financial successes and challenges in their family of origin and in their own experiences), personal characteristics (e.g., tendency to catastrophize, low self-confidence), and current personal circumstances (e.g., a pile-up of financial and nonfinancial stressors in the person's life). Couple conflict can arise from differences in partners' levels of financial strain experienced from a shared financial stressor (one is more distressed about the problem than the other).

Research across cultures has indicated that financial stressors negatively affect not only individuals' own mental health but also the quality of couple relationships. When members of couples are concerned about financial problems, they are likely to experience depression (Falconier, 2010; Helms et al., 2014; Mistry, Vandewater, Huston, & McLoyd, 2002; Robila & Krishnakumar, 2005), anxiety (Falconier, 2010), and/or general emotional distress (Aytac & Rankin, 2009; Kinnunen & Feldt, 2004; Neppl, Senia, & Donnellan, 2016). In turn, this individual psychological distress affects partners' interactions negatively. A study examining pathways of influence among stressors, subjective responses, and couple interactions (Falconier & Jackson, 2020) analyzed findings from research conducted in countries around the world (e.g., Argentina, Czech Republic, Finland, Greece, Romania, South Korea, and the United States) involving a total of 34,007 participants. Falconier and Jackson found that partners' subjective financial strain about family finances was associated with greater negative interactions (e.g., psychological aggression such as criticism and name-calling, hostile behavior, demand–withdraw communication, arguing), and fewer positive exchanges (e.g., supportive messages, warmth, intimacy, constructive communication). Those couple interaction behaviors in turn were associated with lower relationship satisfaction and stability. Given that money is a common source of conflict and distress for couples, therapists are highly likely to encounter couples in their clinical practices for whom finances are significant presenting problems. Consequently, therapists need to be prepared to understand sources of financially related stress and conflict, and know how to provide assistance in resolving financial concerns.

SOCIOCULTURAL FACTORS IN COUPLE FINANCIAL PROBLEMS AND COPING

There is wide sociocultural variation in assumptions, standards, and behaviors regarding aspects of individual and family finances such as earning money, generating a profit, managing money, distributing financial roles, tasks, and control in a relationship, independent versus total or partial pooling of partners' financial resources, and coping with financial stress and solving problems. Sociocultural variations may reflect religious influences as well as local political and economic conditions. For example, based on one's family and broader cultural background, it may be acceptable to speak openly about money and celebrate making profits in business, whereas individuals with different cultural backgrounds may consider such disclosures socially undesirable. Growing up in a country with chronic severe economic conditions versus one with a stable economy can affect individuals' money management attitudes and behavior. Gender identity and sexual orientation also may also affect financial cognitions and behaviors. For example, same-sex couples have been found to have less gendered division of financial roles (Solomon, Rothblum, & Balsam, 2005) and manage their finances more independently rather than pooling their resources (Burgoyne, Clarke, & Burns, 2011). Immigrants' lack of familiarity with the financial system of their host country may lead couples to avoid entrusting funds to financial institutions or to make unwise decisions about use of credit. In many developing countries, some aspects of financial management (e.g., building credit, investing in retirement plans) that are critical in developed countries such as the United States with more complex financial systems may not be necessary, so immigrant couples may need some financial education in order to be better prepared to establish financial security.

As a result of sociocultural influences on financial cognitions and behaviors, therapists should expect differences to be present to varying degrees within couples and between the therapist and each partner. The *money genogram*, described in the assessment section of this chapter, is useful for exploring how partners' sociocultural backgrounds and identities have shaped their cognitions and behaviors about financial matters. Therapists need to take a curious and nonjudgmental stance when exploring sociocultural differences and should refrain from conveying any notion that a particular financial cognition or behavior is universal. In order for therapists to decrease their likelihood of working with implicit biases, they should reflect on their own beliefs regarding the financial behaviors and well-being of their clients who belong to various cultural groups and social identities before addressing their financial stress.

RISK FACTORS FOR FINANCIAL STRAIN

Within a stress and coping view of risk factors for problems in couple relationships (Epstein & Baucom, 2002), identifying factors at the societal level (the broader environment within which the couple lives), the relationship between the partners, and the characteristics of each individual partner is essential in constructing a treatment plan designed to reduce them. At the *societal level*, economic conditions commonly create problems for vast numbers of people. Thus, the negative economic effects of the COVID-19 pandemic took a major toll on the well-being of families around the world. Those stressors have been among the financial concerns that couples have brought to our clinical practices. Previously, the major economic downturn in the early 2000s triggered by the collapse of financial investment institutions had similar effects. Such major shifts in national and global economic conditions commonly create specific stressors for individual families as they result, among other things, in job insecurity and shrinkage of savings accounts. In contrast to stressors resulting from actions that individual couples have taken (e.g., failing to build "nest egg" savings), societal level economic stressors can be abrupt and so pervasive that they leave partners feeling disoriented and helpless.

In addition to macroeconomic downturns, individuals and families from different sociocultural groups do not have equal access to the same financial resources and opportunities. Structural racism, discrimination, legal barriers, lack of job opportunities, housing restrictions, and inability to afford good education, child care, and/or healthcare are some of the many reasons why income and wealth distribution are not equal and equitable across a society such as the United States, with less privileged members experiencing ongoing financial hardships and strain. Resources at the societal level to assist those who are not financially privileged include national programs such as social security, financial counseling resources within the community, food pantries, and other social support services for families experiencing financial need. However, such resources can vary considerably from one locale to another.

At the *couple relationship level*, financial stressors that may be risk factors can include joint debt, conflict between partners' approaches to managing money, financial demands from assisting extended family members, and expenses regarding education and health needs. Couple-level risk factors involving deficits in resources include insufficient income to meet financial demands, lack of accumulated wealth that can provide a buffer in the event of new expenses or unemployment, and inadequate dyadic coping, communication, and problem-solving skills, as well as limited cohesion between partners and commitment to the relationship.

At the *individual partner level*, examples of risk factors for financial stress include a family background of financial hardship that produced chronic insecurity and limited or no accumulation of wealth, past financial setbacks in prior couple relationships, money "habitudes" that foster unwise spending and inadequate money management, and factors contributing to unemployment, job instability, and difficulty earning sufficient income. Characteristics interfering with reliable employment may include forms of psychopathology, limited education and skills training, and long periods out of the job market due to illness, caregiving responsibilities, or incarceration. In addition, immigration-related barriers to obtaining education and/or securing a job that meets family economic needs can include issues such as limited language fluency, lack of local recognition of education credentials earned in another country, and immigration legal status barriers to employment. Limited personal resources such as coping, problem-solving, and communication skills, as well as a social support network, also may be risk factors for developing financial problems.

A stress and coping view of life stressors such as financial problems at the societal, couple relationship, or individual levels also considers individual differences in people's cognitions—*perceptions and inferences about potential stressors* (Epstein & Baucom, 2002). The ways that members of couples think about finances can be risk factors for financial stress by exacerbating the individual's subjective experience of danger. For example, some individuals may selectively pay attention to negative aspects of their financial circumstances (e.g., unpaid bills) and overlook positive aspects (e.g., a partner's recent salary raise at work). Similarly, some individuals may tend to "catastrophize" with negative expectancies of dire financial outcomes such as becoming homeless. Such negative cognitions can serve as risk factors for subjective financial strain and should be assessed as potential targets in a treatment plan.

FINANCIAL CIRCUMSTANCES AND STRAIN FROM A CBCT PERSPECTIVE

Within a CBCT framework, stressors associated with finances are among the significant life stressors that can disrupt the stability and well-being of a couple and its members. The success of a couple's relationship over time depends on their ability to cope effectively with such stressors (Epstein & Baucom, 2002). Within that framework, the couple's *resources for coping* with the financial stressors also come from characteristics of the two individuals (e.g., beliefs regarding the use of money, financial behavior patterns, problem-focused and emotion-focused coping styles), the dyad (e.g., dyadic coping skills; shared goals for financial security), and the couple's environment (e.g., social and financial support network).

The factors involved in financial stressors and couple resources commonly have cognitive, affective, and behavioral components, which can be taken into account in understanding a couple's financial problems and in planning relevant interventions. The following are brief descriptions of those cognitions, affective responses, and behaviors.

Financial Cognitions

In Chapter 1, we described a typology of cognitions that commonly occur in couple relationships, and those cognitions readily apply to the area of finances. Based on various life experiences in one's family of origin and other social contexts, individuals develop relatively stable cognitive schemas about money and its place in relationships, including *assumptions* and *standards*. For example, whether or not it is accurate, many people hold an assumption that accumulating wealth leads to happiness. For many people one's income is a key indicator of a person's social status. We have worked with some heterosexual couples whose conflict was fueled by the male partner's strong standard that men should earn more than their female partners or that the partner with the higher income has a stronger voice in the couple's financial decisions. Thus, it is important that the assessment investigate partners' assumptions and standards regarding finances and that any information regarding their origins (for example, beliefs espoused by their parents) can be incorporated into planning interventions to soften rigid beliefs.

Partners' *selective perceptions* about finances may play roles in couple distress and conflict. For example, an individual who is insecure about finances, perhaps based on prior life experiences, may monitor a partner's spending, selectively notice instances of spending and failing to notice when the partner is behaving frugally. Skewed views of one's partner can lead to negative emotions (anxiety, anger) and adversarial behavior toward the partner.

Similarly, when individuals make *negative attributions* about a partner's traits and motives regarding money from observing the partner's actions, those negative inferences can elicit negative affect and behavior toward the partner. For example, if an individual observes their partner spending money on a personal item (e.g., clothes, a personal hobby) and attributes it to the partner being a selfish person, or to the partner having no respect for the individual's concerns about the couple's finances, the individual may berate the partner and trigger an argument. *Expectancies* about future events also can contribute to couple distress regarding finances, as the predictions influence how the individual behaves toward a partner. Thus, if an individual has observed staff cutbacks in their workplace and is worried about losing their job, the individual may keep their distress a secret if they have an expectancy that their partner would express little emotional support if they disclosed those concerns.

Emotional Responses to Financial Issues

Because financial issues have significant meaning for people, in terms of their self-concept, perceived respect from their partner and society, degree of power within their couple relationship, and sense of security, it is not surprising that they elicit strong emotional responses. Therefore, therapists explore themes in the cognitions individuals attach to financial events in their couple relationships, identifying associations between themes and particular emotional responses. The following are descriptions of common financial issues, associated cognitions, and emotional responses. It is important to note that these are not exclusive links among financial events, cognitions, and emotions, and individuals may have other idiosyncratic experiences that trigger emotional responses, so therapists need to approach assessment of emotions with a curious perspective and probe carefully to understand each person's subjective responses.

Within a cognitive-behavioral perspective (Beck, Emery, & Greenberg, 1985; Leahy, Holland, & McGinn, 2012) and stress and coping theory (Lazarus & Folkman, 1984), individuals commonly experience anxiety when they perceive danger to their well-being, especially if they view the danger as severe, unpredictable, and uncontrollable. Because people typically view financial resources as a core aspect of security in their lives, it is not surprising that events they interpret as threatening those resources trigger anxiety. Threatening stressors can include those associated with the individual (e.g., an injury that reduces one's work productivity and learning that one's job is at risk), those associated with the couple relationship (e.g., arguments regarding saving money), and those originating in the couple's environment (e.g., massive job layoffs nationally due to a health pandemic). In turn, anxiety may elicit dysfunctional behavioral responses that can contribute to relationship conflict and exacerbate financial problems. For example, Samantha became quite anxious when Maria told her that she felt burned out at her job and wanted to quit and find a new one. Samantha expressed her distress by severely criticizing Maria as being selfish and unreliable, resulting in Maria leaving their home to stay with a friend and cutting off communication. Thus, therapists who work with couples experiencing financial stressors need to assess partners' levels of anxiety and how they cope with it.

Because financial issues commonly involve partners' relative degrees of control over money decisions and use, including judgments regarding lack of equity, individuals can experience anger toward each other, which may be expressed constructively or in inappropriate ways. Their ability to regulate and manage anger has a significant effect on the adequacy of their individual and dyadic coping. Consequently, it is important that therapists assess the degrees to which partners are aware of their experiences of anger associated with finances, the degrees to which they regulate its intensity, and ways they communicate it to each other (see Chapter 5).

Experiences of financial losses can contribute to perceptions of loss of one's dreams of a good life and bright future, a sense of competence and accomplishment, and respect from one's partner and others. Cognitions regarding loss, especially involving hopelessness that the future will bring improvement, commonly are associated with sadness and even depression ranging from subclinical levels to diagnosable disorders. Because symptoms of depression (e.g., low mood, self-criticism, sense of hopelessness, loss of motivation, social withdrawal, difficulty making decisions) can disrupt coping and problem solving with stressors, as well as contribute to couple relationship distress, therapists need to be alert to signs of depression when working with couples experiencing financial problems. When significant depression is identified, the therapist should integrate interventions for it (described in Chapter 10) within the treatment plan.

Shame is another powerful emotion that individuals may experience regarding financial problems, involving *condemnation of the self as a person* for what one considers financial failure. As we have noted previously, shame tends to shut down motivation and lead the individual to withdraw rather than engaging in problem solving to resolve the financial stressors.

On the one hand, individuals may induce shame in themselves when they violate their own personal standards for how they should perform financially. On the other hand, an individual may blame their partner for the couple's financial problems and induce shame in the partner (e.g., "You are a failure as a spouse for spending recklessly and getting us into debt!"; Epstein & Falconier, 2011). Because individuals who experience shame commonly avoid disclosing their distress, as doing so can exacerbate the focus on the behavior that led to the shame, members of couples who are experiencing shame regarding financial problems often fail to mention it to a therapist. It is therefore up to the therapist to uncover instances of shame when assessing a couple. Sometimes particular nonverbal behaviors (e.g., becoming silent in a session when the topic of finances is raised, nonverbal forms of withdrawal such as downcast eyes, and slumped posture) can be clues to shame experiences the therapist can ask about tactfully.

These four emotional responses are not the only ones that may be associated with couples' financial problems. Consequently, therapists need to inquire about a range of emotions that each partner might experience and explore both the events that trigger them and their effects on individual and dyadic coping with problems.

Behavioral Factors in Financial Issues

A number of forms of behavior are relevant in couples' experiences with financial stressors. First, each person's behavioral patterns for relating to money include actions such as ways of keeping records of income, expenses, and budgeting (e.g., entries in an online checking account record), as well as degree of structure used when shopping (e.g., having a predetermined shopping list and avoiding impulse purchases). Second, the couple's communication regarding finances and financial problems involves the extent to which each person expresses their beliefs and emotions regarding money topics, as well as how well they use active listening to understand each other's experiences and convey that empathy to each other. Third, the couple's individual and dyadic forms of emotion-focused and problem-focused behavioral coping with financial stressors (e.g., avoidance, distraction, seeking emotional support from others) include those for which the partners have similar approaches and those on which they differ. Specific problem-solving skills involving collaboration should be identified.

SCREENING AND ASSESSMENT FOR FINANCIAL PROBLEMS

Information regarding financial issues is collected through joint interviews with the couple as well as individual interviews with the partners, supplemented with specific questionnaires and direct observation of how the partners behave toward each other when discussing money. The following are descriptions of those assessment methods.

Financial History of the Partners and Their Relationship

During their initial meeting with a therapist, when asked to describe their reasons for seeking therapy, some couples spontaneously report conflict and distress regarding money-related matters, whereas others reveal it when the therapist surveys their areas of concern via interview or a questionnaire such as the *Relationship Issues Survey* (see Chapter 3). In either case, it is important that the therapist identify aspects of the couple's experiences with money that need to be addressed in therapy, and decide whether a referral to a financial specialist also is needed. Assessment interviews should identify whether distress and conflict are related to (1) financial stressors that are taxing the couple's coping abilities; (2) the adequacy of individual and dyadic stress management skills; (3) differences between partners' cognitions and/or behaviors ("habitudes") for interacting with money; (4) dissatisfaction with the distribution of financial roles and tasks; (5) ways in which conflict about money reflects broader issues regarding autonomy, power, and control in the relationship; (6) the couple's communication skills for sharing thoughts and emotions; (7) problem-solving skills; and/or (8) level of mastery of financial management skills. Money issues often are related to difficulties in several of these areas, not just one. For example, a couple's financial problems may be exacerbated by their poor stress management and problem-solving skills, as well as differences in their money "habitudes."

Whenever the couple's presenting concerns are related to financial matters, it is important to conduct an interview to gather background information about the *financial history* of the couple and of their respective families of origin in order to contextualize the couple's current challenges. This information can be gathered during the interviews through the *couple's money history* and the *money genogram*. These guides to partners' financial backgrounds do not gather specific objective information about their current finances (e.g., joint income, debt level), but they help the clinician understand individual and joint experiences in partners' lives that may have shaped their financial cognitions, behaviors, and emotions.

• **The couple's money history** consists of interview questions designed to gather historical and current information about the couple's financial journey together (see Figure 8.1). These questions invite clients to share when their joint financial history began (e.g., when they bought their first car together), any difficult financial times they faced, coping strategies, moments of resilience, experiences of success, current strengths and challenges, partners' current financial roles and tasks, and so on. It also identifies areas of couple conflict regarding financial matters for further assessment and treatment planning. The questions typically elicit the partners' cognitions about their joint experiences with finances (e.g., viewing each other as "teammates" versus adversaries), their emotional responses during those experiences (e.g., pleasure at saving together for a dream house, anger toward each other for perceived unfair behavior, anxiety about perceived financial dangers), and their behavioral interactions associated with money (e.g., coercive strategies used to try to control their joint finances).

The following questions focus on how the members of a couple have handled money together over the course of their relationship. These questions can be considered initial probes, and therapists should feel free to ask follow-up questions to reveal more details about the partners' cognitions, emotional responses, and behaviors regarding ways in which they manage finances together.

- In describing your financial history as a couple, your experiences dealing with finances together, when and how would you say that history began?
- Imagine drawing a timeline of your financial history together, with one end being the very beginning and the other end being where the two of you are right now.
  - What can you identify as critical events and moments? When did they happen, and what happened?
  - In what way did each event affect your decisions about each of your financial roles in your relationship, and how finances would be handled?
  - What if any major financial stressors occurred, and when?
- What are some of the things that you agree on regarding your finances?
  - How did you come to understand what each of you wants financially (financial goals) and how you prefer to manage your finances?
- How do you manage your finances?
  - Do you pool all of your financial resources or do you keep them completely or partially separated?
  - Have you always had this arrangement? If you have not, when did it change? What contributed to the change?
- Does each of you have specific financial roles and tasks? If so, what are they?
  - How did the roles develop?
  - What, if any, changes would you like to see in the roles?
- Please describe for me your process for coming to financial agreements/decisions together? If I was watching you talk about making a decision, what would I see?
  - How do you handle disagreements?
- Have differences or similarities in your individual financial resources (e.g., income, personal wealth) played any role in your relationship such as in decision making and independence?
- Resilience is the ability to experience problems and stresses and to bounce back from them, even making you stronger. In what ways have you built resilience as a couple in managing financial difficulties?
- What strategies have you developed individually and as a couple to handle stress associated with financial issues? How well do your individual ways of coping work out together as a couple?
- What do you appreciate in your partner regarding financial management attitudes and skills?
- What do you consider to be your strengths/challenges as a couple regarding financial management?

FIGURE 8.1. Couple's money history interview questions.

• **The money genogram** (Mumford & Weeks, 2003) helps the therapist and couple understand family-of-origin experiences, cultural factors, and individual life experiences that shaped their financial cognitions, behaviors, and emotions. It can be used for both assessment and intervention purposes. Similar to other types of genograms, the money genogram is a family tree diagram that includes at least three generations, but it specifically is intended to identify family-of-origin patterns, involving strengths and challenges regarding financial experiences. It not only taps specific financial events that affected the family; it also captures beliefs (e.g., that financial success is a key indicator of one's value as a person) and behaviors (e.g., spending and saving patterns) that may have been passed down from generation to generation. It also should include each partner's past couple relationships, so that financial experiences and patterns in those relationships can be identified. If the couple has any adult children who manage their own finances, it may also include information about them. The genogram may generate some historical information about the couple's money history together, but for an in-depth exploration, the couple's money history is likely to provide a more comprehensive picture.

The therapist introduces the money genogram to the couple with a rationale that individuals' approaches to finances commonly are shaped at least in part by experiences in their family of origin. The therapist notes that each person probably will have clear memories, allowing answers to some of the questions, but perhaps not others. The questions ask how each person's parents or other adults who raised them handled finances as a couple (e.g., separate vs. conjoint accounts), messages the parents conveyed about the importance of money, any periods of financial stress the family experienced, and how they affected the family (including residual effects on the individual such as worry about financial security), financial roles each partner's parents played in their family, and to what extent any differences in the financial resources of the partners' families of origin (e.g., income and wealth) played a role in their family experiences. Similar questions can be asked in regard to any memories that each individual has about the financial experiences of grandparents and other family members (e.g., an uncle who was seriously in debt and pressured the individual's parents for financial help). Money genograms can highlight particular family members for their exemplary or problematic financial behavior, as well as key events that created changes in family relationships with finances (e.g., bankruptcy, inheritance, lottery winnings, job loss). The goal is to uncover links between family-of-origin messages, experiences, and relationships with money and financial issues in past romantic relationships with each partner's present cognitions, emotions, and behavior regarding money. The therapist also may begin to uncover cultural beliefs and traditions regarding money that were present in each person's family.

After constructing a standard genogram that depicts the family tree across three generations (McGoldrick, Gerson, & Petry, 2020), the therapist adds information regarding financial patterns by asking questions such as those listed in Figure 8.2. The therapist can think of these questions as initial probes and follow them up with inquiries regarding details about each person's family experiences.

As we describe in the Intervention section of this chapter, the money genogram can also be used as an intervention method to help partners increase their understanding of factors that shaped each other's assumptions, standards, and expectancies about financial roles and tasks, the value and meanings they associate with money, their financial coping and problem-solving strategies, and how they communicate about money. These insights may increase mutual empathy for each other's personal responses to money issues and pave the way for discussions regarding ways to bridge differences between partners' patterns.

The following questions are used to probe for information about experiences that each member of a couple had regarding ways in which members of their family-of-origin managed finances, and how observing those money dynamics may have influenced the individual's own cognitions, emotions, and behavior regarding money. The interviewer should feel free to ask follow-up questions in order to achieve an understanding of the person's family-of-origin money experiences.

- What messages about money (things people said or did) did you receive from family, relatives, friends, and the community when you were a child? How did they affect your personal thoughts, emotions, and behavior with money?
- How often did you observe your parents (or other adults who raised you) talking about money? What were their conversations like?
- How well matched were your parents (or other adults who raised you) in their values regarding money? On what topics did they have different values?
- How were the major decisions about money made in your family of origin? What financial roles and tasks (e.g., wage earning, keeping a budget, making purchases, paying bills) did each person have, and how satisfied was everybody with their financial roles and tasks?
- When a conflict about money arose in your family, such as between your parents, what aspect of money led to the conflict? How was the conflict resolved? How did observing the conflict affect your own relationship with money (how you think about money, the emotions that you experience regarding money, and how you behave with money)?
- What were the best and worst examples of money management in your family? What consequences did they produce?
- Describe any worries or fears about money among members of your family. How did observing those worries affect your own relationship with money?
- What were your first experiences in managing your own money (for example, a parent having you open your own bank account)? How did those experiences affect your relationship with money?
- What significant experiences have you had during adulthood that have shaped your views about money and your relationship with money?

FIGURE 8.2. Individual Family-of-Origin Money Interview questions.

Assessment of Current Financial Stressors

When partners identify finances as an area of conflict, the therapist should assess the degree to which the conflict is related to objective financial stressors, such as reduced or insufficient income to meet economic needs, unexpected large expenses, and increased debt, theft, or bankruptcy. Therapists also need to understand the *severity* and *chronicity* of financial stressors. In evaluating the severity of the couple's financial stressors, the therapist needs to differentiate between objective events (e.g., insufficient income to meet basic needs, a partner who has been the primary wage earner just lost their job) and the partners' subjective financial strain. Rather than quickly drawing a conclusion about the severity of a particular stressor, the therapist needs to inquire about the specific effects it is having on the couple's life. Thus, although it might seem that the couple's sudden loss of a major source of income would constitute a severe stressor, perhaps the couple will reveal that the individual had been unhappy in that job, both partners were looking forward to an opportunity for her to find a more satisfying position, and they have sufficient savings to provide a buffer for at least several months. Unless the therapist has good reason to believe that a couple is denying the reality of the problems they face, judgment of the severity of their financial stressors is based largely on the couple's perceptions. However, sometimes partners do not agree about the severity, which may be a source of conflict.

Whether the partners agree or disagree, it is important to explore with each person aspects of their experience that influence how severe they find a financial stressor. A number of factors may influence individual differences in experiences of severity, such as past experiences of being traumatized by financial hardships that leave the person feeling vulnerable to dangers of current stressors, an overall tendency to be emotionally reactive to stressors (i.e., temperament), or a tendency to engage in catastrophic thinking. The therapist's ability to identify such factors will be helpful in treatment planning, which may require interventions to address them.

The therapist also should identify whether the couple has struggled with financial stressors over a long period of time, or whether their current stressors are acute and created by a sudden change such as an unexpected job loss, a large new expense (e.g., a medical treatment not covered by insurance), or a change in societal-level economic conditions (e.g., inflation, a major drop in the stock market that devalues investments). This information is critical to evaluate whether the couple may benefit from referral for expert financial advice. When appropriate, the therapist can refer clients to an agency that offers job and career support services (e.g., to find a job) and/or financial counseling (regarding budgeting, debt management, etc.). Couples who face difficult financial circumstances may benefit from a combination of financial advice and couple therapy that protects their relationship from the negative effects of financial stress. Without such financially focused assistance, a couple's improvement in communication, coping, and problem-solving skills through therapy may be insufficient to help them.

Even when a therapist refers a couple to a financial professional, the partners may still see the value of staying in therapy to address the emotional impact of the financial issues. They can benefit from improving individual and dyadic coping with financial stress, their communication skills for discussing money matters, their problem-solving skills, and their ability to resolve couple differences in ways of thinking and behaving about money. This option for concurrent intervention for financial stressors and the couple relationship should especially be explored when it appears that resolving their financial problems may take considerable time. They will likely need assistance in developing ways to cope with the stressors in the meantime and protect their well-being from the detrimental effects of financial stress.

Differences in Partners' Current Money Cognitions and Behavior

Sometimes conflict about money stems from differences in partners' cognitions and behaviors regarding dealing with money. It is very common for members of a couple to have different cognitions and behavioral patterns about earning, saving, and spending money. Partners may vary in their standards about how money should be earned, how much money one should earn in order to meet basic needs and/or live comfortably, how funds should be allocated in a budget (e.g., proportions allocated to children's educational expenses, clothing, or recreational activities), what proportion of income should be saved, how much money an individual can spend without first checking with their partner about it, whether and what level of debt is acceptable, the extent to which members of a couple should pool their financial resources or keep separate financial resources, and the like. Sometimes these differences do not become obvious to a couple until they play out in daily life—for example, when one member surprises the other by buying an expensive gift for themselves without mentioning the plan to the partner.

Partners' attributions about each other's money-related behavior also may be sources of negative emotion and conflict. For example, whereas one partner may consider taking out a loan for a purchase to be a wise decision to build the couple's credit rating, the other partner may attribute the individual's desire to do so as a reflection of irresponsibility. Another example is a person attributing their own desire to plan a joint vacation as based on a need for periodic vacations to maintain mental health, whereas their partner may attribute it to the individual's tendency to focus too much on frivolous fun rather than security that comes from saving money.

Partners' differences in financial cognitions are also linked to differences in financial behaviors regarding, among other things, spending, saving, taking on debt, budgeting, and providing financial assistance to relatives. For example, partners may differ in the degree to which they keep records of income, expenses, and savings via a budget, depending on the degree to which each person holds a standard that financial security depends on monitoring and controlling the flow of funds, versus a standard that adults should be allowed spontaneity and freedom as long as they do not make what the individual considers foolish spending decisions. Furthermore, cognitions may influence variation in each individual's financial behavior across situations and across time. For example, a partner may spend liberally on their children's clothing but be less inclined to spend money on clothes for members of the couple, based on different standards regarding the needs of children and adults. A couple may have agreed on having separate bank accounts for their earnings and expenses during their first years together, when their expenses were limited to the couple's own activities, but may come to disagree about having separate accounts once they have children.

As we have noted, differences in partners' money cognitions and behavior, as well as emotional responses such as anxiety, are common because they tend to originate from experiences in each person's family of origin (e.g., observing money as a source of conflict between one's parents), cultural beliefs and prescribed behaviors about money (e.g., money provides one power), and adult experiences (e.g., poverty, bankruptcy) with or without the present partner. Because members of a couple may lack empathy for roots of the other's way of functioning with money, it is important for a therapist to identify the degree to which partners understand each other's life experiences with money, as well as any negative attributions they make about causes of differences in their money management. Figure 8.3 lists questions a therapist can ask each member regarding their ways of thinking about and managing money.

Questions can be asked about budgeting, saving, earning money, or other aspects of financial behavior for which the partners reported differences. It is important for the therapist to convey a nonjudgmental stance when asking these questions, posing them in a curious way that helps each partner describe how they experience the couple's similarities and differences. Partners should be discouraged from criticizing the other's money cognitions and behavior, and the therapist should emphasize that each person is offering personal perceptions of each person's patterns. Each member of the couple has an opportunity to disagree respectfully with the way the partner described their patterns, with the therapist emphasizing that it is useful to uncover any differences in their perceptions, for further exploration. This approach emphasizes the message that people vary in the ways they think and behave with money, and a variety of approaches to managing money have potential to be successful.

It also is important for a therapist not to assume that similarity between partners' cognitions and typical behavior will consistently result in good money management. For example, we have worked with some couples, both of whom had an inattentive approach to budgeting and keeping

- Please describe your spending habits.
  - What types of things do you spend money on by yourself, and what things jointly with your partner?
  - How much is your spending planned in advance, and how much is it spontaneous (e.g., seeing something online that you would like to have and deciding to buy it)?
- Do you think that in general you spend too much, too little, or neither too much nor too little? Why?
  - Does that judgment vary depending on the type of expense?
  - What other factors do you tend to keep in mind when making decisions about spending?
- Have your spending habits changed over time? If so, in what way?
  - Please describe any life experiences that have resulted in you changing the way you spend money (e.g., changes in your income).
- To what extent do you think that your spending habits are similar or different from your partner's habits? Please describe the similarities or differences.
  - To what extent do the similarities or differences in spending between you and your partner seem to be helpful or create challenges in your relationship and in your family? Has it always been that way?

FIGURE 8.3. Questions for individual partners regarding spending.

track of expenses; for example, both often withdrew cash from ATMs without recording it, resulting in insufficient funds available to pay some bills.

An alternative approach to assessing couples' cognitions and behavior is a card game called *Money Habitudes* (Solomon, n.d.), which allows the therapist to talk with them about their typical responses in a nonthreatening, nonjudgmental way. Each card has a statement about a financial behavior (e.g., "I have fun money to spend the way I want"), and each partner decides the extent to which it represents them individually. After the couple sorts the cards in this way, the cards are turned over, revealing a category of "habitude" that each statement they selected reflects: *spontaneous* (money encourages you to enjoy the moment), *security* (money helps you feel safe and secure), *status* (money helps you create a positive image), *planning* (you use money to achieve your goals), *carefree* (money is not a priority at this point in your life), and *giving* (money helps you feel good by giving to others). This game may be particularly useful when partners need assistance in describing the functions money serves in their lives or when they are critical of each other. The Money Habitudes game can be used in combination with a money genogram (Mumford & Weeks, 2003) to explore cultural and family-of-origin messages that shaped partners' money cognitions and behavior.

Dissatisfaction with Financial Roles and Tasks

Whether it was the result of explicit negotiation, partners automatically carrying on family-of-origin traditions, or a pattern the couple developed implicitly over time through their interactions regarding money, all couples have established some distribution of financial roles and tasks. In terms of financial contributions to the relationship, partners may be main providers, secondary providers, co-providers, or nonproviders. In addition, they may have one or multiple unique or shared roles, such as managing family wealth and/or retirement investments, making saving and/or major spending decisions, and managing debt/credit, managing taxes/flex accounts/benefits, and estate planning. Roles usually include specific tasks such as paying bills, obtaining insurance reimbursements for medical expenses, making savings fund transfers, making ATM cash withdrawals for daily expenses, making purchases, bookkeeping, and filing taxes. Financial roles and tasks may become a source of conflict when one or both partners do not feel satisfied with the distribution. An individual may judge the distribution to be inequitable in terms of the workload and/or decision-making control over the couple's resources. Partners may perceive that the distribution of financial roles and tasks limits their financial independence and/or control over finances. Some partners may perceive that the couple never explicitly agreed on their current roles. The actual distribution and partners' satisfaction with their financial roles and tasks are influenced by their cognitions (e.g., standards) as well as their personal behavioral tendencies with money, which may have been influenced by internalized family-of-origin and cultural messages, as well as their past personal experiences with managing money.

Thus, when a couple presents financial disagreements, a therapist should assess the extent to which the conflict is based on partners' dissatisfaction with the distribution of their financial roles and tasks, one of the areas in the *Couple's Money History* interview. The therapist should ask follow-up questions about the source of their dissatisfaction and conflict, and how the present distribution of financial roles and tasks originated. Another measure that can provide useful information about the distribution of financial roles and tasks is the *Financial Management Roles* survey (Archuleta, 2013), which asks each partner about their level of involvement in financial management roles and tasks, as well as their level of satisfaction with their involvement. A therapist may need to administer this survey before interviewing the couple in detail about their financial roles when one or both partners appear uncomfortable about discussing dissatisfaction with their roles. Discomfort with addressing this topic may be based on a variety of factors, such as an individual not being satisfied with the couple's role distribution but reluctant to express it due to role expectations within their culture (e.g., that a male has primary responsibility as a provider in a heterosexual relationship). Alternatively, an individual's characteristics (e.g., a general conflict-avoidant style) may inhibit expression of unhappiness with roles. In addition, an individual may have an expectancy that it is not safe to disclose unhappiness with financial roles because their partner controls financial resources as a form of partner aggression (see Chapter 5). The Financial Management Roles survey (Archuleta, 2013) allows individuals to reveal concerns about financial roles more privately and safely to the therapist, and the therapist must use clinical judgment to decide when and how to inquire about more details, taking into account sources of partners' reluctance to disclose.

The therapist also can use the couple's money genogram to understand family of origin and other past relationships, including cultural influences that shaped each partner's standards about how financial roles should be distributed. For example, when constructing the genogram, the therapist can ask to what extent the couple's distribution of financial roles and tasks is similar or different from those modeled by couples in their families. When one or both partners express dissatisfaction with their roles, the therapist can inquire regarding whether any efforts to change them would involve acting in opposition to their family cultural background (e.g., establishing egalitarian financial roles when couples in their families have tended to be patriarchal).

Issues of Control, Power, and Autonomy/Dependence

Control over financial decisions and access to financial resources are associated with power and autonomy/dependence in relationships. When partners do not have equal access to money and/or say in financial decisions, there is likely to be an imbalance of power that can affect each partner's level of autonomy in making decisions, including acting on a desire to leave the relationship. Even though a gender-based power imbalance may be acceptable in some heterosexual couples based on their cultural traditions, it can create conflict for partners who value equality and independence. Conflict may be related to different standards about the extent to which partners should consult each other when making financial decisions, as well as the extent to which partners' incomes are pooled or kept separate. In addition to cultural influences, standards regarding financial decision making may be determined by a belief that a partner who earns more money or has more experience with managing money should take leadership. Disagreements may lead to arguments over the fairness and equity of each partner's control and access to financial resources. This may occur especially when one partner is the sole or main financial provider and tends to make decisions beyond financial ones. In cases in which partners pool all of their income and financial assets, they still may disagree about the extent to which they should consult each other regarding purchases or investments, or how much each person should contribute to expenses if their incomes are unequal.

Considering the potential presence of issues of autonomy, power, and control whenever a couple has financial disagreements, therapists should routinely ask about access and control over financial resources and assess each partner's level of comfort and satisfaction with such arrangements. However, it also is important for clinicians to identify whether an imbalance in financial decision-making power is part of a broader pattern in an abusive relationship, in which a partner restricts the other's freedom by dominating access to money. Exploration of potential coercive control must be conducted carefully to protect victims of partner aggression.

Styles of Coping with Financial Stress

Partners may describe feeling overwhelmed by their financial problems, noting how the problems affect their emotional and physical health, family relationships, and their productivity. Even if partners do not complain about financial stress, the therapist should always ask those who describe financial issues whether they are experiencing personal financial stress. This assessment can be aided by administering the *Family Economic Stress Scale* (Hilton & Devall, 1997) or the *In-Charge Financial Distress/Financial Well-Being Scale* (Prawitz et al., 2006), self-report instruments that ask about the level of stress individuals experience about their finances. When members of a couple report financial stress, the therapist should inquire about the effects of stressors on each of them individually and on their relationship, as well as how they are coping with the stressors individually and as a couple. Improving individual and couple coping strategies for financial stressors is critical to protect individual and relational well-being.

Effects of Financial Stress on Health, Relationship(s), and Productivity

The therapist needs to assess the negative impact of financial stress on each partner's individual mental and physical health, relationships with family, friends, and others, and productivity. This helps determine whether strengthening individual and dyadic coping strategies should be a focus of the treatment plan and whether referrals to other providers (e.g., individual therapist, physician, financial counselor) should be made. When one partner has been open about experiencing financial stress, the therapist should ask about the effects of financial stress on both partners, as research has shown that when one partner is affected, the other commonly is as well (e.g., Falconier & Epstein, 2010). The therapist should ask each partner what changes they have noticed since their concerns about finances increased: individual physical health and health behaviors (e.g., smoking, decreased exercise, increased alcohol use, changes in eating, sleep problems, fatigue, headaches, hypertension); mental health issues (e.g., depression, anxiety, irritability); deterioration in the couple relationship (e.g., less intimacy, more conflict, relationship dissatisfaction); problems in relationships with children, other family members, and colleagues/co-workers (e.g., more conflict, disengagement, aggression); and personal productivity (e.g., difficulty completing tasks). The negative effects of financial stress in any of those areas should signal that individual and dyadic coping strategies should be assessed to determine which aspects of coping could be improved.

Individual Coping Strategies

When financial stress is present, the therapist should evaluate the coping strategies that each partner is using individually, either to manage or reduce the negative cognitions (e.g., hopelessness, or helplessness) and emotions (e.g., anxiety, anger) associated with stress or to resolve the financial problem that is causing the negative subjective distress (Lazarus & Folkman, 1984). Individual partners' *emotion-focused coping* involves *cognitive strategies* such as reframing or decatastrophizing financial stressors as less threatening, distracting oneself from distressing thoughts; or mindfulness exercises; *behavioral strategies* that induce a different emotional state, such as recreational (e.g., walking, singing) or relaxing activities (e.g., breathing exercises, progressive muscle relaxation); and *problem-focused strategies*, which may involve getting advice, seeking information or skills to resolve financial problems, or generating solutions (Lazarus & Folkman, 1984). The therapist can administer a self-report questionnaire that taps various emotion-focused and problem-focused coping strategies. The Brief COPE (Carver, 1997), the Ways of Coping Questionnaire (WCQ; Folkman & Lazarus, 1988), and the Coping Strategies Inventory (Tobin, Holroyd, Reynolds, & Kigal, 1989) ask repondents how frequently they use strategies such as planful problem solving, confrontive coping, seeking social support, religion, positive reframing, venting, problem avoidance, social withdrawal, seeking instrumental support, humor, action, denial, and so forth. Because these surveys ask about individual coping with stress in general, therapists should ask partners to think about financial stress in particular when responding.

Some coping strategies (e.g., drinking, distraction) may provide immediate short-term relief, but they eventually have undesirable consequences or may have limited effectiveness. Often, some individual strategies may create challenges for the other partner and the relationship. For example, one person's use of distraction to cope with negative moods created by financial stressors may interfere with their partner's preferred way of coping through focusing on generating solutions to the problem. Conversely, the partner's problem-focused strategies may exacerbate anxiety in the partner who prefers to cope through distraction. Identifying such problematic dyadic effects is important for treatment planning.

Dyadic Coping

In the presence of financial stressors, therapists also should assess the couple's dyadic coping skills (see Chapter 3). This assessment should include an evaluation of how partners communicate their experiences of stress to each other, how they provide support to each other, and to what extent they engage in joint coping strategies.

STRESS COMMUNICATION

How much a partner provides support to the other or engages in joint strategies to cope with financial stressors depends on the partners' ability to communicate their stress experiences to each other and understand each other's experiences. On the one hand, partners may fail to communicate that they are seriously concerned about a financial matter, try to hide their level of stress, and/or do not feel comfortable asking for support. This may be due to personal standards that it is undesirable to express distress and/or ask for support, but it may also be due to the fact that sometimes partners are unaware that they are experiencing financial stress or may reject the notion that they could truly be stressed over financial issues. On the other hand, individuals may not support a stressed partner if they fail to observe verbal and nonverbal indicators of financial stress in the partner (e.g., frequently asking about expenses, often checking bank account balances, limiting purchases, increased drinking, restless behavior). Therefore, before asking about ways that partners support each other during times of stress, the therapist should inquire about the extent to which members of the couple can identify when they are feeling stressed in general and over financial issues in particular, and the degrees to which they explicitly communicate about and understand stress in each other.

The couple's stress communication can be assessed by asking each person to what extent they can tell that they are stressed over financial matters, how they communicate those feelings to their partner, and how they know when their partner is experiencing financial stress. Therapists should be sure to assess not only verbal indicators, but also paralinguistic (e.g., raised voice, rapid speech) and nonverbal indicators (e.g., tense body posture, agitation, excessive sleeping, change in eating habits).

PROVIDING SUPPORT

Within couple relationships, partners can benefit from receiving emotional support (e.g., understanding and validation, a positive reframe about a stressor's danger) and/or instrumental support (e.g., having practical guidance, seeking information together to solve a problem, generating solutions, and a partner taking over some of a stressed person's tasks to lighten their load) to cope with financial stressors. However, this support may sometimes be superficial or insincere (e.g., "Don't worry, everything is going to be all right"), or it may be accompanied by a blaming and/or unsupportive remark (e.g., "It will be fine, but you should learn from this experience and use better judgment in the future"). Sometimes the support provided may not align with the partner's needs. For example, a person may need to feel different (e.g., less shame over a financial setback) before being ready to seek a new solution, but their partner may only offer advice and no emotional support. Consequently, their therapist should assess the kind of support partners offer each other for financial stress and the extent to which it is helpful for the recipient, with discrepancies becoming targets for intervention.

CONJOINT COPING

Financial problems tend to be common dyadic stressors because they typically affect both partners. Research has indicated that when one partner is concerned about financial problems, so is the other (Falconier, 2010). As with other dyadic stressors (e.g., problems regarding a couple's children), partners can use conjoint strategies to cope with them. These common strategies can be *emotion-focused*, such as relaxing together or talking about the financial problem in a way that helps them remain hopeful, or *problem-focused*, such as gathering information and discussing potential solutions together. An extensive body of research has shown the benefits of coping with stressors conjointly as an "our" problem, even with stressors that seem individual in nature, such as one member's medical condition (for a review of studies, see Falconier & Kuhn, 2019). When partners engage in conjoint strategies, their bond strengthens. Considering the benefits, therapists should assess the extent to which partners rely on this type of coping to manage financial stressors by inquiring about how they perceive the stressors (as an individual or as a shared problem) and what, if any, conjoint strategies they use.

Even though stress communication, providing support, and conjoint coping can be assessed during a couple assessment interview, a therapist also can administer the Dyadic Coping Inventory for Financial Stress (DCIFS; Falconier, Rusu, & Bodenmann, 2019). The 23-item self-report DCIFS is an adaptation of the Dyadic Coping Inventory (Bodenmann, 2008) and asks participants about their own and their partner's communication regarding financial stress, positive and negative support, conjoint strategies to deal with financial stress, and their overall satisfaction with their financial stress-coping strategies as a couple.

Couple Communication Skills

When couples seek therapy for disagreements and arguments over financial matters, their communication styles are likely contributing to conflict. Partners commonly report feeling misunderstood, emotionally distant, and frustrated for not resolving their financial problems. Ineffective communication can severely limit a couple's ability to cope with financial stressors. Poor use of expressive and listening skills create challenges in partners' ability to understand differences in their money cognitions and behavior, including their standards about financial roles and tasks, as well as issues of control of financial resources. Poor communication also interferes with discussion of each person's financial stress, ways of providing each other positive support, and strategies for conjoint coping. It also may lead to escalated conflict and risk of psychological and physical partner aggression. As described in Chapter 3, couple communication regarding finances is assessed both via partners' self-reports and the therapist's direct observation of the couple's interactions in the therapy room. It also includes identification of cognitions and emotional responses that contribute to communication difficulties.

Problem-Solving Skills

Some couples feel overwhelmed by their financial stressors, which may block them from active problem solving or which result in a disorganized approach. In such cases, the therapist should assess the couple's current approach to problem solving, including the extent to which it is collaborative rather than adversarial. To what extent do they set clear goals, brainstorm possible solutions, evaluating the pros and cons of each potential solution, decide which solution(s) to try, implement the solution in daily life, and evaluate the results? The therapist also should probe for barriers to financial problem solving, such as a lack understanding of causes of their financial problem, poor financial management knowledge, or difficulties with executive function planning ability. Interventions to reduce such barriers become an important part of the treatment plan.

Financial Management Knowledge and Skills

Even though therapists can address the emotional impact of financial difficulties and help couples develop ways to communicate effectively about money problems, some couples lack basic knowledge regarding finances and can benefit from becoming more educated and/or skillful in managing their finances. Improving financial literacy and skills may be useful to the couple beyond dealing with a particular financial stressor. In general, couples may benefit, for example, from learning to prioritize expenses, develop budgets and saving plans, manage banking and credit effectively, plan for children's college expenses and/or retirement, understand taxes and employer benefits, and consider the pros and cons of joint or separate investment and bank accounts.

Improving financial management knowledge and skills may be critical for immigrant couples who come from countries with economic rules and contexts different from those of the U.S. model. Given that financial management is not within the expertise of many couple therapists, therapists need to be prepared to make appropriate referrals. In order to determine whether a referral to a financial counselor or a financial education program is needed, the therapist may ask the couple if they think they might benefit from getting expert financial guidance, or ask how confident each partner feels about their financial knowledge and skills. Even if only one partner reports low financial self-efficacy, the therapist should strongly recommend obtaining more financial education and guidance as a couple. Attending financial education sessions together will ensure they receive the same information and can work jointly on improving their household financial management. While pursuing financial education, the couple can meet with the therapist to work on the psychological impact of their financial problems and ways of coping together with them.

GOAL SETTING AND SOCIALIZATION TO TREATMENT

The goals of treatment follow from factors that the therapist's assessment identifies as contributing to the couple's financial problems. The therapist gives the couple feedback regarding patterns identified through the assessment and presents a case formulation that links their presenting concerns with aspects of their cognitions, emotional responses, coping responses, and financially related behavioral interactions. The therapist provides feedback about each area covered in the assessment:

- financial history of the partners and their relationship
- current financial stressors
- differences in partners' current money habits
- dissatisfaction with financial roles and tasks
- issues of control, power, and autonomy/dependence
- styles of coping with financial stress
- couple communication and problem-solving skills applied to finances
- financial management knowledge and skills
- cultural factors in couple financial problems and coping

The therapist also gives the couple a brief overview of a *stress and coping model* showing how financial issues affect individuals and couples, including not only the objective financial events they face but also their subjective cognitions about the financial stressors, emotional responses, and the ways they cope with stressors individually and as a couple.

Based on the information the couple provided during the assessment, the therapist and couple collaborate to set treatment goals. When dealing with couples who present with acute and severe emotional distress and conflict over financial stressors, the therapist tends to initially prioritize deescalation interventions, such as anger management strategies, expressive and listening skills, dyadic coping patterns, and financial advice. Beyond initial crisis intervention, frequent goals are helping partners understand each other's money cognitions and behavior better and manage their differences, increasing their ability to talk about financial matters constructively, and managing financial stress more effectively through improved coping, especially as a team.

Most couples who present with conflict regarding finances benefit from working on most areas covered in this chapter, but the primary focus of the treatment plan for each couple depends on the areas identified as needing more attention. For example, whereas some couples may need an immediate referral to a financial expert to be able to make decisions about their finances (e.g., refinancing, consolidating debt) or because they have low confidence in their financial management knowledge and skills, others may seek financial counseling later. The next section describes a number of interventions that help address financial concerns in couple therapy.

PLANNING TREATMENT

As we emphasized in Chapter 1, within a CBCT framework, therapists integrate interventions that target behavior, cognitions, and emotional responses because all three realms typically influence each other in partners' responses to each other. For the purpose of clarity, we describe interventions for behavior, cognitions, and emotions regarding finances in separate sections below, with examples of how one realm commonly is influenced by the other two.

Interventions to Modify Behavior

Modifying Problematic Financial Behavior through Psychoeducation

An individual's financial behavior, such as strategies used to keep records of income and expenses, commonly seem so routine to the person that they give little thought to using a different approach. In addition, if a partner, friend, or therapist suggests a different approach, the person's anticipation of awkwardness and potential difficulties may interfere with motivation to experiment. Furthermore, if the individual has been shamed for contributing to financial problems, their tendency to withdraw may interfere with trying a new behavior. Consequently, it is crucial that the therapist convey information about different money management actions in a nonjudgmental way and convey empathy for how "moving out of one's comfort zone" can be daunting. Although psychoeducation regarding the advantages of particular money management behaviors such as systematic recordkeeping are more appropriately conveyed by financial counselors, therapists can encourage clients to seek such professional consultation to learn about new approaches. They can frame such attempts as "experiments" that individuals need not continue.

Communication Training and Deescalation Strategies

For couples who can benefit from improving their expressive and listening skills, the therapist can follow the communication training procedures presented in Chapter 4. When the therapist is providing psychoeducation about the benefits of using expressive and listening behaviors, they need to emphasize that communication about money is difficult for many couples. The therapist may explain that some challenges in talking about finances are related to the meanings that partners assign to money, income differences between partners, and conflict regarding control over financial resources. Thus, the therapist will be monitoring how the couple interacts while discussing financial issues and will point out any instances of counterproductive behavior, such as blaming, criticism, name-calling, or defensiveness. The therapist will also explore the partners' thoughts and emotions that may contributing to those negative actions. For example, the therapist might interrupt when an individual who is in the empathic listener role responds to a partner's expression of feeling dominated in decisions about money by exhibiting signs of agitation and defending themselves rather than reflecting back the speaker's thoughts. In addition to reminding the partner of the listening guidelines, the therapist can explore the partner's cognitions and emotional response that led to their defensive behavior and emphasize that when the couple switches roles, the partner will have an opportunity to share thoughts and emotions about the couple's financial decision making. Given that arguments over money tend to escalate quickly, the therapist should apply deescalation techniques as needed, such as the negotiated time-outs discussed in Chapter 4. Handout 8.1 (available on the book's web page at *www.guilford.com/epstein-materials*) lists the financial topics a couple could focus on when practicing communication skills.

Problem-Solving Skills for Resolving Financial Issues

When couples present conflict and distress over financial matters, the therapist can guide them through the problem-solving steps outlined in Chapter 4. It is critical to have the relevant financial information to be able to set appropriate goals and brainstorm solutions, as well as to identify criteria for evaluating the effectiveness of solutions the couple attempts. It is important that the therapist avoid venturing into financial counseling without adequate training and should instead be prepared to refer the couple to a specialist. Nevertheless, the therapist and couple may determine that some specific problems can be addressed in couple therapy through generic problem-solving skills. For example, a couple may argue because they have different standards for how much each person should consult with the other before making purchases. Because this problem is based on issues regarding control and sharing information, rather than on the logistics of managing finances, the therapist can guide the couple in generating, evaluating, and experimenting with alternatives to their present arrangement. Intervention by a couple therapist can help reduce relational problems that interfere with some couples' abilities to make good use of advice from financial counselors.

Behavioral Homework

Once a couple has devised a mutually acceptable new approach to their joint money management, the therapist should collaborate with them to plan homework to implement the new behavior. This guided behavior change may involve practicing behaviors individually or as a couple. For example, an individual who tends to make impulse purchases may agree to go grocery shopping at least once before the next therapy session and stick to a written list of items the couple agreed they needed. For another couple whose conflict stems from one member dominating management of their investments, the partners may agree to meet for at least 30 minutes in the coming week. At this time, the person who had unilaterally made financial decisions will explain their investment strategy and methods to their partner, as a first step toward sharing the decision-making role and balancing power in the relationship.

Interventions to reduce cognitions that are interfering with a couple's ability to devise new, mutually acceptable approaches to financial problems commonly must be integrated with coaching a couple in problem solving. Those interventions focused on partners' cognitions are described in the next section.

Interventions to Modify Financial Cognitions

When a couple's financial conflict is based on their different standards regarding financial roles and tasks, the therapist needs to facilitate a cognitive shift involving partners' increased understanding of their differences before assisting them in ways to manage them. However, increasing mutual understanding is not possible if partners are not motivated to hear each other's internal experiences, such as traditions from their family of origin or anxiety based on painful financial experiences in a prior relationship. When significant differences in money cognitions and behavior exist, partners often are critical and judgmental about each other's patterns. Criticism and judgment build resentment and distance between partners, preventing them from feeling understood and valued. Coming to associate discussions of finances with aversive behavior and emotional pain can contribute to a desire to avoid each other. Therefore, it is important to move partners from judging each other's financial cognitions, behavior, and emotional responses to actually understanding them, thereby allowing partners to be empathic and supportive with each other. This can help them collaborate to find ways of managing their different styles by acknowledging the strengths and challenges each style brings to the process.

Psychoeducation Regarding Managing Differences

In order to increase partners' openness to discussing differences in their approaches to finances, therapists usually need to begin with psychoeducation about the benefits of mutual understanding of factors in each person's life that shaped their financial standards, expectancies, emotional responses, and behaviors. This focuses on exploring their differences rather than viewing them as insurmountable. For example, a therapist might encourage a member to describe their experience in which their former partner's poor management of investments resulted in them losing a significant portion of their savings, leaving them vulnerable to perceiving danger anytime the present partner showed interest in making even a minor impulse purchase. The partner's expressed anger at what was perceived as unjustified criticism and financial control on the other partner's part exacerbated such anxiety and anger that the partner exhibited no empathy for the other party's distress, forming a couple pattern of mutual negative emotion and criticism. The therapist provides psychoeducation about how the individual's need for security and the partner's need for respect and trust contribute to adversarial interactions. Instead, what is needed are mutual empathy and creative problem solving about how to manage differences between their financial cognitions and behavior that are based on their different life experiences.

As noted previously, the money genogram can serve as an intervention to increase partners' understanding of each other's standards and emotional responses regarding financial roles and tasks. While the therapist asks one partner about their family's beliefs, major financial events, and distribution of financial roles and tasks, the therapist is also modeling for the other person how to learn about one's partner from a stance of curiosity. The therapist asks the individual who is sharing information about ways in which they think patterns in their family shaped their current standards, expectancies, emotions, and behaviors regarding finances. Whenever the individual discloses such information, the therapist should ask the person's partner (1) what they heard that was new to them; (2) what they were able to hear that they were not able to hear before; (3) what factors may have prevented them from listening and understanding more about their partner's experiences; (4) how the information they heard has helped them understand the partner's thoughts and emotional reactions regarding financial roles and tasks better; and (5) how the information from the partner is helpful in dealing with differences between the two of them. Thus, this approach uses a behavioral intervention of teaching the couple how to communicate better regarding their life experiences that shaped their personal relationships with money to produce cognitive change involving increased mutual understanding that is likely to foster greater empathy for each other and less blaming.

For example, a Latina's insistence on helping her brother financially to open a store instead of encouraging him to ask for a bank loan had led to conflict with her partner whose ethnic background placed less emphasis on collectivist values. When the therapist guided the couple in constructing their money genogram, the woman described a long-standing tradition in her family of origin and community of family members helping each other financially and experiencing a sense of pride in being able to do so. Exploring the beliefs and emotions associated with assisting other family members helped her partner evaluate her behavior less critically. Her partner now seriously reconsidered his view:

> "In her cultural background, family members supporting each other is important, and as I think about it, she has made a variety of sacrifices for me and our kids. She's consistent about trying to help *all* of her family members."

When exploring differences in partners' approaches to finances, the therapist emphasizes that understanding each other's relationship with finances does not imply agreeing with everything a partner thinks and does. The therapist provides psychoeducation that reducing conflict over differences requires a balance between modifying some behaviors (e.g., increasing joint problem solving regarding financial decisions) and challenging one's own cognitions that fuel conflict, including each person ultimately accepting their differences (i.e., modifying one's standards for what differences are acceptable). This psychoeducation is a cognitive intervention for socializing the couple into a collaborative relationship in which each member accepts the importance of taking responsibility for reducing conflict.

The therapist discusses how pathways to managing differences can involve realization that the couple can find collaborative behavioral solutions rather than attempting to coerce the other person to change. However, if partners continue to escalate arguments with mutual accusations and criticism, the therapist should focus on a three-pronged approach involving strengthening communication skills, improving emotion-regulation strategies, and exploring each person's cognitions that are interfering with acceptance of the other's preferences (e.g., a belief that accepting the value of a partner's ideas means admitting flaws in one's own ideas).

Providing psychoeducation regarding the advantages of developing more flexible standards for acceptable management of finances can be quite productive. However, when partners continue to disagree about the distribution of control regarding money (especially when one member is unhappy while the other seems content with the status quo), this may reflect a significant broader issue in their relationship. As we noted previously, control of finances is common in relationships in which one member engages in psychological aggression, restricting the partner from access to resources that would facilitate personal autonomy (Murphy & Hoover, 1999). Thus, if a therapist attempts to induce an individual to reveal dissatisfaction with the distribution of control of finances in their relationship, there is some risk that the disclosure will result in a controlling partner retaliating after the session. It is wise for therapists to be cautious when they are assessing aspects of finances that may be influenced by power dynamics.

Not all dissatisfaction about financial tasks is based on one partner attempting to dominate the other. Another pattern that couple therapists observe involves one member taking responsibility for managing finances as the other partner has avoided financial roles, for reasons such as feeling incompetent regarding money management. In some cases, both members of the couple are satisfied with the arrangement, but in others the person responsible for budgeting, banking, investments, bill-paying, and like functions resents the burden. This issue likely poses little risk for partner aggression, but it may create conflict between partners about equity. Exploration of both partners' cognitions, emotional responses, and behaviors regarding this type of pattern can pave the way for collaborative problem solving to identify a more equitable division of labor and to reduce an issue that may have a corrosive effect on the quality of the relationship.

Identifying Steps toward Change in Financial Behavior, Based on Modification of Problematic Cognitions

Once partners' differences in financial cognitions, emotional responses, and behaviors have been delineated and they have worked on understanding each other's experiences regarding the differences, the therapist can ask each partner to identify areas in which they believe they can make behavioral changes. For aspects that partners identify as changeable, the therapist should encourage small steps rather than radical changes. For example, an individual might believe that it would be acceptable for him to shift toward keeping a family budget rather than making purchases without considering their financial resources. However, because he holds a standard that partners should not control each other's decisions, the therapist coached him in considering that a shift toward setting up a written budget with his partner and discussing income and expenses on a weekly basis might trigger discomfort on his part. The therapist guided him in identifying a sequence of steps toward formal budgeting, so that he could gradually increase his comfort with the change, beginning with each partner keeping a log of expenses on their phones and entering them in a joint record.

The therapist also had the couple anticipate any other personal, interpersonal, and environmental factors that could facilitate the change or that might create barriers. For example, the man who was open to taking steps toward budgeting reported an expectancy that his partner would "micromanage" him, a prediction that had some basis in the couple's history. Consequently, the therapist engaged the couple in discussing how the partner could contribute to change through a conscious effort to do minimal checking.

Although a therapist might choose to begin this work individually with the partners if they seem entrenched in their standards for how their finances "should" be managed, the goal is to conduct it as much as possible with each partner in front of the other. The other partner is invited to identify ways in which they can support the process of change. As illustrated by the example above, this usually involves behavioral interventions focused on guiding partners to avoid criticizing and correcting each other, looking for opportunities to encourage each other to make and sustain change. However, the therapist must be on the alert for cognitions and emotions elicited during work on resolving differences in financial behavior. In addition, the therapist may need to use any of the interventions for cognition and emotion described in Chapter 4 to facilitate couple collaboration on devising a new mutually satisfactory pattern of managing finances together.

Interventions to Modify the Experience and Expression of Financially Related Emotions

Partners' failure to manage negative emotions such as anxiety, anger, depression, and shame can interfere with a couple's joint management of financial stressors. Consequently, a number of cognitive-behavioral interventions for inhibited or poorly regulated emotions can be included in the treatment plan. The following are descriptions of useful interventions.

Enhancing Awareness and Expression of Emotion

Regarding enhancement of awareness and expression of emotional experiences, therapists can begin with psychoeducation that emotional responses to financial stressors are normal and can alert individuals that they are reacting to meaningful events in their lives. The psychoeducation also can increase partners' ability to differentiate among various positive and negative emotional states, as well as enhancing individuals' ability to use their emotional responses to identify their needs that are affected by financial issues. For example, an individual's anxiety may indicate that an overdrawn checking account has threatened their need for security. While coaching an individual to identify emotional responses to money issues, it is important for the therapist to attend to the other partner's reactions to the self-disclosure, which may interfere with the insight. For example, if a person is expressing anxiety associated with an expectancy that the couple's current spending will lead to problematic debt, the partner might respond, "That's ridiculous! You worry about everything! We have lots of savings, and neither one of us is an impulsive shopper." Even if the partner's perception is at least somewhat valid regarding the couple's resources and the individual's tendency to worry, the criticism and denigration are likely to upset the individual more and block their examination of their negative expectancy or any constructive joint problem-solving discussion ("As usual, you couldn't care less about my feelings! It's useless to try to talk to you!"). Pointing out the negative dyadic pattern can facilitate each person's exploration of their cognitions and emotions regarding finances as well as the couple's ability to use mutual empathic listening and collaboration to address their conflict and financial stress.

Improving Partners' Abilities to Moderate the Experience and Expression of Intense Emotions

As we have emphasized in this chapter, finances commonly take on significant meaning for members of couples and elicit strong emotions. For example, an individual who has a tendency toward catastrophic thoughts of financial insecurity, perhaps based on prior life experiences, may perceive a threat whenever their partner spends money beyond the amount they budgeted. The negative automatic thoughts may result in fear, criticism of the partner, and controlling behavior, all of which will elicit anger and criticism from the partner. Although behavioral interventions focused on reducing negative interactions and improving couple communication about approaches to money are important, a variety of interventions also can be used to improve partners' abilities to moderate strong negative emotional responses. In addition to coaching them in monitoring internal feelings (awareness of physical cues that they are becoming emotionally aroused), the therapist emphasizes the acceptance of one's emotions as useful information about one's goals and needs. Thus, the individual who automatically perceives danger and becomes fearful can identify the underlying need for security, whereas the individual who becomes angry can identify their underlying need to perceive respect and trust from their partner. However, the therapist also emphasizes balancing acceptance of one's own emotions and empathy for those of one's partner with efforts to moderate intense affect. This may involve countering some individuals' belief that venting anger is a good way to get others' attention. The therapist provides psychoeducation and practice with self-talk to prepare oneself to cope with stressors regarding money and to self-soothe to reduce strong emotions (e.g., muscle relaxation and mindfulness methods), use constructive skills to communicate about emotions with one's partner, and engage in problem solving to resolve the issue that triggered the strong emotions.

Integrated Interventions to Enhance Coping with Financial Stressors

Because both individual and dyadic coping with stressors involve cognitive, emotion-regulation, and behavioral components, we describe them together here and demonstrate how therapists can integrate them. The following are interventions for coping with financial stressors.

Individual Coping Skills

The three main interventions commonly used to improve individual coping with financial stress are: (1) identifying and removing unnecessary financial stress; (2) increasing use of effective emotion- and problem-focused financial coping strategies; and (3) enhancing physical and mental health.

With regard to identifying and removing unnecessary financial stress, individuals sometimes add to their subjective financial strain by adhering to unrealistic financial goals. For example, based on unrealistic standards for financial achievement, members of some couples set goals such as accumulating substantial savings or taking on unnecessarily large expenses (e.g., an expensive house), given the reality of their income. They place inappropriate financial demands on themselves, failing to differentiate between things they want and things they and their family need. Furthermore, individuals may exacerbate their financial strain by having catastrophic expectancies about their financial situation (e.g., that they will lose all of their assets during a national economic downturn), and making negative attributions regarding a financial stressor (e.g., "I didn't get that higher-paying job because I'm incompetent"). When therapists identify negative cognitions that are increasing distress regarding finances and in some cases are leading individuals to make spending choices that increase that distress, they can use a variety of cognitive interventions. Examples of these interventions are guiding partners in weighing the advantages and disadvantages of living according to unrealistic standards for financial success, coaching them in evaluating and modifying their catastrophic expectancies, challenging negative attributions regarding causes of their financial problems, and gaining a broader perspective when they have selectively overlooked instances of their financial successes.

The therapist also should help partners identify sources of unnecessary stress in other areas of their life that may add to the impact of financial stressors. The pile-up of stressors in stress and coping theory (Bodenmann et al., 2016; Price, Price, & McKenry, 2010) refers to the process in which various simultaneous stressors have an additive (and perhaps even a multiplicative) effect on individuals' subjective stress. Thus, a stressor that in itself may have a modest impact may combine with others to overwhelm their coping abilities. Therapists should encourage members of couples to notice whether some financial stressors could be targeted for elimination, reducing part of the pile-up. One useful method (Falconier & Kim, 2015) is to provide partners with rocks of different sizes and weights and ask them to label the rocks with names of the financial stressors they are experiencing. Heavier rocks should represent more severe stressors that are more difficult to avoid, whereas smaller rocks represent milder stressors that the individuals may impose on themselves through unrealistic standards (e.g., paying high monthly fees to belong to a popular gym rather than using a neighborhood recreation center). Partners are asked to feel the total weight of the bag that represents the total financial stress they carry. The therapist then asks the partners to remove the rocks that represent unnecessary sources of financial stress, until the bag feels lighter. This experiential exercise can facilitate a discussion with the couple about surveying all of their financial stressors, taking a realistic look at which may be optional, and feeling how decreasing the pile-up even by removing some relatively small stressors can result in a meaningful improvement.

Identifying and increasing the use of effective emotion- and problem-focused financial coping strategies initially is conducted during assessment of the couple when partners are asked about the strategies they use to reduce emotional distress and those they use to actually resolve the financial problems that cause the stress. The therapist should encourage each partner to use the individual coping strategies they have found effective in improving how they feel in the short term and have no untoward effects (e.g., cognitive restructuring to reduce upsetting thoughts about financial problems, talking to a friend whose empathy feels good, relying on spirituality/religion) or that help them solve the problem (e.g., financial planning, asking for temporary financial support from extended family). Coping strategies that have a negative effect either immediately or subsequently on the individual's health or their relationship (e.g., substance use, excessive escape into watching television) should be avoided. The therapist can coach partners to engage in the effective strategies as homework, logging when they use each strategy and how helpful it was.

Therapists also can help partners improve their coping with financial stress individually by guiding them in carrying out activities that enhance their general physical and mental health. The therapist begins with psychoeducation regarding the benefits of such health enhancement for managing stress because some clients may not realize the degree to which overall health influences one's executive functioning and motivation to persevere in the face of life stressors. Partners then can be asked to describe their current activities that contribute to physical and mental health and to brainstorm additional feasible healthy activities (e.g., creative and expressive activities such as drawing and singing, outdoor activities such as walking and biking, and leisure activities with others). The therapist and clients collaborate on planning such health- enhancing activities as homework.

Dyadic Coping

Interventions for improving dyadic coping skills for financial stress focus on stress communication, providing support, and engaging in common dyadic coping.

Interventions to improve stress communication between partners may include identifying when one's partner is stressed about finances or asking for support. In order to increase a person's ability to tell when their partner is stressed, the therapist should encourage each member of the couple to observe the other between sessions. They should pay attention to what their partner says, how they say it (e.g., tone), and what they do (nonverbal behavior) when they believe the partner is experiencing financial stress. The observations should be recorded in a journal and brought for discussion during the couple's therapy session. In session, partners should report what they observed about the other person who in turn can confirm or not that they were experiencing financial strain. The therapist needs to convey to the couple the benefits of communicating to one's partner what is causing financial stress, the emotions one experiences about the stressor, and the distressing meaning the stressor has for oneself. For example, an individual may report, "I feel incredibly frustrated and sad because we won't be able to afford to have our children attend college because we are already in debt. I am disappointed with both of us." The therapist can coach each partner in expressing their financial stress during sessions and ask the listening partner to reflect back what they heard. Partners should be encouraged to follow the speaker and listener rules for good communication at all times and to continue practicing between sessions.

Once partners have practiced observing signs of stress in each other and expressing their financial stress to each other, the therapist can focus them on providing mutual support. Therapists should encourage them to be specific about the type of support (emotion-focused or problem-focused) they need. After one person expresses financial stress and a specific need for support, the other is encouraged by the therapist to try to provide the requested type(s) of support. In case the partner feels limited in providing this support, the therapist can provide some ideas and modeling. The person who requested support then is invited to share how useful the support was in terms of helping them feeling any reduction in emotional distress and hopeful that steps can be taken to resolve the stressful financial problem. The feedback should not involve criticism of the partner who attempted to provide support, but rather an opportunity to help the partner obtain a better understanding of what type of support would be most helpful to the person in need. The therapist should describe positive and negative forms of dyadic coping to guide the couple in practicing mutual provision of support. Homework in which the couple continues practicing dyadic coping in daily life between sessions is critical.

Based on the benefits of dyadic coping we described earlier and because financial stressors commonly affect both members of a couple, clinicians should always encourage use of those forms of coping. As is true of any other intervention, partners should receive psychoeducation regarding the benefits of dyadic coping to manage financial stress and to strengthen their relationship. Therapists should discuss what they can do together to reduce emotional distress (e.g., relaxation exercises, breathing exercises, mindfulness strategies, engagement in spiritual practices, mutual encouragement, focusing on positives of the situation), as well as concrete steps they can initiate to resolve the financial problem (e.g., gather information, search for feasible solutions, seek instrumental support from financial experts, plan changes in money management). Therapists should also address any factors that have interfered with the couple's use of a particular dyadic coping strategy (e.g., a belief that seeking help is a sign of personal weakness) and troubleshoot ways to reduce those barriers.

Referral to a Financial Counselor or Expert

A referral to a financial expert should be made initially if the assessment indicates that the couple needs help in understanding options for solving their financial problems or if the partners have low confidence in their financial management skills. However, referrals frequently are made later in therapy whenever the therapist and couple agree on the need for expert advice and both members of the couple have provided written authorization to exchange information with the financial counselor. On the one hand, the financial counselor may share information about ways in which negative couple interaction patterns (e.g., mutual criticism, defensiveness) are preventing constructive work to solve financial problems. On the other hand, the couple therapist may share evidence revealed during therapy sessions of gaps in the couple's financial knowledge and skills.

TROUBLESHOOTING PROBLEMS IN COUPLE THERAPY FOR FINANCIAL STRESS

Couple therapists may encounter challenges with assessments and interventions regarding financial issues when one or both partners exhibit difficulty in examining and possibly modifying their cognitions and behaviors regarding the role of finances in their lives. Because money takes on significant symbolic meanings for many people (e.g., self-worth, security, power/control), attention to finances during sessions can trigger strong emotions and self-protective behavior. The following section describes common issues that may arise and presents suggestions for managing them.

Defensive Responses to Perceived Threats to Needs for Security and Control

Therapists need to recognize that individuals have developed patterns for protecting themselves when they perceive that their needs for security, control, and the like are in jeopardy. Clients who react defensively must be approached with a balance between respect for their fears and interventions to increase their motivation to take what they perceive as risks in order to better meet their own and their partner's needs.

- The couple therapist may need to hold individual sessions to focus on each person's perceived dangers regarding finances, negative emotions, and counterproductive coping styles. The therapist may also assess for possible individual mental health problem (e.g., clinical depression, an anxiety disorder) that may be exacerbating a person's responses to financial issues. This assessment may result in a referral for individual therapy.

- In some cases, couple therapy might be discontinued temporarily during a referral for individual therapy, but often it is useful to use concurrent couple and individual therapies, with couple sessions focused on improving their ability to interact constructively when a partner becomes distressed about finances.

Financial Power Imbalance between Partners

When there seems to be a power imbalance in access to financial resources but the individual with little power seems reluctant to talk about it or to challenge the status quo, the therapist should consider the possibility that this reflects a pattern in which financial control is part of partner aggression.

- It is important to carefully evaluate whether partner aggression is occurring. It may be unsafe to continue couple therapy if it increases the risk to a victimized partner, even if neither partner mentioned aggression during the assessment.

- Even though partners have not explicitly described a power imbalance in their relationship, the therapist can look for signs that one exists and can work to develop collaboration among the three of them in addressing whatever patterns they did describe as relevant to sharing influence, as long as the risk of intervening is judged to be low. For example, both partners may have described tension associated with "poor communication" and an inability to make decisions together about various issues. Although the therapist may avoid describing the pattern as a power struggle or point out an evident imbalance, it may be possible to engage both members of the couple in working toward a goal labeled as "improving communication and decision making." By focusing on skills for expression and empathic listening, as well as collaborative brainstorming of solutions during problem-solving discussions, the intervention may begin to gradually shift the power imbalance.

Financial Secrets

Another common challenge arises when one of the partners is holding financial secrets (e.g., gambling, debts unknown to the other partner, current or impending loss of a source of income). Such secrets interfere with progress in couple therapy, as the unsuspecting partner and therapist lack important information about the factors that are contributing to the couple's financial stress.

- Therapists may suspect the presence of secrets when an individual seems to be avoiding steps to make changes in how the couple manages finances (e.g., is reluctant to provide details about investments when the partner requests them, avoids scheduling a meeting with the partner to plan a budget). The therapist can initiate an individual session with each partner to discuss their approach to finances, with the goal of probing for any financial topics that each person has felt uncomfortable sharing with their partner. As we emphasized in Chapter 2, it is crucial for the therapist to preface individual sessions by emphasizing the goal of not holding secrets about finances or any other topic that affects the clients' relationship and treatment, but this also may inhibit an individual from sharing a financial secret. If the therapist suspects that a partner is withholding a secret, the therapist can make a statement such as

> "I've noticed your hesitation to discuss some aspects of your finances with your partner, and it makes me wonder whether there are things you feel uncomfortable sharing with your partner. As I have emphasized, I do not want to keep any secrets between the two of you, but it seems to me that in order for the two of you to work well together in managing your finances now and in the future, the teamwork will depend on your being open with each other about all aspects of your finances. I encourage both of you to communicate openly with each other, and if you are fearful of being open with your partner, you and I could discuss any negative reactions you are concerned you would get from your partner, and how you could handle them."

• If an individual does reveal a secret to the therapist, the therapist should encourage the person to reveal it to the partner. As in the above example, the therapist should explore the barriers that have blocked the individual from disclosing the information to the partner (e.g., fear of the partner's reaction, including anger and rejection; shame about how the individual has managed funds) and offer the individual support in preparing how to reveal the secret in a couple session.

• Because financial problems are a common cause of shame experiences for individuals and couples, the strong inhibiting effects of shame can pose a challenge to discussing financial issues in therapy. Couple therapists need to be prepared to identify and address individual partners' internal experiences of shame regarding what they consider terrible personal failures, as well as dyadic patterns in which one member of a couple actively attempts to shame the other member for creating financial problems.

KEY POINTS

- It is important for therapists to be attuned to multilevel sources of financial stress in couple relationships.

- Money issues commonly take on significant meanings to the partners regarding basic needs for security, fairness, control, identity, and caring.

- Treatment planning requires assessment and selection of integrative interventions that address partners' financial cognitions, emotional responses, and behavioral patterns.

- Therapists need to establish collaborations with financial counselors to whom they can refer couples whose needs fall outside therapists' professional expertise.

CHAPTER 9

Co-Parenting Problems

Of the responsibilities a couple may face together, raising children is among the most demanding of their time, energy, and emotional investment. Although being a parent can be a source of great pleasure, it is inevitable that parents will experience stressors in the process. Some stressors are normative and predictable (e.g., a significant loss of sleep with newborns and young children, fatigue from the combined demands of child care and other roles; disruption of familiar and pleasant patterns in the couple relationship). In contrast, other stressors come on suddenly and without warning (e.g., a child's acute serious illness or injury, violence at a child's school). Whereas some stressors can be relatively brief (e.g., an illness that remits), others are long-term (e.g., diagnosis of a cognitive disability). Furthermore, some stressors directly involve the relationship between a child and their parent(s) (e.g., oppositional behavior in response to parental requests). Given how common parenting challenges are, ranging from mild and temporary to severe and chronic, the likelihood that couple therapists will encounter clients struggling with managing them is quite high.

Each individual parent is faced with learning and applying a variety of skills, and a wealth of resources is available for them to enhance their knowledge and skills (e.g., parenting books). Although the adults in two-parent families may make use of such resources jointly, such as reading a parenting book together or attending a parenting program together, the emphasis in psychoeducation and skills training is on each parent–child dyad. Less attention is paid to challenges and strategies for couples (or other dyads such as a parent and grandparent) trying to work as a team. Some couples may naturally mesh their parenting beliefs and behavior smoothly, but others experience difficulty in forming a united team. Given the extensive resources available for enhancing one's individual parenting abilities, this chapter has a different focus; namely, enhancing a couple's capacity to co-parent smoothly and effectively. Thus, we focus on the couple as a parenting team, including strengths that contribute to teamwork, barriers to teamwork, and strategies to strengthen that aspect of the couple's overall relationship.

Thus, although the term *co-parenting* has been used to denote ways in which separated or divorced couples can continue to raise their children cooperatively between two homes, that is not our focus here. Of course, issues and strategies described in this chapter can be relevant for separated and divorced parents as well, but we are emphasizing work with clients who have sought conjoint couple therapy and who identify parenting issues as being among their concerns. We do address diversity in couple relationships (e.g., couples who have formed a blended family, LGBTQ+ couples, intercultural/racial couples) that must be taken into account in treatment planning. Again, co-parenting also may involve two individuals who are not in a couple relationship (e.g., a biological parent of a child and a grandparent; McHale & Lindahl, 2011; Sainii, Pruett, Alschech, & Suchchyk, 2019). Although this chapter focuses mostly on co-parenting for couples who have sought therapy, many of the principles and procedures we apply to couples also are relevant for those other parenting teams.

Sometimes a couple brings up co-parenting issues in the context of family therapy, such as regarding a presenting problem pertaining to a child (e.g., ADHD, behavior problems), and the therapy focuses on interactions among the adults and child. In some cases, the family therapy sessions are sufficient to address co-parenting difficulties. However, in other cases a referral for couple therapy may be needed to treat severe relationship issues that interfere with co-parenting.

Research has found a bidirectional relationship between quality of the couple relationship and quality of the co-parenting relationship (e.g., Belsky & Hsieh, 1998; Christopher, Umemura, Mann, Jacobvitz, & Hazen, 2015; Durtschi, Soloski, & Kimmes, 2017; McHale & Irace, 2011; Zemp & Bodenmann, 2018). Conflict and distress in the overall couple relationship can interfere with the partners working as a team to raise their children; in turn, conflict regarding parenting can erode overall relationship satisfaction. Therefore, co-parenting can be a major presenting problem in couple therapy, and programs that are designed to improve parenting skills may uncover underlying couple relationship problems that will continue to impede collaborative parenting unless they are addressed.

There also is substantial research evidence not only that parental couple distress and conflict are associated with a variety of negative child mental health and social outcomes, but also that co-parenting conflict itself has a direct influence on child well-being (Davies, Martin, & Cicchetti, 2012; Murphy, Jacobvitz, & Hazen, 2016). In addition, a causal pathway has been found from couple relationship conflict and distress to individual parents' negative behavior toward their children (emotional unavailability, insensitivity, irritability, use of aversive control), which in turn predicts child behavioral and psychological problems (Gao, Du, Davies, & Cummings, 2019; Holland & McElwain, 2013). In other words, the conflict in the couple's overall relationship has a negative spillover effect on their parenting, which affects children's well-being. There also is evidence of a reverse spillover process in which the degrees to which parents support versus undermine each other's co-parenting efforts predict their level of couple relationship satisfaction (Schoppe-Sullivan, Mangelsdorf, Frosch, & McHale, 2004). Consequently, direct therapeutic intervention to improve co-parenting interactions may improve the overall quality of the parents' relationship as well as children's functioning.

In spite of the evidence that overall couple conflict interferes with positive parenting, research also has shown that a couple's ability to co-parent effectively has positive effects on child adjustment, even after controlling statistically for the couple's relationship satisfaction (Teubert & Pinquart, 2010). Thus, if partners who are experiencing distress in their couple relationship are able to compartmentalize their issues and still collaborate well in parenting their children, the children will fare better. It is possible to make constructive improvements in a couple's co-parenting without fully addressing their overall relationship issues, which is the goal of interventions for improving the co-parenting of separated parents who have residual anger toward each other (Pruett & Donsky, 2011). Nevertheless, persistent relationship conflict and distress in intact couples with children seems to pose a risk for relapse in co-parenting problems, so it behooves couple therapists to focus on both aspects of the relationship in the treatment plan.

Parenting roles are among a variety of roles that members of a couple develop in the course of sharing life together. Some couples explicitly discuss and negotiate roles, but many slide into them without discussion (Stanley, Rhoades, & Markman, 2006), shaping each other's behavior. Aspects of parenting that both people may share or that may be addressed primarily by one parent include attending to children's emotional needs, managing socialization processes (e.g., teaching social skills, good manners, impulse control and emotion regulation; dealing with racism, heterosexism, and other forms of discrimination), transmission of cultural and family/personal values, and managing child behavior. The distribution of these roles between parents varies from family to family, but the pattern that a couple establishes early in their relationship tends to be stable over time (McHale, 2011; Schoppe-Sullivan et al., 2004).

One potential source of conflict in co-parenting involves partners having different standards for their roles and lacking adequate communication and problem-solving skills to resolve their differences constructively. It is important to consider possible cultural influences on role responsibilities (e.g., in some cultures, mothers in heterosexual couples might be more involved in children's daily lives, and fathers might focus more on discipline). Intercultural couples (see Chapter 11) may differ in their beliefs about the role of children in the family (e.g., whether children are allowed to express disagreement with parents) and about what discipline methods are acceptable. Personal standards regarding roles may be formed by exposure to prominent models in the general culture within which each parent grew up, and more specifically through the roles exhibited by the parental figures in their own family of origin.

Unresolved differences in partners' standards regarding parenting roles are widespread. For example, a survey of U.S. couples conducted by the Pew Research Center (2019), before the COVID-19 pandemic profoundly increased the amount of time many parents spent at home with their families, reported time spent in parenting within families with children younger than 18 in their household. Findings indicated that 78% of married or cohabiting mothers reported doing more parenting than their spouse/partner regarding management of children's schedules and activities, and 62% of the fathers agreed with that view. The survey also found that 56% of married fathers and 42% of married mothers were very satisfied with their spouse's approach to parenting. In spite of evidence that fathers' involvement in parenting increased during the past generation, these findings suggest that father underinvolvement in parenting still is common and may be a stressor in the couple's relationship, depending on the partners' personal standards.

RISK FACTORS FOR CO-PARENTING PROBLEMS

We use terms such as *teamwork, collaboration,* and *dyadic* coping throughout this book to emphasize the importance of partners functioning well as a system that is greater than the sum of its parts. Co-parenting is a key example of integrating the knowledge, skills, creativity, and energy of two adults in meeting children's emotional and physical needs while guiding them toward healthy development. When partners can integrate their efforts well, they provide resources for their children to flourish. However, if various factors interfere with their teamwork, parent–child conflict, parenting stress, couple relationship distress, and psychological adjustment problems within both the parents and children can result.

External Stressors Affecting Co-Parenting Problems

Stressors both internal and external to parent–child relationships often influence a couple's ability to co-parent. A stressor that negatively affects one individual may have spillover effects on the couple's overall relationship or specifically their co-parenting relationship. For example, in a couple with a child with developmental delays that require multiple forms of evaluation and treatment, a parent who has taken a major responsibility for managing those interventions often is highly stressed by the demands of that role and the sacrifices it produces for the parent's personal life. The negative effects on the parent's emotional and physical well-being can reduce their capacity to engage in parenting individually and with their partner. Furthermore, external stressors such as job demands, financial problems, demands of caretaking for extended family members, discrimination, social injustice, and neighborhood unsafety can produce a pile-up of stressors by either affecting the couple indirectly through their impact on one member or by interfering directly with couple functioning (e.g., eliminating time and energy for shared leisure activities). If a couple also is in conflict over different approaches for trying to resolve stressors, the conflict itself becomes a significant stressor that can spill into co-parenting.

Stressors take a toll on parenting especially when a couple has insufficient resources for coping with them. Limited financial resources for accessing medical and mental health professionals for a child's needs, insufficient funds to pay for child care that can provide respite for burdened parents, limited or no availability of culturally sensitive and affirming health care, educational institutions, and social service agencies, and the absence of a social support network such as friends, extended family, and welcoming communities are common examples of deficits in tangible resources. In addition, limitations in each partner's personal psychological resources can limit the capacity for parenting. Examples are chronic depression, anxiety disorders, overall emotion-regulation difficulty, and low self-confidence as a parent. Therefore, assessment and treatment planning must include resources both within the couple and beyond their family unit.

Cognitive Factors in Co-Parenting Problems

Partners' cognitions about themselves, each other, and their children may influence their ability to collaborate in parenting. Regarding personal *standards*, an individual may apply harsh or unrealistic criteria in judging their own performance (e.g., "I let my son ignore me and get away with everything. I'm incompetent as a parent"), a partner's actions (e.g., "He knows he should always check with me before letting the kids watch TV"), or the couple's co-parenting relationship (e.g., "We agree that our daughter needs to work harder to get good grades, so we should agree about how to motivate her to do it"). In addition to issues with an individual's own standards, a couple may hold conflicting standards regarding child-rearing practices, such as discipline methods, the degree to which children should be allowed to disagree with their parents, who should be responsible for aspects of child care, and so on. Those differences in standards may be based on differences between the partners' family-of-origin experiences, cultural standards for appropriate parenting, and each person's past parenting experiences (e.g., in a prior couple relationship). In addition, different standards might be based on a difference in partners' personal characteristics. For example, one parent may have stronger organizational skills and flexibility in shifting to a new strategy if their initial approach to a problem is ineffective, whereas the other parent may compensate for personal difficulty in organizational skills by holding strict standards for authoritarian parenting. The therapist's understanding of factors shaping parents' standards that contribute to co-parenting conflict is important for treatment planning.

Partners also may hold disparate *assumptions* about children and parenting that contribute to co-parenting problems. Some assumptions involve characteristics of children and appropriate methods of child rearing for those characteristics. Thus, one parent may assume that young children, especially those who seem highly intelligent, will understand and comply readily with logical explanations about their misbehavior, whereas the other parent may assume that children are by nature impulsive and only respond to consequences such as punishment. These different assumptions can result in co-parenting conflict regarding management of children's behavior.

If parents have similar assumptions about children and discipline, that does not guarantee that their joint child management efforts will be smooth and effective. They may share an unrealistic assumption, which leads to counterproductive co-parenting. For example, parents, perhaps based on their similar family-of-origin experiences, may endorse the belief that oppositional behavior by an adolescent must be met with firm control. When their adolescent ignores school homework or the curfew they set for getting home from outings with friends, their joint responses may include harsh parenting consisting of escalating punishments (e.g., grounding for the next month) combined with not allowing the adolescent to express feelings. During a therapist's assessment, it may become clear that the parents are frustrated with the reciprocal negative behavior between them and their child but have not engaged in any problem solving to identify alternative discipline approaches. The rigidity of their approach may be due to a lack of information about effective child-rearing strategies or assumptions that other approaches are ineffective.

Individuals' *attributions* for each other's parenting behavior also can affect their co-parenting. For example, an individual might observe their partner allowing their child to behave in a way the couple previously agreed was inappropriate. The individual may become angry based on an attribution, "My partner let Mark get away with that behavior and clearly doesn't respect my opinions." In addition, parents may disagree about the appropriate way to respond to a child's negative behavior based on their different attributions for the cause of the child's behavior. Thus, if the child has a tantrum when told to stop watching TV and come to the dinner table, one parent may attribute the tantrum to disrespect by the child, whereas the other may attribute it to emotion-regulation difficulty when the child was frustrated. Although the parents might agree that the child's tantrum was inappropriate, the first individual may become angry and punitive with the child, while the second individual tries to coach the child in self-regulation.

Partners' *expectancies* about each other's parenting behavior can limit their flexibility in co-parenting. Some couples who discover that one of them tends toward strict discipline whereas the other tends to be relatively lenient will develop polarized expectancies about each other, with the stricter one predicting overly lenient responses to child misbehavior from their partner and the more lenient one predicting overly strict responses. In order to compensate for the behavior they predict from each other, they "double down" and increase their own approach when a child violates their behavioral standards. For example, a parent may state, "When the kids ask for extra play time, I know my partner is going to give in. Somebody has to set limits, so I jump in and tell the kids they need to do chores or homework." The partner reacts to this description by stating, "I know my partner is going to be harsh with the kids, so I'll interrupt, pointing out that they have been keeping up with their chores and homework and deserve some fun time." Allowing this type of exchange in front of the children can increase the partners' upset feelings and polarization in their co-parenting.

Parents' *selective perceptions* of each other's and their children's actions can interfere with co-parenting, as partners who notice different events are likely to respond differently both emotionally and behaviorally. They may differ in the degrees to which they selectively attend to positive versus negative child behavior, perhaps based on their attributions about a child's underlying motives and personality. For example, an individual may attribute child misbehavior to a trait (e.g., "She's an oppositional kid and loves to control everything"). Parents who have developed beliefs that their children have negative traits tend to notice misbehavior and overlook positive behavior. Educational and therapeutic parenting programs include interventions to reduce such selective perceptions and guide the parent in reinforcing positive behavior. A co-parenting framework also focuses on discrepancies between two parents' perceptions.

These examples of cognitions that influence co-parenting can help therapists to become attuned to standards, assumptions, attributions, expectancies, and selective perceptions occurring in a couple's interactions regarding parenting. Therapists are likely to encounter unrealistic or inaccurate cognitions that should be targets for intervention.

Emotional Factors in Co-Parenting Problems

Effective co-parenting requires that partners be able to regulate negative emotions that contribute to internal distress and overt conflict. Among those emotions are anger, anxiety, and depression. The cognitive and emotional distress that parents often experience from the challenges involved in raising children are different from clinical psychopathology symptoms of depression and anxiety disorders (Deater-Deckard, 2004; Kwok & Wong, 2000). Therefore, therapists must differentiate between a situation-specific emotional state such as anxiety that one's child will do something harmful and a diagnosable clinical disorder such as Generalized Anxiety Disorder. Similarly, the exhaustion that results from sleep deprivation and unrelenting child care responsibilities can produce symptoms that need to be differentiated from those of depression. However, although the burdens and stresses of parenting will more likely result in situation-specific emotions, they do have the potential to elicit a clinical disorder such as a major depressive disorder (American Psychiatric Association, 2022). A parent may present with both conditions, and both may influence their co-parenting, but the interventions for them may be different; for example, a clinical disorder may require individual treatment as well as couple or family therapy.

Conflicts arising from differences between partners' standards and assumptions have potential to elicit frustration and some degree of anger. Anger can occur rapidly as one individual sees the other engaging in parenting behavior that is counter to their own standards or assumptions about the appropriate management of children. Based on that anger, the individual may escalate conflict through behavior such as contradicting the partner's instructions (e.g., "No! It is not okay for you to play when you haven't cleaned your room") or criticizing the partner's actions.

The challenges of parenting often elicit anxiety, especially when parents have expectancies that uncorrected child behavior will lead to worse child functioning and negative consequences such as academic problems, antisocial behavior, and a child's eventual inability to mature and live independently. Anxiety often begins when parents of a newborn fear that they are incompetent to keep their infant healthy and safe, and there are many sources of parenting anxiety throughout the child's development. Other examples of co-parenting challenges that may elicit anxiety and conflict between parents include managing a child with a disability such as ADHD or autism, responding to a child's coming out regarding gender identity or sexual orientation, helping a child with the complex process of applying to colleges, deciding on appropriate courses of action when an adult child wants to move back in with the parents and is not pursuing employment, and providing emotional support when an adult child is coping with a major life stressor such as job loss or the breakup of a couple relationship.

Often there is anxiety underlying anger that parents express about their children's behavior or the frustrations of trying to intervene appropriately with developmental challenges such as those listed above. However, vulnerable feelings such as anxiety may not be expressed to their partner. Parents may attempt to cope with their anxiety by imposing firm control over their children, using an authoritarian parenting style, as well as by arguing with their partner about each other's approach. A parent may experience anxiety when they have expectancies that the other's approach will be harmful (e.g., predicting that their partner's welcoming an adult child to move into their home will enable the child's passive approach to life; fear that their partner's preference to let a child write their college application essay without parental editing will lead to the child being rejected), although they may express anger more directly than anxiety to each other. Given the influence that anxiety can have on co-parenting, it is essential that therapists probe for it during assessment of a couple who present with parenting issues.

An individual's depression, ranging from mild to clinical levels, can interfere with their individual parenting ability as well as with the co-parenting relationship. Depression commonly is associated with thoughts of helplessness and hopelessness, and it may contribute to a negative self-concept and low self-efficacy as a parent. In turn, chronic parent–child conflict can contribute to a parent's low self-efficacy and depression (Kim et al., 2022). Helplessness and hopelessness can be influenced by both the challenges of raising a child and chronic difficulty co-parenting with one's partner. As with anxiety, it is important to differentiate between relatively mild situational depression elicited by experiences such as pervasive burdens of managing children's behavior and a depressive disorder that predated parenthood and affects other areas of the person's life.

Behavioral Factors in Co-Parenting Problems

A couple's co-parenting interactions with each other have been described as being either supportive or undermining (Ambrosi, Kavanagh, & Havighurst, 2022). Supportive co-parenting involves communicating respect for each other's style and collaborating (Feinberg, 2003; Margolin, Gordis, & John, 2001; McHale, 2011; Van Egeren & Hawkins, 2004), whereas undermining co-parenting is characterized by belittling, criticizing, and interrupting the other's parenting (Feinberg, 2003; Van Egeren & Hawkins, 2004). Another dynamic that can undermine co-parenting occurs when one of the parents triangulates a child into a coalition against the other parent—for example, by complaining about the other parent and encouraging the child to take sides. Such cross-generational coalitions are commonly addressed by structural family therapists (e.g., Fishman, 2012), but they are also within the scope of a cognitive-behavioral model and can be addressed in couple therapy sessions.

Behavioral factors that influence a couple's ability to resolve parenting issues and engage in supportive co-parenting include communication skills, problem-solving skills, and dyadic coping skills. The quality of a couple's skills can determine whether they can collaborate versus engaging in conflict or distancing from each other. Negative patterns include demand–withdraw, mutual escalation of conflict, or mutual avoidance (see Chapter 1).

Effective expressive and empathic listening skills are necessary for partners to understand each other's parenting perspectives and to provide supportive co-parenting. Constructive problem-solving skills are critical for finding mutually acceptable solutions to their differences and parenting challenges. Patterns of undermining co-parenting such as criticism, belittling, and blaming each other for child problems must be eliminated and replaced by collaborative negotiation. The collaboration inherent in good problem solving not only increases the likelihood that the couple will devise effective solutions to parenting challenges; it also creates a positive emotional atmosphere in their relationship.

Effective dyadic coping skills also are crucial for managing parenting stressors. For example, parents may be dealing with a child with significant needs or challenges (e.g., a developmental or medical condition, behavioral problems such as conduct disorder), or with child stressors such as discrimination (on the bases of gender, sexual orientation, religion, race, ethnicity) or immigration challenges in school, with peers. All these conditions add stress to the normal taxing tasks associated with parenting. Although it is important that parents engage in self-care practices to reduce the negative effects of stressors, partners can support each other by providing understanding (supportive dyadic coping), practical solutions (problem-focused dyadic coping such as seeking assistance from mental health professionals), or taking over a stressed partner's parenting tasks (delegated dyadic coping). Because many parenting stressors affect a couple jointly, parents can benefit from viewing a stressor as a "we" problem and engaging in dyadic coping, a process that can strengthen their bond. In contrast, when parents engage in negative dyadic coping (acting indifferent, hostile, blaming, or providing insincere or superficial support), negative effects on the couple bond, co-parenting behavior, and child well-being likely ensue.

COUPLE THERAPIES FOR CO-PARENTING

The extensive professional and self-help literature on improving parenting skills focuses on the context of an individual parent–child relationship rather than co-parenting, including psychoeducation about child development and parenting styles, as well as parenting skill enhancement. Books meant for clinicians and those intended for parents typically apply evidence-based interventions that improve an individual parent's interactions with their child(ren). For example, the widely used and empirically supported Parent Management Training—Oregon Model (PMTO; Forgatch, 1994; Forgatch & DeGarmo, 1999) includes components of giving good directions, teaching through encouragement, setting limits, monitoring, and problem solving (family negotiation). Another extensively used evidence-based parenting program is parent–child interaction therapy (PCIT; Eyberg & Members of the Child Study Laboratory, 1999; Niec, 2018). PCIT coaches parents in using authoritative parenting: a combination of warm communication/nurturance toward one's child and calm, firm control that involves clear instructions, selective attention to and reinforcement of positive behavior, and safe time-out procedures. Parental consistency is emphasized to foster a secure parent–child relationship.

Parenting programs and their dissemination through books for lay audiences most commonly have been based on research with primarily white, middle-class samples (Coard, Wallace, Stevenson, & Brotman, 2004), although they present their concepts and methods as relevant for any parent. Increasingly, the need to adapt evidence-based generic programs for use by diverse cultural, racial, sexual orientation, and gender identity groups has been stressed (e.g., Coard et al., 2004; Rodriguez, McKay, & Bannon, 2008; Parra Cardona et al., 2009). For example, the PMTO and PCIT programs have been adapted for application with culturally diverse parent populations, such as Latine families (McCabe & Yeh, 2009; Parra Cardona et al., 2012). They provide Latine parents, including those who are immigrants, with psychoeducation regarding ways to cope with common challenges they may face while raising their children, such as acculturation stresses (e.g., regarding language, traditions, values) and barriers to accessing support from community services (Gonzales, Deardorff, Formoso, Barr, & Barrera, 2006; Parra Cardona et al., 2009). Foci include discrepancies between parents' values and those of their children who are acculturated more in their host country's predominant culture, and parents' desire to teach their children values of *familismo* (strong bonds with others rather than independence), *respeto* (respect for elders and decorum in public), and *educación* (responsibility and moral conduct; Ayon, Williams, Marsiglia, Ayers, & Kiehne, 2015; Calzada, Huang, Anicama, Fernandez, & Brotman, 2012; Halgunseth, Ispa, & Rudy, 2006). Cultural sensitivity also involves therapist awareness that models that attempt to minimize authoritarian methods may fail to capture parenting by other cultural groups that is intended to keep children safe. Thus, Latine immigrant parents commonly have been found to use methods of control that blend authoritative and authoritarian aspects (warmth, restricted autonomy) to protect children from discrimination (Domenech Rodríguez, Donovick, & Crowley, 2009). A major goal of Black parents' racial socialization methods is keeping children safe in a racist environment (Voisin Berringer, Takahashi, Burr, & Kuhnen, 2016).

In addition to programs that adapted evidence-based parenting protocols for application in groups beyond the white middle-class populations in which they were developed, other programs have been designed from their inception to be culturally relevant for such applications. For example, programs that prepare Latine parents to use generic evidence-based parenting skills based on their cultural values and traditions and have demonstrated efficacy in improving parenting—for example, *Familias Unidas* (Prado & Pantin, 2011), *Bridges/Puentes* (Gonzales et al., 2012), and *Padres Informados Jóvenes Preparados* (Allen et al., 2012). In addition, parenting programs have been developed to enhance the skills of ethnic and racial minority parents for implementing racial socialization for their children and adolescents. Bo, Durand, and Wang (2022) conducted a review of outcome studies of such programs targeting Black and Latine parents—for example, Anderson, McKenny, Mitchell, Koku, and Stevenson's (2018) Engaging, Managing, and Bonding through Race program; Anderson et al.'s (2020) Family Learning Villages program; and Stein, Coard, Gonzalez, Kiang, and Sircar's (2021) One Talk at a Time program. Those programs commonly include components of cultural socialization, development of positive racial identity, preparation for bias, and overcoming school-based racial stressors, often combined with elements from evidence-based parenting programs such as giving effective directions, managing child noncompliance, monitoring, positive involvement with one's child, and family problem solving. The results indicated positive effects on outcomes such as parents' ethnic and racial socialization behavior, improved racial stress coping for both the parents and youth, and increased adolescent self-concept (Bo et al., 2022).

In addition, self-help parenting books for LGBTQ+ parents (e.g., Lev, 2004; Shelton, 2013) incorporate generic parenting skills with discussion of challenges commonly experienced by sexual minority parents, such as coping with discrimination as a parent and socializing one's children to deal with discrimination; finding physicians, mental health professionals, adoption agencies, legal assistance, day care facilities, and schools that provide affirmative services; and in some cases lack of support from families of origin. Furthermore, therapists can guide parents of LGBTQ+ children, adolescents, and young adults to online resources such as the *Child Welfare Information Gateway* within the U.S. Department of Health and Human Services, Administration for Children and Families (*www.childwelfare.gov/topics/systemwide/diverse-populations/lgbtq/lgbt-families*) and *A Practitioner's Resource Guide: Helping Families to Support Their LGBT Children* within the Substance Abuse and Mental Health Services Administration (*www.store.samhsa.gov/sites/default/files/d7/priv/pep14-lgbtkids.pdf*).

In spite of research demonstrating the importance of co-parenting, the major parenting programs have involved one parent from a family, either in group or individual sessions. Studies have indicated that couple counseling or therapy focused on partners' overall relationship (without a specific component on parenting) has a positive effect on general relationship satisfaction but not on co-parenting, in spite of findings linking overall relationship and co-parenting quality (Darwiche, Carneiro, Imesch, Nunes, & de Roten, 2022; Le, Treter, Roddy, & Doss, 2021). In contrast, couple therapies that explicitly include co-parenting have shown some improvements in the partners' parenting relationship (Darwiche et al., 2022; Gattis, Simpson, & Christensen, 2008). Gattis et al. (2008) used behavioral couple therapy that included interventions for parenting, whereas Darwiche et al. (2022) used a six-session integrative brief systemic intervention (IBSI) that focuses on improving the couple's romantic alliance as well as their co-parenting collaboration, for their children's benefit. Partners are encouraged to envision goals for improvement in both aspects of their relationship. Although differences in the dynamics of their overall and co-parenting relationships are noted, changes the couple can achieve in co-parenting (e.g., improved validation of each other's parenting efforts) are framed as evidence of their overall ability to resolve problems together. Psychoeducation also is provided regarding the negative effects of couple and co-parent conflict on children, to motivate the couple to work on their relationship. Parents are guided in empathizing with their children's stressful experiences in the family, which may be expressed through negative behavior because children commonly are not skilled at or comfortable sharing vulnerable feelings with their parents.

Thus, it is important for therapists to be attuned to differences in diverse families that need to be taken into account when using generic parenting programs that commonly reflect white heterosexual middle-class parent–child relationships (e.g., encouragement of development of child independence, verbal expressions of love). They need to supplement generic programs that may overlook parenting tasks that are central for other populations (e.g., racial socialization, gender and sexual orientation affirmation).

Some other research has found that couple relationship treatment can have positive effects on co-parenting. Based on the value of brief interventions in attracting clients, Doss, Cicila, Hsueh, Morrison, and Cahart (2014) conducted a randomized controlled trial for new parents, comparing brief interventions for couple relationships problems, co-parenting problems, and a control condition. The couple relationship protocol was based on Integrative Couple Behavior Therapy (Christensen et al., 2023) combining the building of communication and problem-solving skills with interventions to enhance partners' acceptance of behavior that may be difficult to change. The co-parenting intervention included couple discussions of their expectations for the transition to parenthood, expectancies of how disagreements would be handled, development of a co-parenting behavioral plan, and use of problem-solving skills to modify the plan as needed. Doss et al. (2014) found that both interventions improved both the overall couple relationship and the co-parenting relationship. It is unclear whether the equivalent effects of the two interventions would be similar for couples with older children whose characteristics and behavior pose more complex parenting challenges.

Studies have demonstrated that relationship education programs that focus on communication and problem solving to enhance parental teamwork have positive effects on a variety of outcomes, such as positive co-parenting behavior, family violence, parental mental health, and child psychological functioning (Feinberg et al., 2016; Gattis et al., 2008; Vaudan, Darwiche, & de Roten, 2016). These findings support the concept that couple therapy intended to improve co-parenting problems should include interventions specifically targeting the co-parenting relationship and factors that interfere with collaboration. Those factors that impede collaboration often include conflict in the overall couple relationship, but they also tend to involve other issues that we address in this chapter.

Ambrosi et al. (2022) adapted a program that focuses on teaching parents about skills for recognizing, understanding, and managing their own and their children's emotions to include co-parenting content. The original Tuning in to Kids program, whether delivered in a group format or to individual parents, focuses on noticing the cues of a child's emotional responses, validating and empathizing with them, and helping the child resolve upset feelings and engage in problem solving. It has received empirical support in a number of outcome studies (e.g., Mastromanno, Kehoe, Wood, & Havighurst, 2021). However, because most parents who attend parenting programs such as theirs are mothers, Ambrosi et al.'s (2022) goal is to increase the involvement of both parents by including co-parenting in the protocol. This is consistent with the trend in the field toward focusing on the co-parenting relationship because it emphasizes the advantages of teamwork and guides partners in developing patterns of collaboration that are not necessarily addressed in parenting programs for individual parents or in general couple therapy.

SCREENING AND ASSESSMENT FOR CO-PARENTING PROBLEMS

During the initial assessment of a couple, screening for co-parenting problems can be through brief questionnaires, interviews with the couple and individual partners, and direct observation of couple interactions. Within cognitive-behavioral assessment, the clinician is focused on information about how the partners behave within their co-parenting relationship, their cognitions (assumptions, standards, attributions, expectancies, and selective perception) regarding parenting and their co-parenting relationship, and their associated emotional responses. We rely on all three methods of self-report scales, interviews, and direct observation of couple interactions to gather information about co-parenting behavior. In contrast, we explore each individual's internal cognitions and emotional responses much more through interviews that allow the clinician to follow leads to uncover each individual's unique experiences.

Self-Report Scales

The Relationship Issues Survey (RIS; Epstein & Werlinich, 1999) (see Chapter 3), on which each partner reports the level of couple conflict in 28 areas of their relationship, includes the item "Child-rearing/parenting approaches." An individual's report that parenting is slightly, moderately, or very much a source of disagreement or conflict provides no details about the process between the partners. It is only a screening question that requires inquiry during interviews. Reports from members of some couples will be similar, whereas in other cases one member will report conflict regarding parenting while the other does not. Although care must be taken in exploring discrepancies regarding some sensitive RIS topics, such as partner aggression and sexual problems, asking tactfully about partners' different perceptions of parenting conflict generally is less risky. However, some partners will report that co-parenting issues produce significant conflict. In such cases the therapist can preface the inquiry with a statement that parenting is a big responsibility that can bring both pleasure and stress, and that many couples have some disagreements. The therapist can emphasize that couple therapy can be a good place to explore parenting experiences and ideas about ways to manage this stage of family life.

Even if neither member has indicated couple conflict over child rearing and parenting, during the assessment interviews the therapist should inquire about that topic as one of the possible sources of stress in one or both partners' lives. Lack of couple conflict does not mean that parenting is stress-free, and a couple may agree about parenting stresses but be ineffective both individually and together in managing those challenges. Thus, interviews can begin with questions about child functioning and any associated challenges, followed by questions about how the couple has tried to cope with child issues individually and jointly. This chapter focuses primarily on the co-parenting relationship rather than on improving each person's parenting skills, but knowing the specifics of the child-rearing challenges a couple faces is still relevant.

Differences between partners' skills for dealing with particular child issues, as well as differences in their levels of parenting self-efficacy, can contribute to ineffective co-parenting. Consequently, even though administration of questionnaires assessing areas of child functioning is not a standard part of couple assessment, when a therapist learns that parents are struggling with child problems, having them complete measures of child symptoms can be useful. Goodman's (2001) Strengths and Difficulties Questionnaire (SDQ) is a brief behavioral screening questionnaire that parents can use to describe areas of a child's problems with emotions (e.g., "often unhappy, depressed, tearful"), conduct (e.g., "often fights with other children or bullies them"), hyperactivity (e.g., "constantly fidgeting or squirming"), and social relations (e.g., "rather solitary, tends to play alone"), as well as prosocial behavior (e.g., "shares readily with other children"). The SDQ also allows the parent to report the degree of burden the child problem places on the individual parent or family. A more extensive measure is the widely used Child Behavior Checklist (CBCL), with versions for rating the behavioral symptoms of young children and school-age children. The version for parents of school-age children (CBCL/6–18; Achenbach & Rescorla, 2021) has subscales for eight clinical syndromes (anxious/depressed, depressed, somatic complaints, social problems, thought problems, attention problems, rule-breaking behavior, and aggressive behavior) that comprise two higher-order internalizing and externalizing factors, plus six subscales that are consistent with DSM diagnoses (affective problems, anxiety problems, somatic problems, ADHD, oppositional defiant problems, and conduct problems). Aside from identifying types of child behavior that pose challenges for parents, these types of rating scales can reveal instances in which partners' different perceptions of a child's behavior contribute to co-parenting difficulties and need to be addressed in treatment. Furthermore, when the therapist conducts a follow-up interview with a couple regarding their ratings of their child, it may become clear that one or both members lack confidence as well as knowledge in their ability to parent a child with particular problems. Their different ways of thinking about the task they face can elicit different emotions; e.g., as when a parent with low parenting self-confidence experiences more anxiety than their more confident partner. Because the child is not included in the therapist's work with the couple, these scales do not contribute to plans for particular parenting methods (e.g., methods for working with a child with ADHD symptoms). However, information from the parents' ratings could lead to a referral to a family therapist who specializes in teaching skills for managing particular child problems.

There also are questionnaires that assess qualities of the co-parenting relationship. For example, the Coparenting Relationship Scale (CRS; Feinberg, Brown, & Kan, 2012) is designed for intact families (rather than separated or divorced couples) and includes seven subscales (co-parenting closeness, exposure to conflict, co-parenting support, co-parenting undermining, endorsement of partner parenting, co-parenting agreement, and division of labor). Those subscales tap individuals' descriptions of behavioral interactions between partners. Members of a couple may describe different perceptions of those co-parent behaviors, based on different personal standards for co-parenting and different selective perceptions. Thus, the assessment can shift from descriptions of behavior to exploration of each partner's cognitions and emotional responses to the couple's co-parenting behavioral patterns. The therapist can use discrepancies between members' perceptions to stimulate discussion regarding the patterns that a good co-parenting relationship between them "should" exhibit; that is, their personal standards. Overall, self-report scales are used to identify problems and conflicts, but the assessment typically proceeds to more in-depth exploration through interviews about personal cognitions and emotions.

Couple and Individual Interviews

If a couple's stated reasons for seeking therapy are unrelated to parenting or co-parenting, the therapist still can ask about any effects of other presenting concerns on their individual parenting and co-parenting relationship. Examples of such effects are being distracted from co-parenting by other life stressors or feeling too tired from other life demands to have sufficient discussions as a couple about parenting.

When one or both members of a couple indicates on the RIS that child-rearing/parenting is a source of conflict, the therapist should ask for examples of how the conflict tends to play out in daily life (i.e., couple behavior and upset feelings triggered by issues regarding child care responsibilities). If one member reports greater stress regarding child rearing than the other, the therapist can first ask about the aspects of parenting that are stressful for that person, exploring the individual's cognitions about it (e.g., a negative expectancy that one's efforts will have minimal impact on a child's misbehavior) and associated emotions (e.g., anxiety, anger). The therapist also can inquire about how that individual's parenting stress may spill into the couple relationship. Thus, the distressed individual may yell at the child, exhibiting behavior that angers the other partner, who then criticizes the person. The other partner also can be encouraged to provide their observations of any spillover effects.

Because co-parenting issues can exist in the absence of significant couple conflict (e.g., both parents feel ineffective and overwhelmed by parenting), some couples may not mention co-parenting as an issue they would like to address in therapy. Consequently, it is important to routinely inquire about parenting and co-parenting concerns during couple assessments. The therapist might learn that partners commiserate with each other about their children's behavior and jointly feel ineffective as parents but seek couple therapy for other types of concerns, such as decreased feelings of intimacy. The therapist can acknowledge that parenting was not an issue they had in mind for couple therapy, but that parenting stresses have potential to detract from a couple's overall relationship and may be worth exploring. The therapist then can ask the couple to describe specific aspects of parenting that led them to consider themselves as incompetent and overwhelmed (cognition), their emotional responses, and what occurs between them behaviorally in those situations.

If working as a parenting team is a presenting concern, the therapist should ask for each partner's perspective on when the issue began (during early discussions while still childless, when they became new parents and experienced the realities of parenthood, when a child reached a developmental stage that produced new parenting challenges, when a threat to a child's well-being such as a serious illness occurred). Each partner should be asked about their views on the effects that the parenting issue had on their individual well-being, their couple relationship, and their children. What solutions have they attempted, and what were the consequences? What emotions (e.g., low mood, irritability) have the parenting issues elicited, and what effects have those emotions had on co-parenting?

When a couple describes co-parenting conflict, the therapist can inquire whether it stems from the fact that they have different assumptions and standards regarding child functioning and appropriate parenting methods. During the couple assessment interview, the therapist can collect information about each person's past parenting experiences, as well as the couple's co-parenting history. The individual assessment interviews provide an opportunity to gather more information on each individual's exposure to parenting models in their family of origin and elsewhere (e.g., portrayals in movies), any parenting experiences they had in prior couple relationships, and any concurrent parenting roles they have with children from a prior relationship.

Figure 9.1 lists topics that can be explored regarding partners' parenting experiences, both within their individual histories and in their relationship. Although the therapist can ask these questions during both the joint and individual assessment interviews, covering them in a joint interview provides an opportunity for members to increase their understanding of experiences that shaped each other's cognitions, emotions, and behavioral patterns in their current co-parenting relationship. These questions are intended to be starting points, and the therapist should be prepared to ask follow-up questions to uncover more in-depth information about the clients' personal experiences. When deciding how much detail to pursue in the joint interview, rather than more privately in the individual interviews, the therapist should gauge individuals' comfort levels with revealing information in front of their partner. When a person reveals historical information during an individual interview that seems to be influencing the current co-parenting relationship, the therapist can ask the individual to share their experiences of parenting in a subsequent joint session so that the therapist and couple can discuss the similarities and differences, and the implications for their ability to co-parent smoothly now.

In addition to interviewing the couple about their parenting and co-parenting histories, assessment includes an inquiry into the current state of their co-parenting. Figure 9.2 includes sample questions. As with the history interview questions, the therapist should use their judgment in selecting topics that can be discussed comfortably in the joint session versus those that at least initially might best be discussed with each member of the couple individually.

DIRECT OBSERVATION OF A COUPLE'S CO-PARENTING BEHAVIOR

In couple therapy, the clinician does not have opportunities to observe how the partners behave toward each other while interacting with their children. However, during joint assessment and treatment sessions, the therapist often can notice specific aspects of couple behavior related to co-parenting. Behavioral observations during sessions may produce an underestimate of the extent to which those co-parenting behaviors occur during a couple's daily interactions because couples may censor themselves in the presence of a therapist. Nevertheless, our experience is that as couples become more comfortable with their therapist or more emotionally engaged in a discussion of issues, they reveal a considerable amount about their relationship patterns.

Note: When a parenting dyad involves a dyad other than members of a couple (e.g., a biological parent and their adult sibling, a parent and a grandparent), the therapist should inquire about many of the same co-parenting aspects that are relevant, including historical development of the relationship and challenges that have been experienced.

- What parenting behavior did they observe from their own parents, both individually and as a team, when they were at various ages?
- What values and principles defined their parents' parenting and co-parenting style? Did their cultural/racial/religious/gender or other factors shape their values and principles? If so, how?
- What parenting challenges did their parents experience (e.g., a child with ADHD)? How did they deal with those challenges?
- What aspects of their parents' parenting and co-parenting styles did they consider positive and attempted to enact themselves as parents?
- What aspects of their parents' parenting and co-parenting styles did they consider negative and have attempted to avoid themselves as parents?
- What are each partner's standards for good parenting and the degrees to which they view both themselves and each other as living up to those standards?
- If the members of the couple have different cultural backgrounds, in what ways have those backgrounds influenced their parenting beliefs and styles? If the cultural differences have created some conflict, how has the couple managed it?
- How did this couple become co-parents together (e.g., unplanned pregnancy, planned pregnancy but with one partner desiring it more, planned pregnancy that they desired equally, surrogacy, adoption, forming a family with a partner who already had children)? Have those circumstances had any long-term effects on the quality of their co-parenting relationship or overall couple relationship?
- In same-sex couples, how did the partners reach agreements about each person's degree of involvement and responsibility in raising a child, and how satisfied has each person been with each other's childrearing behavior? For lesbian couples in which one partner is the biological parent of a child, how did they work out each of their parenting rights, including legal issues of parental rights?
- In blended families, to what extent have the partners defined a stepparent as playing a role in raising the children, and how well has that role worked (e.g., the quality of the relationships between the stepparent and stepchildren)?
- What significant events in the couple's parenting history influenced them positively or negatively as individual parents or their co-parenting relationship (e.g., a child's physical or psychological diagnosis, a child's accomplishment)? When did those events occur?
- At what times was each individual most satisfied with their own individual parenting, with the other's parenting, and with their co-parenting? What contributed to their feeling of satisfaction?
- In what ways has the quality of the couple's overall relationship influenced their co-parenting relationship, and vice versa?
- What factors outside their own relationship (e.g., input from their own parents, oppositional child behavior, a pile-up of life stressors, work–life imbalance, gender/racial/ethnic or other types of discrimination toward them or their children) have influenced their co-parenting relationship positively or negatively?
- What challenges have they experienced with their individual parenting, their partner's parenting, and their co-parenting relationship?
- What, if any, sources of information about child functioning and parenting skills have they consulted individually or together? How much have they discussed and applied the information in their family?
- What other strategies have they tried in order to improve their co-parenting relationship, and to what degree were the strategies effective?

FIGURE 9.1. Parenting history topics.

- In their co-parenting relationship, what roles and responsibilities is each person carrying out? If they share particular roles, how do they coordinate their efforts?
- If a member of the couple has joined the partner's family as a stepparent, how has the stepparent shared their thoughts about the biological parent's parenting style, and if the two people have some disagreements, how do they manage them?
- Have they noticed any differences in the ways their children respond to each of their parenting styles? If so, what do they think may be contributing to the difference?
- How satisfactory does each person think their current co-parenting roles are? What, if any, changes would they desire?
- How much confidence does each member have in their own ability as a parent and as a co-parent?
- To what extent do they have discussions about their co-parenting, to share their experiences, try to solve problems, and so on? How would they describe their skills for communicating with each other about parenting and other challenges?
- Fairly recently, when the couple faced a problem with parenting and felt that they handled it well, what did they do that was successful?
- In what ways is their overall couple relationship currently influencing their co-parenting relationship, and vice versa?
- What challenges are they currently experiencing with their individual parenting, their partner's parenting, and their co-parenting relationship?
- What resources do they have individually and as a couple (e.g., extended family and friends, finances to pay for assistance) to help them with the responsibilities of parenting? To what extent do they feel comfortable asking for assistance from those resources? Which, if any, resources are they using now?
- Currently, what factors outside their own relationship (e.g., input from their own parents, oppositional child behavior, when one parent says "no" a child pursues the other parent to obtain a "yes," a member's job demands, a member's health problem) are affecting their co-parenting relationship positively or negatively? How do those factors influence their co-parenting?
- Some couples' co-parenting relationships are affected by discrimination that the couple themselves experiences in society, based on race, culture, sexual orientation, gender identity, and other characteristics. If this couple has had such experiences, how have they dealt with possible spillover into their co-parenting?
- For parents in minority families and parents of transgender, gender-fluid, gay, lesbian, and bisexual children, how do they address socializing their children regarding discrimination, social injustice, and other difficult issues? How do they resolve any disagreements they may have about ways to parent their children regarding those issues?
- What are each partner's priorities and goals for working on co-parenting issues in their couple therapy?

FIGURE 9.2. Current co-parenting relationship topics.

Repond, Darwiche, El Ghaziri, and Antonietti's (2019) system for coding couple behavioral interactions when discussing parenting issues is a good guide for observation of a co-parenting relationship. *Positive relationship* codes are warmth and empathy in the dyad, nonverbal displays of positive affect (e.g., smiles), and shared positive emotion between partners regarding enjoyment of their child. *Cooperation* codes include behaviors indicating that partners were listening to each another, demonstrations of validation (e.g., encouraging a partner's participation in discussion of parenting, mutual investment of the partners in the discussion of parenting, and partners' agreement on their perspectives regarding child rearing. Codes for *elements of problematic interaction* include dismissal of a partner's ideas, disparagement of the partner's input, competition between partners about their expertise about their child, defensive behaviors, and interference with the discussion by negative emotions such as anger. Finally, codes for *role imbalance* include either parent's resisting or relinquishing the co-parenting role (e.g., withdrawing from taking responsibility for a child) and either parent behaving to restrain the other's co-parenting. The codes developed by Repond et al. (2019) are consistent with supportive and undermining forms of co-parenting (Ambrosi et al., 2022) we described earlier.

There is no need for a clinician to conduct detailed coding of a couple's interactions regarding co-parenting because being familiar with the types of positive and negative co-parenting behavior can help the clinician to notice them during a session. Beyond obtaining samples of a couple's behavior for assessment purposes, a therapist can apply the codes in interventions. This can include teaching the couple about the types of co-parenting behavior, briefly interrupting an interaction to point out the occurrence of particular acts, and guiding the couple in monitoring their own behavior. Monitoring also should include attention to each person's cognitions (e.g., "My partner's way of handling our child's misbehavior will make it worse") and emotions (e.g., anger) associated with their actions. As described in Chapter 3 on assessment, a therapist can briefly interrupt couple interaction to probe for the thoughts and emotions an individual experienced just before exhibiting a negative behavior such as dismissing the partner's idea about how they should response to problematic child behavior. In turn, the therapist can ask about the partner's thoughts and emotions regarding the individual's dismissive comment.

THERAPIST DECISIONS REGARDING APPROPRIATENESS OF COUPLE THERAPY FOR CO-PARENTING

The primary reasons why a therapist may decide against couple therapy for a co-parenting problem tend to be generic issues that make conjoint treatment inadvisable. These issues include evidence of partner aggression that places one or both members at risk of physical or psychological harm, substance use or individual psychopathology that interferes with an individual's ability to interact constructively with a partner and benefit from parenting interventions, and evidence that one or both members of the couple are unmotivated to collaborate as parents. During the assessment, the therapist also may discover that other people are having major effects on the couple's ability to function as a co-parenting team and that proceeding without involving those individuals in the treatment would likely be ineffective. For example, a household may include a dual-income couple, their young child, and one partner's parents who provide extensive assistance with child care and household chores. On their own, the partners have similar beliefs about appropriate child rearing that differ from those of the grandparents. However, the individual whose parents live with them feels pressure to honor their preferences, leading to couple conflict over parenting. Although the therapist initially thought it may be possible to help the couple develop their ability to establish their authority as the parental subsystem, it became clear that cultural factors in this three-generation family posed a strong barrier to shifting the family's power dynamics. The clinician discussed with the couple the option of a referral for family therapy that could include the grandparents. The therapist noted that family therapy could have more potential to find a balance between respecting the grandparents' roles and validating the importance of the young couple developing their own expertise and confidence as parents of a young child. Other factors in a couple's life that affect their ability to co-parent and cannot be addressed sufficiently in couple therapy interventions (e.g., unilateral physical aggression that resulted in one member's injury) also may lead to decisions for referrals, for concurrent treatment, or in place of couple therapy.

GOAL SETTING AND SOCIALIZATION TO TREATMENT

Difficulties in a couple's co-parenting relationship and problems in their overall relationship often influence each other. Consequently, when a couple seeks therapy for one area but not the other, it is important for the therapist to discuss with the partners how it would be wise to explore any possible spillover effects. We explain that our assessment is designed to identify any factors regarding the histories and characteristics of each partner, characteristics of the couple's overall relationship, and aspects of the couple's environment that are contributing to their parenting issues. Conversely, the therapist also considers it important to rule out the possibility that co-parenting problems have influenced the couple's overall relationship. Because co-parenting conflict also can affect the children's well-being, another goal that addresses parents' desire to raise happy, healthy children is to achieve a parenting atmosphere that contributes to children's sense of safety and security. Handout 9.1 (available on the book's web page at *www.guilford.com/epstein-materials*) lists goals we suggest a couple consider pursuing regarding co-parenting.

PLANNING TREATMENT

In clinical practice, therapists tend to integrate interventions for cognition, emotion, and behavioral patterns because these three core aspects of relationships continuously influence each other. However, for clarity of presentation, we describe the three types of intervention in separate sections. For all three domains, it is important to take into account diversity among individuals' prior life experiences that may have contributed to their parenting and co-parenting cognitions, emotional responses, and behavioral patterns. For example, two partners may have formed a blended family following the end of prior relationships due to divorce or death, and the co-parenting patterns they were accustomed to from those relationships may contribute to uncomfortable differences between them now. The treatment plan must take variations in past experiences into account. In the case of a blended family, differences in parenting standards and methods, as well as the quality of couple communication, problem solving, and dyadic coping may necessitate discussions of partners' different experiences, mutual empathy for each other's parenting background, and flexibility in experimenting to find mutually comfortable approaches.

Interventions to Modify Behavioral Patterns

When the therapist reviews with the couple information gathered regarding their co-parenting behavioral interactions, the three of them collaborate on identifying targets for change. This may involve reducing a tendency to interrupt each other when giving directions to a child, exhibiting conflict in front of children, expressing thoughts and emotions with vague and aversive verbal and nonverbal behavior, being adversarial and competitive rather than collaborative in trying to generate solutions to a parenting problem, or engaging in a demand–withdraw pattern regarding discussion of parenting issues. Some behavioral interventions (e.g., communication and problem-solving skills) are relevant for most couples, but other interventions will be selected and tailored to the needs of each couple. Some couples need more structure and guidance than others to establish a safe and collaborative co-parenting relationship. In setting treatment goals together, the therapist describes the clinician's role, including ongoing feedback to the couple to maintain a mutually supportive atmosphere in sessions. Devising a plan of how they will create a similar constructive atmosphere at home also is essential.

Psychoeducation is a prime example of the integration of cognitive and behavioral interventions. Providing a rationale for a type of behavior change and the steps involved in implementing it is a cognitive intervention that focuses on clients' executive function abilities, facilitating their motivation to try new behaviors and their abilities to carry them out. By the time couples seek assistance from a professional, they often feel inept as parents, and although they want to learn more effective ways of relating to their children, the therapist's expertise also is intimidating. Therefore, the therapist's conveying empathy for each individual's concerns about change in parenting behavior, which can reduce the person's worry that the clinician has judged them to be an incompetent parent, is important in developing a strong therapeutic alliance.

Improving Communication and Problem-Solving Skills

Communication skills training focuses on creating a safe environment for discussing parenting concerns and preferences, addressing disagreements constructively. This involves expressing one's ideas and emotions clearly, avoiding blaming and adversarial behavior, and listening respectfully to each other, especially when partners disagree. We emphasize mostly having these conversations without the children present, in order to achieve a common parenting approach before sharing it with them. However, it also is essential to be able to discuss disagreements in front of the children, because conflict situations often arise unexpectedly. For example, a couple and their young children may be sharing an enjoyable day at an amusement park, when the children begin to argue. At that moment, one parent may intervene in a particular way that the other parent believes is inadvisable. Perhaps the couple has a preexisting agreement that one will not interrupt the parent who has initiated a particular response to the children but will raise the issue later when the couple are alone. However, a partner may have difficulty restraining themself from interrupting and proposing a different approach, which may lead to an argument. A therapist can work with the couple on either improving their original strategy for handling in-the-moment disagreements or improving their ability to communicate about their disagreement in the children's presence. The therapist can present a rationale for open communication that emphasizes the "teaching moment" in which their children would observe their parents managing conflict well. Focusing on expressive and empathic listening skills (Chapter 4) will help the couple address conflicts better, whether privately or in front of their children.

Closely linked to expressive and listening skills is the couple's ability to collaborate in solving a variety of parenting problems (e.g., a child who argues with parents, noncompliance with family rules regarding chores, siblings who frequently argue, academic and school conduct issues, parents' different preferred discipline methods). In addition, partners often need to collaborate in solving problems their children face in the outside world, such as racial discrimination or being bullied at school. Therapists can guide a couple in using problem-solving communication (Chapter 4) to identify a specific problem, brainstorm possible solutions (including roles the partners would play in carrying out each solution), evaluate the pros and cons of each solution in terms of feasibility and acceptability to each person, select a solution to try, implement the solution on a trial basis, evaluate its level of success, and modify or replace it as needed. When partners begin with different ideas regarding how they are to solve a problem (e.g., a child being bullied at school), one parent may emphasize standing up for oneself, whereas the other may favor withdrawal in order to stay out of trouble and avoid conflict with peers and teachers. The therapist would guide the couple in respectfully listening to the advantages that each sees in their preferred approach, discussing potential disadvantages and agreeing on a solution that has good potential to have predominantly positive consequences.

Improving Dyadic Coping Skills for Parenting Problems

Couples can be coached in the dyadic skills they need to cope with the stressors of parenting. As described in Chapter 4, forms of dyadic coping involve behavioral interactions between the members of a couple that reduce the existence of a stressor (problem-focused coping) or decrease the negative emotional impact of the stressor (emotion-focused coping). The therapist provides psychoeducation regarding the value of dyadic coping in the co-parenting process, as well as forms of positive and negative dyadic coping, with examples tailored to the present couple's parenting stressors. For example, an individual might disclose to their partner that the stressors associated with providing for the needs of a child with a developmental delay have become overwhelming and emotionally exhausting. Emotion-focused supportive coping might involve the partner expressing empathy and caring, and arranging times when the individual can engage in stress-reducing recreation and relaxation. Problem-focused delegated coping might involve the partner offering to take on some of the individual's child care tasks (e.g., appointments with therapists) and household chores. The therapist and couple also can identify any instances when the partner engaged in negative forms of dyadic coping (e.g., ambivalent coping involving half-hearted efforts to share the individual's tasks accompanied by complaints about the extra work).

Improving Specific Behavioral Parenting Methods

Many couples whose co-parenting efforts have been ineffective benefit when a therapist teaches them about alternative methods that can be effective when they use them consistently as a team. It is important that the therapist remember that the partners likely feel incompetent regarding their parenting and will be sensitive to feedback from a professional they perceive as criticism. For example, a therapist may learn that both partners have relied on a coercive, authoritarian parenting style with threats and severe punishments (extensive grounding, taking away a child's favorite possessions for an extended period, corporal punishment). Explicit disapproval from the therapist can interfere with the therapeutic alliance and the clients' openness to new ideas. Instead, the therapist can note the clients' own reports that their parenting methods have had limited success, can tactfully provide psychoeducation that some alternative parenting approaches have been found to work well, and propose experimenting with those methods to see how well they may work with their children. If the couple also revealed that there has been inconsistent parenting between them rather than teamwork, the therapist can emphasize a "strength in numbers" approach in which children receive a clear message that their parents are strongly united.

Psychoeducation about effective co-parenting must take into account beliefs about appropriate child behavior and parent–child relationships that are based on cultural backgrounds or social location. For example, we have noted that parents from various minority groups who have experienced discrimination commonly use aspects of what is typically defined as authoritarian parenting (e.g., a focus on respectful behavior, restriction of autonomy) to protect their children from discrimination in the community. Consequently, giving them feedback that their behavior is harsh and inappropriate can alienate them. Similarly, some parents, especially from collectivist cultures, may be opposed to behavioral contracts in which children are rewarded for compliance with parental requests (e.g., for completing chores) when parents hold a standard that children need to learn that contributing to one's family is a responsibility.

Thus, when a therapist provides a couple with information about behavioral parenting methods and encourages them to use these approaches, which were developed in Western cultures, it is important to explain the rationales for the methods, ask about the parents' views about them, and collaborate with the parents in finding a version of each method that is palatable to them. For example, some parents view rewards provided to children for compliance with parental requests in behavioral contracts as bribery and counter to instilling collectivist values in their children. For these parents, the therapist can focus on rewards that involve positive activities between parent and child that enhance the child's self-esteem and attachment security without compromising the lesson that contributing to one's family is essential.

In co-parenting, it is crucial that the partners agree on the child behaviors they want to increase or decrease, as well as the consequences they will provide, and that they collaborate in monitoring child behavior and following through on those consequences. Therapists need to be vigilant of situations in which a behavioral contract has been ineffective primarily because the parents have failed to do their part. Therapists should explore with the parents what factors have interfered. Other behavioral parenting skills that can be included in the treatment plan are giving clear directions to children (rather than vague descriptions such as "clean your room"); communicating interest in a child's thoughts, emotions, and activities; making effective use of "time-out" procedures; and coaching a child in thought processes for good decision making. The parenting books we listed previously include detailed descriptions of interventions to develop those parenting skills and other books, such as Kennedy's (2022) parenting guide for lay audiences, emphasize building a strong emotional bond with one's child as a foundation for gaining compliance. However, therapists may need to supplement those guides with coaching on how partners can collaborate to carry them out jointly.

The core interventions for modifying co-parenting behavior are summarized in Figure 9.3. Interventions for modifying partners' standards, assumptions, attributions, expectancies, and selective perceptions regarding co-parenting commonly are integrated with interventions for behavior, due to the influence that cognitions have on individuals' parenting behavior, as well as their emotional responses. The following are interventions for modifying cognitions regarding co-parenting that are contributing to negative behavior and emotions.

Psychoeducation

Psychoeducation is used to increase partners' knowledge about child functioning, constructive and problematic parenting methods, factors that interfere with parenting, and qualities of an effective and satisfying co-parenting relationship. Other than the focus on co-parenting, the psycho-

- Monitor the partners' behavioral interactions in sessions, interrupt negative interactions, and coach the partners in substituting more constructive ways of behaving when discussing co-parenting issues. The foci are on interrupting each other's instructions to their child, expressing conflict negatively in front of the children, expressing their thoughts and emotions to each other with vague or aversive behavior, behaving in a competitive manner, engaging in a demand–withdraw pattern regarding discussion of parenting issues, and so forth.
- Use psychoeducation to provide a rationale for each new type of parenting/co-parenting behavior and the steps involved in implementing it (see Handout 9.2 for psychoeducation topics regarding behavioral interactions).
- Tailor the amount of structure and direction from the therapist to each couple's demonstrated need for it.
- After teaching parents about ways to collaborate on a co-parenting skill, rather than each person using it independently, and exploring adaptations that may be required based on parents' cultural beliefs and traditions, demonstrate it via modeling by the therapist or by professionally produced video presentations, and coach the couple as they practice the skill in sessions, followed by *in vivo* practice with their children at home,
- Build parents' ability to collaborate on setting up a behavioral contract to decrease specific negative child behaviors and increase specific positive actions, taking into account cultural adaptations that may be needed, based on parents' beliefs (e.g., about child responsibilities to their family and the implications of giving a child rewards).
- Guide parents in the use of collaborative communication skills for sharing their thoughts and emotions associated with co-parenting, again taking into account cultural variation in individuals' comfort with expressing themselves.
- Teach and coach parents in collaborative problem solving to respond effectively to parenting challenges.
- Build parents' skills for collaborative emotion-focused and problem-focused dyadic coping with parenting stressors.

FIGURE 9.3. Interventions for modifying co-parenting behavior.

education material is similar to protocols used in empirically based parenting programs that traditionally have been attended by only one parent (most often mothers). Details of the educational components of those programs are too extensive to be described in this chapter, so we recommend that therapists consult publications on programs such as PMTO (Forgatch, 1994; Forgatch & DeGarmo, 1999) and PCIT (Eyberg & Members of the Child Study Laboratory, 1999; Niec, 2018) and incorporate the material in discussions with couples.

As we noted previously, those programs provide information regarding normal child development (cognitive, emotional, and behavioral responses typical of children at various ages), the consequences of using coercive discipline methods versus more authoritative ones, and constructive ways of communicating with one's child. Information about constructive parenting methods such as giving clear positive directions, listening respectfully to a child's thoughts and emotions, setting clear limits consistently, and teaching through encouragement is intended to broaden each parent's assumptions and standards about children and parenting. All of this information should be tailored to parents' cultural beliefs and normative behavior. The psychoeducation is integrated with direct coaching and feedback to parents as they practice parenting skills, as described in the next section. Examples of other books for parents that include extensive "user-friendly" psychoeducation material as well as guidelines for improving parenting skills for particular child problems are Barkley's (2020) volume on ADHD; Barkley and Benton's (2013) text for parents of defiant children; Barkley, Robin, and Benton's (2014) book on parenting defiant teens; and Kazdin's (2009) book on parenting defiant children.

Although those sources of psychoeducation regarding parenting provide a wealth of information, there is limited coverage of the variety of factors that can interfere with individual parenting or co-parenting, which we have described in this chapter. In addition, only limited psychoeducation material is available that focuses on strategies to build a strong co-parenting relationship. Consequently, therapists need to be prepared to provide psychoeducation on co-parenting as part of the treatment plan for couples experiencing co-parenting problems. Handout 9.2 (available on the accompanying web page at *www.guilford.com/epstein-materials*) lists some topics that can be included in psychoeducation regarding the co-parenting relationship, which can be given to couples so they can refer to it in sessions and at home.

Helping Partners Modify Their Inaccurate Attributions about Each Other's Parenting Behavior

A collaborative co-parenting relationship is based on members of a couple viewing each other as having positive intentions and shared goals in raising their children. If an individual attributes their partner's actions to negative intent and goals that are in conflict with their own, it is likely to elicit negative emotions (e.g., anger) and negative behavioral (e.g., arguing with the partner). CBCT focuses on guiding members of a couple in evaluating the accuracy and appropriateness of their attributions about each other's parenting behavior and considering alternative causes for each other's actions.

With co-parents, it also is important to guide partners in sharing similar insight into the causes of their children's behavior, thereby facilitating a united approach to parenting. If one parent attributes a child's disobedience to disrespect for parents, whereas the other attributes it to the child's anxiety about life stressors, those different inferences may lead to different emotional responses (anger versus warmth) and behavior toward the child (punishment versus empathic listening). Nunes, Pascual-Leone, de Roten, Favez, and Darwiche (2020) describe how parents' empathy with their children's experiences involves understanding the child's motives in terms of thoughts and emotions and demonstrating openness to modifying their initial view of the child based on new information. Insight into children's experiences is linked to high-quality co-parenting (Marcu, Oppenheim, & Koren-Karie, 2016).

This does not rule out the possibility that a negative attribution about a partner or child might be accurate. For example, an individual told a child to stop watching television and observed their partner telling the child it was okay to continue. The individual attributed the partner's action to the partner intentionally giving the child permission to disregard the initial instruction, thereby undermining the individual's parenting authority. This attribution resulted in the individual venting anger at the partner in front of the child. When the angered individual recounted this incident to their couple therapist the next day, the therapist asked how certain the individual was that the partner's behavior was based on intentionally invalidating the individual's instructions to their child. The individual reported a high degree of belief in the negative attribution. The therapist then turned to the partner, stating:

"I can see your partner was upset that you contradicted her instruction to your son and is concerned about why you did that. In the interest of good communication between the two of you, and to be sure that she has a good understanding of your actions, please describe to me and her what you were thinking and feeling when you told your son it was fine to continue watching TV."

Perhaps the partner's self-disclosure actually was consistent with the other's negative attribution:

"We both want our kids to be serious about school work, but I think she's overly harsh and controlling when it comes to balancing some leisure time with all of their homework. When I saw her abruptly stop our son from watching TV, I just couldn't let that happen, so I stepped in and told him he could keep watching."

Thus, the individual's upsetting attribution was accurate, and it became clear to the therapist that they needed to focus on differences between the partners' beliefs regarding management of their children's school work and leisure activities, as well as how they can communicate to resolve conflicts directly rather than through incidents involving a child.

In some other cases, feedback from a person's partner provides information that may contradict and weaken a negative attribution. The therapist also can use other cognitive interventions such as guiding the individual in recalling past experiences with the partner that may reinforce or contradict their negative attribution. For example, the individual who made a negative attribution about their partner's undoing their instruction to turn off the television might report:

"I know we both want the children to value education and get their work done, and I often see my partner getting after them to do homework. So, it's not like I'm the strict parent and he's the lenient one. So, I was surprised and upset that he told our son it was fine to keep watching television, and I am confused as to why he did it. The first thing I thought was that he wasn't respecting my decision and was fine with undoing it in front of our son."

The therapist then turned to the partner and said:

"Your partner says the two of you have a history of being on the same page about school work, and she was taken aback when you contradicted her in front of your son. Please help her (and me) understand by saying more about how you decided to do that. What were your intentions, and how did they fit in with the way the two of you generally work on parenting together."

Thus, this exchange in the session combined gathering information relevant to an upsetting attribution and communication between partners regarding their co-parenting.

Helping Partners Modify Their Polarized or Unrealistic Assumptions and Standards, and Associated Expectancies, Related to Co-Parenting

Partners with different assumptions and standards regarding appropriate child behavior and appropriate discipline often develop polarized positions if they view each other as unwilling to consider each other's beliefs and preferences. Thus, perhaps one person believes that a parent should set firm rules for children's behavior and need not listen to the children's opinions, thereby teaching the children appropriate behavior and respect for elders, whereas the other person believes that in order to foster children's self-esteem and independent thinking, a parent should listen to the children's opinions and be open to some negotiation. If the partners' standards become polarized and rigid, whereby they convey a lack of respect for each other's beliefs, their ability to collaborate will be limited. Their therapist can explore with them possible advantages they may perceive in maintaining their polarized standards (e.g., a sense of self-righteousness at viewing oneself as wise and correct), but also the disadvantages (e.g., it blocks their ability to share the responsibilities and work of raising children; it detracts from the intimacy and satisfaction in their relationship; their conflict erupts in front of their children, causing the children insecurity about the stability of their family). Given the costs of maintaining polarized parenting standards, the therapist can encourage the couple to brainstorm how they could listen respectfully to each other's reasons for favoring their own standard (acknowledging that both of them are intelligent and both want to raise responsible and mentally healthy members of society) and discuss ways to integrate their ideas. When partners' assumptions and standards have been shaped by their cultural backgrounds, the therapist can emphasize the importance of understanding each other's perspective and honoring each other's cultural values in devising parenting approaches.

In the present example, the couple may agree on their overall goals in child rearing and may attempt to draw on aspects of each person's approach that could contribute to those goals. They might agree that parents should consistently communicate clear rules and guidelines to their children, and promptly give feedback when a child has violated rules. The other parent's role is to validate the point that a rule violation has occurred and requires processing. The purpose of the feedback is to stimulate discussion between parents and child rather than one-way directions from parent to child. On the one hand, the parents can explain the reasons and goals underlying their rule (e.g., keeping the child safe, developing good work habits that can be applied throughout one's life), without criticizing the child, whereas the child's job is to do their best to understand their parents' concerns. On the other hand, the parental feedback about the rule violation is intended to provide the child with an opportunity to express their own ideas about how they can achieve their parents' goals such as staying safe. The couple may then agree that parents should convey caring for their child and foster self-esteem, but still have the final word when a child opposes their rules. The therapist guides the couple in validating the value of each parent's beliefs and in identifying ways of parenting that are consistent with both people's viewpoints.

The therapist can emphasize identifying beliefs partners have in common regarding goals they want to achieve with their children, as this will help them form a strong partnership. The therapist also can emphasize that living with parents who have a positive relationship and are united in their co-parenting will be beneficial for their children's emotional and physical health. Therapists often can uncover partners' shared beliefs, such as the importance of protecting children from harm in the world as much as is reasonable, raising children who will function well as adults, and developing children who are respectful and caring with others. Although partners may vary regarding their standards for respectful behavior, the therapist can focus on their common ground, reducing their perception of each other as adversaries.

Whether partners have different assumptions and standards regarding child rearing or the same beliefs, their therapist can guide them in setting up behavioral experiments that will demonstrate the effects of an alternative approach on child behavior. For those who have negative expectancies about outcomes that would result from their partner's approach or even an approach that integrates their approaches, experimenting with different styles can provide evidence.

Helping Parents Modify Their Selective Perceptions of Child Behavior and Each Other's Parenting Behavior

Sometimes partners' tendencies to take polarized positions on parenting styles result from skewed perceptions of each other's behavior, as well as selective attention to aspects of a child's actions. Parents who are unhappy with particular aspects of a child's behavior often focus on further instances of those acts and overlook their positive behavior. In addition, an individual may selectively notice their partner behaving in a particular way that is counter to their beliefs about good parenting and overlook instances when the partner uses different approaches. The individual also may notice instances when the partner is failing to collaborate on parenting and may overlook instances when the partner is collaborative. When the individual develops an assumption that their partner has an undesirable global, stable parenting style, the individual may try to compensate for the other's parenting by "doubling down" on using an opposite approach (e.g., "My partner's so lax with the kids. I need to be a strong voice for control in our family!"). The therapist can use traditional CBCT methods for reducing selective perception (Chapter 4). For example, the therapist can ask partners to collaborate on making a list of various parenting behaviors that range from very lax to very strict, and then both partners have homework: they must keep a daily log of all those behaviors they themselves used and all the behaviors they saw the other person using with their children during the next week. Even if individuals' perceptions of themselves and of their partner are biased to some extent, the structure of this task puts some pressure on them to be close observers.

Interventions for Emotional Responses Associated with Co-Parenting

Interventions for individual parents commonly include methods for down-regulating one's negative emotions, so anger does not result in punitive behavior (Kazdin, 2009). Interventions for co-parenting also must address partners' tendencies to co-regulate each other's emotions (Greenberg & Goldman, 2008) (Chapter 1). Thus, one parent's anxiety about a child's actions or well-being, or their anger regarding a child's misbehavior, can induce an emotional response in the other parent. The induced emotion may be the same (e.g., one person's anxiety elicits anxiety in the other person) or different (e.g., one person's anxiety elicits anger in the other person). The type of induced emotion depends at least in part on cognition. For example, when an individual interprets a partner's anxiety about child behavior as a sign of weakness, it may elicit anger toward the partner as well as the child.

Interventions also are needed when one or both partners exhibit low awareness or expression of their emotions that may be influencing their parenting behavior. For example, an individual may repeatedly interrupt and contradict their partner's efforts to manage a child's behavior, even after the therapist has worked with the couple on ways to communicate with each other when they disagree. The therapist may notice nonverbal cues that seem to reflect emotional tension when the individual interferes with the other's parenting. When the therapist describes this observation, the individual initially may deny awareness of any emotion. However, the therapist may state that the individual seems to have difficulty controlling their urge to interrupt and suggests paying attention to bodily cues that some emotion may be fueling the strong urge. During subsequent co-parenting interactions, the therapist pauses the couple when the individual exhibits the first signs of tension and seems ready to interrupt the partner, inquiring about any emotions experienced. Gradually, the person notices and discloses some anxiety and anger toward the partner for using what the person considers inadequate child management methods. The therapist emphasizes noticing one's emotions, linking them to one's co-parenting concerns, and using communication and problem-solving skills with their partner to address those issues.

As described in Chapter 4, CBCT includes a variety of interventions to reduce excessive experience and expression of negative emotions, and interventions to increase partners' awareness and constructive disclosure of inhibited emotions. The following are applications of those interventions with emotions associated with co-parenting.

Psychoeducation

Increasing regulation of excessive emotion, as well as awareness and expression of inhibited emotions, both within each parent and between them, begins with psychoeducation. The therapist describes emotions as normal responses that reveal an individual's concerns and have powerful effects on relationships. The therapist also emphasizes that for emotions to be a helpful aspect of a couple's relationship when raising children together, it is essential that they be noticed, communicated clearly and constructively, and their meaning regarding partners' needs be understood. The assumptions, standards, and expectancies individuals hold that either fuel extreme emotion or inhibit emotion must be identified and addressed. Thus, an individual may hold an assumption that forceful expression conveys the importance of an issue, as well as an expectancy that their partner and child will ignore them if they calmly describe feelings. The therapist guides the person in evaluating the validity of those cognitions before implementing emotion-regulation interventions. A combination of psychoeducation about constructive and problematic emotion expression and interventions to challenge unrealistic cognitions (e.g., examining disadvantages of venting negative emotions) can be used.

Mindfulness, Physical Relaxation, and Other Self-Soothing Interventions

Coaching a couple in using mindfulness procedures can increase their awareness of their own emotional states and contribute to down-regulating intense emotion. In addition, the procedures can increase each person's awareness of how their own mindful detachment from upsetting events can reduce the degree to which their own negative emotions increase their partner's negative emotional arousal. For example, a member of a couple might be guided in using mindfulness to state the following:

> "When I express my frustration regarding our child, it makes my partner frustrated and angry, which in turn increases my own anger and frustration, but when I reduce my upset feelings through mindfulness methods, I contribute to both of us staying calm."

The mindfulness procedures can be combined with physical relaxation procedures such as muscle relaxation and breathing exercises that can be used whenever an individual becomes aware of increasing negative emotion, with an emphasis on using them during co-parenting interactions.

Individuals also can practice self-instruction to guide their regulation of strong emotions (e.g., "My partner just contradicted the directions I gave our daughter, which upsets me. I will relax my body and give my partner calm but firm feedback about how that affected me"). In addition, couples can be taught self-soothing procedures such as exercising, taking a shower, listening to relaxing music, and spending time with people who have a calming impact. They also can agree that it is in the best interest of their relationship that each member request a break from couple interaction to calm down. Although it may be impractical to use some of those methods when a couple is actively dealing with a child problem, regular use can contribute to reduction of overall tension.

Communication and Problem-Solving Skills Training

Communication skills for expressing emotions associated with co-parenting issues and listening to a partner's emotions provide individuals with a productive alternative to venting their feelings or ignoring them. Receiving empathic listening also can be a soothing experience for an emotionally aroused individual, as well as create a safe setting for an inhibited individual to experiment with sharing more.

Training in problem-solving skills also provides an outlet for partners to interact constructively regarding co-parenting issues rather than with adversarial behavior that elicits negative emotions. When one or both members of a couple have exhibited low levels of awareness and expression of their emotions, the therapist can emphasize that paying attention to their emotions will help them realize which potential solutions would work best for them.

Dyadic Coping Skills Training

Improving a couple's ability to engage in dyadic coping can reduce the impact of stressful parenting problems. The therapist begins by introducing the couple to types of positive and negative dyadic coping and their effects on decreasing or increasing individuals' stress. Next, the therapist focuses on the initial step of recognizing one's own subjective reactions to a parenting stressor and communicating about it to one's partner, which combines mindfulness and expressive communication skills. If both members of the couple are experiencing distress from a common stressor such as discovering substance use by their adolescent child, the therapist coaches them in taking turns expressing their thoughts and emotions about the stressor and providing empathic listening to ensure mutual understanding. The process then moves to identifying forms of dyadic coping that could reduce the two individuals' stress. The therapist emphasizes that the partners may find different coping approaches helpful, so the goal should be identifying and trying each person's preferences. Both problem-focused and emotion-focused forms of coping should be explored, especially when a parenting problem is likely to require sustained problem-solving efforts as well as some immediate emotional relief. For example, when a parent has shouldered most of the responsibility for pursuing treatments for a substance-abusing child, their partner could engage in delegated supportive dyadic coping by taking on some of those responsibilities. At the same time, the partner could plan some couple leisure-time activities to provide respite from the stress.

Because both members' emotions often are affected by parenting stressors, and partners' emotional responses tend to influence each other, it is important for a therapist to prepare them for co-parenting challenges that place both of them simultaneously in need of coping. The therapist can discuss with the couple the stressful parenting situations they face that require coping for both of them and the approaches they could try to reduce each person's emotional distress, as well as any "emotional infection" between them. The therapist and couple devise a detailed plan they will carry out at home during a trial period, and they evaluate its effectiveness during a subsequent therapy session, revising the plan as needed.

TROUBLESHOOTING PROBLEMS IN COUPLE THERAPY FOR CO-PARENTING ISSUES

Couple therapy for co-parenting issues must simultaneously address each parent's relationship with their child and the partners' relationship with each other. The complexity of intervening in the family system can pose clinical challenges. The following are common challenges in couple therapy for co-parenting and suggestions for dealing with them.

Underlying Couple Relationship Issues That Surface during Assessment and Co-Parenting Interventions

Because the quality of a couple's overall relationship commonly influences their ability to co-parent effectively, therapists should be cautious in accepting a couple's initial report of overall relationship satisfaction and a specific need for assistance with parenting challenges. Some couples with strong overall relationships do encounter problems specific to raising children, but others who have underlying issues may minimize them because they find them more threatening to the stability of their bond than stressors regarding their children. However, as the therapist collaborates with the couple to prioritize treatment goals, devise a treatment plan, and begin co-parenting interventions, signs of broader couple issues may emerge. For example, when discussing the importance of consistency between the partners' parenting behavior with a child, one of them may comment that the other "doesn't back me up with the kids." When the therapist asks the individual for an example, it may lead to more general complaints about the other's "respect for my good sense." Because co-parenting depends on mutual trust, respect, and willingness to seek mutually acceptable solutions to problems, interventions regarding parenting that call for such general qualities may trigger broader relationship issues.

- When co-parenting interventions reveal broader couple relationship issues, it is important to address them but also attempt to minimize how much strengthening their co-parenting teamwork will involve delving into an area that will place the well-being of their relationship at risk. The therapist can emphasize that co-parenting is a special relationship focused on partners' joint concerns about raising their children to be well-adjusted and happy people, and how to work well together toward achieving those goals. They can do this well even if they have some other concerns about their relationship.

- The manner in which the therapist describes the couple's broader relationship issues can make a significant difference. Rather than emphasizing an apparent problem between the partners, the therapist can begin by focusing on the strength the couple has demonstrated in joining as a team in seeking help for parenting challenges. The therapist can state that the partners clearly recognize the importance of their role in their children's development. Moreover, even though it can be uncomfortable seeking assistance from professionals, they have shown they are open to input and to trying some new approaches. The therapist can note strengths the couple has shown regarding their desire to work as a parenting team, such as reading parenting books together. Given their appreciation for teamwork, the therapist would like to give them additional ways to collaborate.

• The therapist can refer to a statement such as "my partner doesn't back me up with the kids" as a sign that a goal for the present therapy could be to figure out together how they might best back each other up (guidelines for possible changes), so that their children will view them as a team. At this point, the therapist could avoid inquiring about the more sensitive issue of how much they feel respected generally by each other, but would continue to monitor whether it is a topic that should be introduced as a therapy goal.

Problems in the Functioning of Individual Partners

At any point in therapy for co-parenting, it may become evident that one or both members of the couple have difficulties with individual functioning (e.g., depression, poor anger management) that likely will continue to interfere with co-parenting.

• The therapist will avoid defining an individual as "the problem" affecting their co-parenting but will note that particular symptoms are making co-parenting more difficult. That person could make a valuable contribution to their teamwork by working on it.

• Referrals for individual therapy to address this goal of contributing to strong co-parenting are made with the caveat that couple therapy for co-parenting can continue. A partner who was not referred for individual work also should make a contribution to teamwork by demonstrating support for their partner's additional therapy.

Parenting Role Conflicts in Multigenerational Families

Finally, if a couple and their children live in a three-generational household with one partner's parents, the hierarchy of parenting authority sometimes is blurred, with grandparents taking on parenting roles that might undermine the couple's parenting. Sometimes this is due to traditions in collectivist cultures in which grandparents have major child-rearing roles, but sometimes it is based on a particular family's dynamics (e.g., a single parent or couple needed to move in with parents due to financial hardship).

• The therapist can coach the couple in communication skills to express thoughts and emotions regarding the intergenerational conflict over parenting and demonstrate empathic listening to each other. They can follow up with problem solving to find new ways of navigating the hierarchy dynamics in their family. This can involve demonstrating respect for their parents' expertise and status in the family while also emphasizing the importance of developing their own parenting skills and relationships with their children.

• Although couple therapy may be sufficient to help a couple resolve generational role conflict, the therapist may at times determine that the family pattern is longstanding and entrenched. Thus, a referral for family therapy may be appropriate.

KEY POINTS

- Co-parenting is influenced by the qualities of the couple's overall relationship, and in turn the quality of their co-parenting is likely to influence their general relationship.

- Positive co-parenting contributes to the well-being of a couple's children, whereas conflictual co-parenting can be a significant stressor in children's lives.

- Partners need to develop parenting knowledge and skills, be attuned to the needs of their children, and understand couple relationship processes and the capacity to collaborate.

- Assumptions and standards partners hold, and their own cultural experiences in their families of origin can influence a couple's ability to co-parent.

- Factors that interfere with co-parenting may require referrals for individual or family therapy. Unless a partner's individual problems or intergenerational conflicts severely impair couple collaboration, couple therapy can continue concurrently.

CHAPTER 10

Couple Interventions
for Individual Psychopathology

Forms of depression (e.g., major depressive disorder, persistent depressive disorder), anxiety disorders (e.g., generalized anxiety disorder, panic disorder, social anxiety disorder), and substance use disorders (e.g., alcohol use disorder), as well as a variety of other psychological disorders (e.g., obsessive-compulsive disorder, posttraumatic stress disorder), are prevalent among people of diverse ages and other demographic characteristics around the globe (Kessler et al., 2005; World Health Organization, 2017). There also is extensive research evidence that individuals' psychological disorders commonly coexist with problems in their intimate relationships. Couple therapists are therefore highly likely to work with dyads in which one or both members are experiencing psychopathology symptoms. The symptoms may exist at a formal diagnosable level or at a degree of severity sufficient to interfere with the individual's daily functioning. For example, it has been found that among couples in therapy for relationship problems, 50% include one or both members with clinically significant depression (Whisman & Baucom, 2012). Conversely, clinicians who conduct individual therapy are likely to learn that relationship issues are one of the major contributors to their clients' emotional distress. The link between relationship distress and forms of psychopathology has been found in both cross-sectional correlational studies (which show a concurrent association between the two problems but do not demonstrate causal direction over a period of time) and longitudinal studies that provide evidence of bidirectional causation over time (Proulx, Helms, & Buehler, 2007; Whisman & Baucom, 2012; Whisman & Uebelacker, 2003).

On the one hand, living within an unhappy and stressful relationship can contribute to the development or worsening of psychopathology; on the other hand, one partner's symptoms can lead to stress, conflict, and dissatisfaction for both members of a couple. Based on evidence that individual psychopathology and intimate relationship problems commonly are linked, clinical researchers have developed couple-focused treatments designed to reduce negative aspects of couple dynamics that contribute to partners' psychological dysfunction and also harness strengths of the couple bond that can help individuals' symptoms improve (Baucom et al., 2020).

PSYCHOPATHOLOGY COMORBIDITY AND TREATMENT PLANNING

This chapter cannot cover treatments for the full range of forms of psychopathology that can appear in couple therapy, but we focus on a set of disorders that therapists commonly encounter in their practices. In particular, we describe couple-based interventions for depressive disorders and anxiety disorders, although we also direct the reader's attention to programs developed for some other forms of psychopathology such as substance abuse, trauma-based disorders, and eating disorders. Furthermore, although we refer to couple interventions that were developed for assisting individuals with specific DSM diagnoses (American Psychiatric Association, 2022), we emphasize the potential for using *transdiagnostic couple interventions* that address common symptoms and processes that occur across many diagnosed disorders.

Clinicians who practice couple therapy and those who practice individual therapy often work with clients who present with complex sets of symptoms (e.g., an individual who has symptoms of depression and anxiety, combined with a level of alcohol use that is troubling to the person's partner). Comorbid (co-occurring) symptoms of multiple disorders present a challenge for the clinician's treatment planning, in terms of where to begin when empirically supported treatments for the specific disorders differ. Existing individual and couple-based protocols for particular disorders identify interventions for specific emotional responses, cognitive content themes, and behavioral patterns typical of each disorder. However, the transdiagnostic model that has emerged in the psychopathology field provides a template for planning a therapy approach for each couple that can simultaneously treat comorbid presenting problems.

We do not have a simple solution to the problem of psychopathology comorbidity for case conceptualization and treatment planning. However, recent developments in understanding the common characteristics shared by many individual psychological disorders and ways in which those characteristics influence (and are influenced by) symptomatic individuals' intimate relationships have provided therapists with a core set of interventions that can be applied with diverse presenting problems. These characteristics involve (1) the types and intensity of individuals' emotional experiences in daily life, (2) the ways the individual thinks about those emotional symptoms, and (3) the behavioral and psychological responses that the individual uses to cope with distressing symptoms. In a couple context, the emotional responses, cognitions, and behavioral responses that the *partner* has to the individual's symptoms also contribute to relationship patterns that can exacerbate or alleviate presenting problems. The transdiagnostic approach described in this chapter has been used widely in individual therapy and can be applied in couple therapy to treat diverse forms of psychopathology. This approach that addresses the emotions, cognitions, and behaviors of both members of a couple as they deal with various life stressors is well suited for helping couples with diverse psychopathology symptoms and for couples with diverse social identities who are experiencing a wide range of environmental stressors in their lives. Focusing on both members' emotions, cognitions, and behaviors produces a dyadic conceptualization of factors that require intervention.

Causal Direction between Relationship Problems and Psychopathology

In addition to the problem that disorder comorbidity poses for treatment planning, couple therapists also need to consider available information regarding the causal direction between relationship problems and individual psychopathology. Sometimes it is clear that psychopathology symptoms predated problems in the individual's intimate relationship; sometimes there is evidence that relationship problems preceded the development of symptoms in an individual with no prior disorder history; and sometimes it is not clear which type of problem came first. The dilemma for treatment planning that addresses individual functioning as well as relationship problems is deciding whether interventions should focus on alleviating symptoms in order to reduce stress on the relationship, improving relationship quality and thus the quality of the symptomatic individual's life, or prioritizing elements of both. Although systems theory suggests that intervening in any component of a system can produce change in the rest of the system, we also know that both negative relationship patterns and psychological disorders can require interventions that specifically target the interpersonal or intrapersonal dynamics.

Cognitive–Behavioral Conceptualization

Although a variety of cognitive-behavioral models have been developed regarding factors contributing to diverse forms of psychopathology, they tend to share foci on four realms: cognitive, affective, physiological, and behavioral. The symptoms associated with each DSM diagnosis can be viewed as forms of cognition, affect, physiological response, or behavior, or a combination of those domains. For example, some common symptoms of a major depressive episode include hopeless thoughts (cognition), low mood (affect), fatigue (physiological), and social isolation (behavior); symptoms of generalized anxiety disorder include excessive worry (cognition), anxious mood (affect), muscle tension (physiological), and restless actions (behavior). We have described these core realms of functioning in Chapter 1. CBT models of individual psychopathology have varied in the degrees to which the four realms are emphasized, but they generally consider all of them to be relevant.

Cognitive components of individual psychological functioning and psychopathology include a variety of aspects of information processing. At some levels, these aspects of information processing are normal and adaptive; they allow individuals to understand and learn from their experiences and to respond in appropriate ways to life situations. However, they are susceptible to distortion and can become dysfunctional when they are inaccurate or extreme. Some aspects of information processing involve momentary "stream-of-consciousness" thinking such as selective perception of the information in one's environment (what one notices or fails to notice), inferences regarding causes of perceived events, and expectancies or inferences about future events. When those cognitions are negative, they can be especially distressing when they take the form of *rumination*—repetitive thoughts about existing distressing symptoms and current or potential problems that cause them, without constructive problem solving (Nolen-Hoeksema, Stice, Wade, & Bohon, 2007). There is considerable research evidence showing that rumination exacerbates psychopathology symptoms (e.g., Marcus, Hughes, & Arnau, 2008).

As described in Chapter 1, another form of cognitive information processing that is inherently normal but can be distorted and contribute to psychopathology involves relatively stable core knowledge structures or schemas that an individual has developed through life experiences regarding characteristics of the world (Fletcher et al., 2018). Schemas can focus on characteristics of other people (e.g., "You can only really depend on yourself"), oneself (e.g., "I'm not a likeable person"; "I don't have the skills and intelligence to make it in this world"), and the nature of the world (e.g., "Some people have all the luck, and others never get a break"). Whereas schemas that are realistic and appropriate help the individual to understand the complexities of the world, including relationships with other people, unrealistic schemas can lead to distress and conflict with others; for example, when they involve unrealistic standards for how partners "should" demonstrate their caring for each other.

Additional forms of information processing that can contribute to various psychological disorders involve "executive functions" such as problem solving, appropriate priority setting, and self-regulation, which have been implicated in many forms of psychopathology (Nezu, Nezu, & Hays, 2019). The abilities to anticipate problems, plan how one can behave to best cope with them, and regulate the intensity of one's emotional responses (which in turn can interfere with cognitive and behavioral problem solving) tend to be developed beginning in childhood via socialization processes, although genetic factors can contribute to attentional and thought disorders (in the extreme, psychotic thinking; Kotov et al., 2011).

Affective components of individual functioning and psychopathology include the level of intensity of an individual's emotions, the extent to which the person is able to *regulate* that intensity, how well the person can tolerate strong emotions, and how well the individual is able to *communicate* with others about the emotions that are experienced (the last involving behavioral skills). People vary considerably in how "in tune" they are with their subjective inner experiences, including emotional states, and their ability to differentiate particular emotions. The capacity for emotion regulation has received extensive attention in the literature on psychopathology from childhood through adulthood and its treatment (Gross, 2014), and we have described strategies used to address it in couple therapy in Chapter 4. Those strategies focus either on *upregulating* emotions in individuals whose experience of emotions tends to be inhibited and *downregulating* overly intense emotions that interfere with constructive functioning. Similarly, behavioral deficits in individuals' abilities to communicate with other people in a clear and balanced rather than overly negative manner about their emotional experiences have been implicated in various forms of psychopathology, such as depression and schizophrenia (Perez, Riggio, & Kopelowicz, 2007; Segrin, 2000).

Physiological components of individual functioning and psychopathology include a variety of somatic symptoms, such as decreased or increased appetite, digestive discomfort, headaches, fatigue, muscular tension and aches, insomnia or hypersomnia, psychomotor retardation, and agitation (World Health Organization, 1993). Because many of these unpleasant symptoms overlap with common symptoms of physical illness but may not respond to traditional over-the-counter or physician-administered medical treatments, individuals and their significant others may have difficulty conceptualizing them as manifestations of psychological problems and may develop a sense of hopelessness about prospects for improvement. Furthermore, physical discomfort associated with physiological symptoms of psychopathology can reduce individuals' motivation to engage in potentially satisfying activities on their own or with significant others, contributing to a pattern of behavioral avoidance that continues or worsens other psychopathology symptoms.

Behavioral components of psychopathology tend to involve excesses or deficits in particular actions that commonly occur in normal functioning, as well as some atypical responses. Among the most common patterns that itself can be a positive form of response to danger and stress is *avoidance*. Theory and research on stress and coping (e.g., Feldman, Cohen, Hamrick, & Lepore, 2004; Lazarus & Folkman, 1984; Peacock & Wong, 1990; Riley & Park, 2014) have emphasized that when an individual encounters a situation that is appraised to involve some degree of personal threat, the individual experiences more subjective distress and physiological arousal. Avoidance is one form of coping with perceived threat that may reduce stress by decreasing the perception of danger. However, any short-term benefit of reduced distress may be outweighed as the individual fails to act in ways that actually reduce or remove the stressors, which have persistent negative effects over time. Behavioral avoidance of perceived threats is a core response across many psychological disorders (e.g., depression, generalized anxiety disorder, social anxiety disorder, panic disorder, specific phobias, PTSD, substance use disorders) that commonly interfere with experiences that could produce therapeutic improvement (Leahy et al., 2012).

Another cluster of behavioral coping responses that can become problematic aspects of psychopathology include antisocial actions in which the individual attempts to exert control over the environment through opposition or aggression (Duarte et al., 2020). In childhood and ado-

lescence, these behaviors have been subsumed within DSM diagnoses of oppositional defiant disorder and conduct disorder, whereas for older individuals the diagnosis of antisocial personality
disorder is used. Severe aggressive acts in couple relationships include intimate partner violence
(Chapter 5). Duarte et al. (2020) note the advantages of assessing the severity of various antisocial
behaviors rather than relying on discrete diagnostic categories. Finally, behavioral patterns in
which an individual clings to other people for nurturance, assistance with decision making, and
initiation of tasks can be normative among children and at lower levels among adults. However,
these patterns can be increasingly dysfunctional with greater frequency and severity. Whereas
some degree of clinging is a common symptom associated with depression and anxiety disorders,
a more persistent pattern is captured by the dependent personality disorder diagnosis (American
Psychiatric Association, 2022; World Health Organization, 1993). Again, assessing the frequency
and severity of clinging behaviors provides more fine-grained information than attempting to clas-
sify individuals into diagnostic categories.

Individual CBT for Specific Disorders

Detailed CBT treatment protocols addressing clients' cognitions, emotional responses, and behavior have been developed for discrete disorders encompassed in the DSM system (e.g., particular
anxiety disorders, types of depressive disorders, forms of eating disorders, substance use disorders).
There is a large body of empirical support for their effectiveness (Dobson & Dozois, 2019; Hofmann & Asmundson, 2017). Therapists who wish to treat a large number of DSM diagnoses have
to become adept in the use of many therapy protocols for specific disorders, even though common
elements are used with many disorders, such as guiding clients in tracking and evaluating negative automatic thoughts associated with their symptoms. In addition, couple therapists who seek
to provide interventions for individuals presenting with specific diagnoses have to learn disorder-
specific protocols, including ways the individual's partner can be involved in treatment of the
disorder. For example, a partner of an individual who attempts to end panic attacks by avoiding
situations the individual associates with risk for these attacks can be coached in encouraging the
individual to engage in graded exposure exercises rather than cooperating with attempts at avoidance (Baucom et al., 2020; Epstein & Baucom, 2002).

   In recent years, the focus on separate treatments for specific disorders, both the interventions involving the individual and those that include significant others, has been supplemented
with development of treatments that can be applied across a variety of diagnoses, based on common elements shared by disorders. This *transdiagnostic* approach to understanding and treating
common factors contributing to symptoms of various disorders has been applied increasingly in
individual psychotherapy. It can be useful to couple therapists treating relationship factors that
influence individual psychopathology.

A TRANSDIAGNOSTIC PERSPECTIVE ON PSYCHOPATHOLOGY

The traditional medical model of psychopathology, which is reflected in the DSM system of the
American Psychiatric Association and the *International Classification of Diseases* (ICD) system of
the World Health Organization, has emphasized identification of discrete disorders that can be
differentiated from each other in terms of syndromes of symptoms. Ideally, each disorder can be

traced to particular causal factors and can be treated with disorder-specific interventions. As a result, clinicians face a challenge of collecting assessment information regarding a client's cognitive, affective, physiological, and behavioral symptoms, identifying the most appropriate diagnosis (or diagnoses) to fit the client's characteristics, and selecting the most appropriate interventions treat the specific symptoms.

Vast evidence of comorbidity among diagnoses, as well as limited reliability of clinicians' diagnoses, has led to the development of *transdiagnostic models* that identify a relatively small number of common characteristics (in statistical terms, latent factors or dimensions that are identified from factor analyses of multiple symptoms) that cut across many traditional diagnoses (Achenbach, Ivanova, Rescorla, & Dumas, 2017; Eaton, Rodriguez-Seijas, Carragher, & Krueger, 2015). Rather than attempting to fit clients into discrete diagnostic categories, transdiagnostic models focus on assessing the degrees to which an individual experiences each symptom dimension. For example, Achenbach and his colleagues (e.g., Achenbach et al., 2017; Ivanova et al., 2015) have accumulated extensive evidence that diverse diagnoses in age groups ranging from children to the elderly can be accounted for by symptoms comprising an *internalizing* latent factor (e.g., symptoms commonly associated with anxiety disorders and depressive disorders) and symptoms comprising an *externalizing* latent factor (e.g., antisocial behavior, impulsivity, aggression, substance abuse). Furthermore, the types of symptoms common to disorders that share a factor such as internalizing disorders can be identified, such as the cognitive symptom of rumination. Research also has differentiated diagnoses associated with the internalizing dimension into two subgroups of *distress* (major depressive episode, dysthymia [persistent depressive disorder], generalized anxiety disorder), and *fear* (panic disorder, specific phobias). Symptoms of eating disorders also fit within the internalizing factor (Forbush et al., 2010). In contrast, borderline personality disorder includes symptoms associated with both the internalizing and externalizing dimensions (Eaton et al., 2015).

In addition to the two major internalizing and externalizing dimensions, research has uncovered a third major factor involving *thought disorder* (or psychosis) symptoms (Eaton et al., 2015). Although differentiating these major symptom dimensions can be helpful in selecting appropriate interventions during treatment planning, it also is important to note that internalizing and externalizing symptoms tend to co-occur, indicating that a general overarching psychopathology factor exists (Eaton et al., 2015). In addition to the commonalities shared by diagnoses within each of the internalizing and externalizing factors, this general psychopathology factor may account for findings that successfully treating one disorder commonly results in improvement in an individual's coexisting disorders.

The research on core dimensions of psychopathology symptoms also has investigated their origins. Nolen-Hoeksema and Watkins (2011) note that the characteristics represented by the transdiagnostic dimensions actually span ranges from low levels that are common and normal in the general population to higher levels that are dysfunctional. For example, noticing negative events in one's environment has problem-solving and survival value, but an extreme degree of negative focus likely produces significant emotional distress and inappropriate coping responses. There is substantial evidence that genetic factors contribute to tendencies to experience greater levels of internalizing and externalizing symptoms (for example, through poorly regulated emotional responses to stressors), although environmental factors, including both early life traumas (e.g., child sexual abuse) and current life stressors (e.g., discrimination on the basis of characteristics such as race and sexual orientation; severe couple relationship problems) also are influential (Eaton et al., 2015; Nolen-Hoeksema & Watkins, 2011).

Thus, many disorders share common types of symptoms that are extreme levels of normal psychological processes, and studies have shown that those common dimensions or factors are similar across genders, ages, races, sexual orientations, and cultures (Eaton et al., 2015). Findings of these factors that many specific diagnoses have in common helps to account for the high degree of comorbidity among diagnoses commonly identified for individuals (Achenbach et al., 2017; Barlow, Sauer-Zavala, Carl, Bullis, & Ellard, 2014; Reinholt et al., 2017). That consistency does not mean therapists can ignore cultural differences among clients that may influence their experiences of psychopathology, their beliefs about causes of psychopathology, and their attitudes regarding therapy. We discuss cultural considerations later in this chapter.

The high degree of comorbidity among diagnoses can be challenging for therapists conducting individual psychotherapy because most interventions in the professional literature have been designed to alleviate clients' distress through protocols tailored to reducing the symptoms of specific disorders, rather than co-occurring disorders with overlapping psychological processes and symptoms. The high degree of comorbidity also is a challenge for therapists working with couples whose members exhibit psychopathology symptoms that correspond to more than one disorder, as well as conflict and distress in their relationship. In treatment planning, this situation leaves the therapist wondering where they should begin.

Implications of Transdiagnostic Dimensions for Clinical Practice

An encouraging implication of the findings regarding transdiagnostic dimensions for clinical practice is that a relatively small set of interventions may be sufficient to reduce common symptoms associated with a variety of disorders. In fact, transdiagnostic treatments have been developed and applied to clients with diverse disorders, through either individual or group therapy, with promising results (Barlow et al., 2018; McEvoy, Nathan, & Norton, 2009; Norton, 2012; Norton & Philipp, 2008). We provide a brief overview of such transdiagnostic therapy procedures in this chapter and describe how couple therapists can adapt them to working with psychopathology within the relationship context.

A transdiagnostic approach does not ignore particular characteristics of specific disorders that should be considered in treatment planning. For example, because significant others commonly become "safety signals" that individuals experiencing panic disorder turn to in order to avoid or reduce distressing panic symptoms, the presence of a panic disorder diagnosis within a couple should alert their therapist to examine interaction patterns between the identified patient and partner. However, a transdiagnostic approach capitalizes on evidence that particular types of interventions can be effective for treating a variety of presenting problems. Nevertheless, it is not a "one-size-fits-all" approach, because treatment planning involves assessing the degrees to which each individual experiences each symptom dimension. Rather than needing to use a different treatment protocol for each diagnosis that a member of a couple has received, symptoms associated with a core transdiagnostic dimension can be targeted with interventions with demonstrated effectiveness for that symptom dimension. For example, one couple's daily interactions may be disrupted by a member's emotion dysregulation shared by generalized anxiety and major depressive disorder diagnoses, whereas another couple's activities are limited by a member's behavioral avoidance associated with social anxiety and panic disorder diagnoses. Even though the therapist considers both couples to be dealing with internalizing symptoms, the decisions about which transdiagnostic interventions should be prioritized may differ.

Transdiagnostic Treatments Involving Cognition, Affect, Physiological Responses, and Behavior

Based on research revealing core dimensions of symptoms underlying various forms of psychopathology, Barlow and his colleagues (Barlow et al., 2018) developed a Unified Protocol for Transdiagnostic Treatment of Emotional Disorders. It is intended to be used with the range of DSM anxiety disorders (panic disorder with and without agoraphobia, social anxiety disorder, generalized anxiety disorder, posttraumatic stress disorder, and obsessive–compulsive disorder), depressive disorders, and substance use disorders with significant negative emotion. The model focuses on three core vulnerability factors/dimensions of individuals' psychological processes that contribute to all of those disorders: (1) *high negative affective reactivity* (considered a form of temperament and often labeled neuroticism in the psychopathology literature), (2) a *tendency to think about their emotions (and other life experiences) negatively*, and (3) *ineffective ways of coping with aversive emotional experiences*, emphasizing efforts to avoid, suppress, or escape from them behaviorally or cognitively. Those coping responses tend to backfire and maintain or even exacerbate the problematic symptoms.

The three core dimensions are highly consistent with a cognitive-behavioral model of psychopathology, involving negative affect, cognition, and behavior. For example, regarding cognitive processes involved in transdiagnostic symptoms, Nolen-Hoeksema and Watkins (2011) point to selective attention and memory for negative events, a negative expectancy bias (typically expecting the worst), emotional reasoning (interpreting one's negative emotions as data regarding reality), and rumination, all of which are common forms of cognitive distortion (Chapter 1). Furthermore, *anxiety sensitivity*, defined as the fear of bodily sensations associated with anxiety and other sources of arousal (McNally, 2002; Taylor, 2014), has been identified as a common form of cognition contributing to the maintenance of anxiety disorders but also a variety of other psychological disorders, including substance use and internalizing disorders such as depression (Leventhal & Zvolensky, 2015; Naragon-Gainey, 2010; Zvolensky et al., 2018). Thus, it has been identified as a transdiagnostic component of internalizing disorders. Anxiety sensitivity is based on the individual's cognitive appraisal that such sensations indicate danger, such as heart palpitations being interpreted as an imminent heart attack (McNally, 2002). Consequently, anxiety sensitivity (perhaps more appropriately considered sensitivity and fear of bodily sensations associated with psychopathology) has become a key target for transdiagnostic therapeutic interventions, such as interoceptive exposure in which the therapist guides clients in participating repeatedly in activities that simulate unpleasant symptoms of psychopathology (e.g., increased heart rate, disorientation) in order to habituate the clients to them. Furthermore, Leahy's (2019) emotional schema therapy is an expansion of cognitive therapy that focuses on challenging individuals' negative core beliefs about emotions (e.g., that they are dangerous and indicate that one is dysfunctional).

Barlow et al.'s (2018) Unified Protocol uses traditional CBT interventions but applies them more broadly to individuals presenting with a variety of diagnoses, focusing on the three major vulnerabilities shared by those diagnoses (high negative affective reactivity, negative thinking about experiences, and counterproductive coping with emotional distress). These interventions are consistent with the CBT interventions described in Chapter 4. The interventions in the Unified Protocol are listed and described briefly in Figure 10.1. Barlow et al. note that clinicians should tailor the number of sessions devoted to each component to the needs of each client.

Session 1: Functional Assessment and Introduction to Treatment

This session focuses on information about the identified patient's symptoms and any formal diagnoses and how the individual thinks about those experiences and attempts to cope with distressing emotions, especially using avoidance or escape strategies. Assessment of emotions involves interviewing and administering questionnaires measuring anxiety, depression, other negative emotions, and positive emotions. Cultural factors are taken into account; for example, in some cultures anxiety is expressed more through somatic complaints than from descriptions of emotional states. In some cultures, individuals who behave unassertively may be adhering to collectivist values rather than being inhibited by social anxiety (Barlow et al., 2018). In this session, the clinician also describes the purpose and procedures of the treatment.

Module 1: Setting Goals and Maintaining Motivation

This module focuses on maximizing the client's motivation to invest time and energy into the interventions (noting the costs and benefits of changing vs. maintaining the status quo), guiding the client in setting concrete goals to overcome presenting problems, and planning manageable steps toward achieving each goal.

Module 2: Understanding Emotions

This module focuses on psychoeducation about emotions—their *components* (thoughts, physical sensations, behavioral expression), their *functions* (e.g., as cues that events important to the person's values and well-being may be occurring), their internal and external *triggers*, the client's *attempts to cope* with aversive emotions, and the *consequences* of coping patterns.

Module 3: Mindful Emotion Awareness

This module focuses on educating clients regarding a nonjudgmental approach to observing their emotional experiences and helping them develop this stance of approaching rather than attempting to avoid emotions. It includes exercises for mindful emotion awareness and mood induction for mindful practice.

Module 4: Cognitive Flexibility

This module focuses on traditional CBT interventions to increase clients' awareness of their cognitions regarding their emotional experiences and how those thoughts influence how they cope with distressing feelings. It includes psychoeducation regarding automatic thoughts, cognitive distortions (e.g., catastrophizing), and approaches to considering alternative (and more constructive) ways of thinking about emotional experiences.

Module 5: Countering Emotional Behaviors

This module begins with psychoeducation regarding "emotional behaviors" (behavioral responses individuals use to try to control distressing emotions such as sadness, anxiety, anger, and shame) and their counterproductive consequences. For example, the client learns how avoidance of anxiety-provoking situations robs the individual of opportunities to discover personal skills and strength in tolerating emotional distress and having rewarding experiences. Next, the client is guided in developing and experimenting with "alternative actions" that produce more positive results, including reduction in negative emotion.

(continued)

FIGURE 10.1. Barlow et al.'s Unified Protocol (UP) for Transdiagnostic Treatment of Emotional Disorders.

Module 6: Understanding and Confronting Physical Sensations

This module focuses on *interoceptive exposure* experiences in which conditions are created in sessions that simulate physical sensations similar to real-life strong emotional experiences (e.g., breathing through a narrow straw to create sensations of difficulty breathing during a panic attack). The goals are increased awareness and tolerance (rather than avoidance) of physical symptoms. In the Unified Protocol, interoceptive exposure is equally relevant for increasing clients' acceptance and tolerance of anxiety and other types of strong unpleasant emotions.

Module 7: Emotion Exposures

This session provides psychoeducation regarding the importance of approaching and staying in situations that elicit strong emotions rather than avoiding or escaping them in order to build confidence in one's ability to tolerate the emotions and carry on with life activities. The clinician guides the client in constructing a hierarchy of challenging situations and using repeated exposures to tolerance for engaging in more challenging levels. These interventions are applicable, with diverse types of emotional symptoms experienced by individuals typically given various DSM diagnoses. It typically involves multiple sessions.

Module 8: Recognizing Accomplishments and Looking to the Future

This final module consolidates therapeutic gains by guiding the client in reviewing and acknowledging gains made toward the initial treatment goals, noting areas for future work and improvement, and planning strategies for relapse prevention. Comparing current improved functioning to the client's status at intake helps increase the client's sense of self-efficacy. Normalizing future setbacks and focusing on renewed efforts to use the skills learned in therapy set reasonable standards for one's progress and counteract potential demoralization.

FIGURE 10.1. *(continued)*

CONJOINT COUPLE TREATMENT FOR PSYCHOPATHOLOGY WITH A FOCUS ON A UNIFIED PROTOCOL

To date, transdiagnostic treatments have been applied primarily in therapy for the symptomatic individual, but there is great potential for implementing them in conjoint couple treatment. Strong evidence of links between individual psychopathology and relationship problems points to a need to address couple processes in treatment.

Couple Relationship Patterns and Individual Psychopathology

Research demonstrating a bidirectional link between individuals' psychopathology symptoms and relationship problems has alerted mental health professionals to the need to take a systemic approach to clinical assessment, case conceptualization, and treatment planning that includes characteristics of the two members of a couple and the dynamics of their relationship. For clients who seek individual therapy for symptoms of various disorders, a thorough assessment of personal history and current functioning is essential to identify life experiences (e.g., traumatic experiences during childhood and later in life) that have contributed to current problems and factors, such as poor ability to regulate one's emotional responses, which interfere with functioning in work and personal relationships. As we emphasized earlier (Chapter 1), a limitation of assessment solely with the individual is the clinician's inability to collect information directly about the client's actual cognitive, affective, and behavioral responses in real-life situations, including interactions with the partner.

Direct assessment of the couple through interviewing them together and observing sequences of responses between partners in the office adds important information about the couple's interpersonal processes. With regard to pathways between individual psychopathology and relationship distress, the therapist can ask the couple about patterns they have noticed in daily life regarding the links between symptoms and couple interactions. During the sessions, the therapist can also observe how one member's actions elicit the other's symptoms or how the partner reacts to the other's symptoms. Such observations create opportunities for the clinician to probe for both partners' cognitions and emotional responses involved in those behavioral interactions. For example, when an individual who experiences excessive worry (whether or not it qualifies for a formal diagnosis of generalized anxiety disorder) vocalizes rumination about a topic, their partner may respond, "Would you please stop that!" in an exasperated tone. This may be related to the concept of expressed emotion (EE), or negative feelings and criticism the partner exhibits toward the identified patient, combined with emotional overinvolvement. EE has been found to be a risk factor for symptom occurrence and maintenance when exhibited by significant others of individuals with a variety of forms of psychopathology, such as depression, anxiety disorders, and schizophrenia (Chambless et al., 2017; Hooley, 2007; Hooley & Miklowitz, 2018). As we describe in Chapter 3 on assessment, the therapist can interject that the partner seems to be having a reaction to the individual's expression of worry and ask the partner to describe the thoughts and emotions involved in that reaction. Similarly, the therapist can inquire of the symptomatic individual what thoughts and emotional responses the individual had when the partner reacted that way. This provides rich information about the processes linking individuals' symptoms and dynamics in the couple relationship. We describe details regarding this assessment and case conceptualization process in the assessment section of this chapter.

Relationship conflict and unhappiness are associated with a wide variety of psychological disorders. Consequently, knowing that an individual is involved in a distressing relationship tells the clinician little about ways in which those negative experiences produce a particular individual disorder, and what couple therapy should focus on to reduce their symptoms. For example, interventions designed to increase a couple's shared pleasant activities might have a positive effect on an individual's relationship satisfaction and reduce the individual's psychopathology symptoms to some extent regardless of their disorder. However, other specific processes in the couple's interactions may lead to one type of disorder more than another. Thus, exposure to a partner's aggressive behavior that instills chronic fear may be more likely to contribute to symptoms of anxiety, whereas exposure to distancing and lack of caring behavior may be more likely to contribute to symptoms of depression. Given the evidence we reviewed that a core set of vulnerabilities underlie diverse forms of psychopathology, as well as evidence for the effectiveness of transdiagnostic interventions such as Barlow et al.'s (2018) Unified Protocol, we propose that treatment planning for couple interventions for partners' psychopathology adapt established transdiagnostic interventions to a dyadic format. However, specific interventions targeting particular characteristics of couple interaction that are salient for development of particular disorders should be considered as well.

Interpersonal Problems Associated with Psychopathology Dimensions

Another line of research that has important implications for couple therapy has identified particular types of interpersonal problems associated with particular symptom dimensions. Girard et al.

(2017) found associations between five transdiagnostic dimensions and DSM diagnoses: detachment (e.g., social phobia, major depression), internalizing (e.g., major depression, panic disorder), disinhibition (e.g., antisocial personality, alcohol dependence), dominance (e.g., narcissistic personality, paranoid personality), and compulsivity (obsessive–compulsive personality). These five transdiagnostic dimensions were associated with types of interpersonal problems; for example, individuals higher on the detachment dimension tended to report difficulties with avoiding other people, whereas those scoring higher on the disinhibition dimension reported engaging in domineering behavior with others. An exception to the specific links between psychopathology symptom dimensions and individuals' problems in their relationships was that those who scored higher on the internalizing dimension had a variety of interpersonal problems (domineering, vindictive, cold, socially avoidant, nonassertive, exploitable, overly nurturant, intrusive). Although these findings do not directly link transdiagnostic symptom dimensions to particular negative patterns in couple relationships, they do suggest that probing for associations between types of symptoms and negative couple interaction patterns could help in planning interventions.

COUPLE-BASED INTERVENTIONS FOR PSYCHOPATHOLOGY

Theory and research identifying how couple relationship quality affects individual psychological functioning and vice versa have led to development of couple-based interventions for psychopathology, particularly protocols tailored to specific DSM diagnoses. Given that many evidence-based individual treatments for psychological disorders involve CBT procedures, the couple-based interventions are adaptations of individual CBT protocols that involve the individual's partner or other significant person(s). The same principles and procedures used in individual therapy are used in the couple context. Three major forms of couple-based interventions are available, depending on what the clinician's assessment reveals about the nature of the link between relationship functioning and the individual's symptoms (Baucom et al., 2020; Baucom et al., 1998; Epstein & Baucom, 2002): (1) partner-assisted therapy for individual psychopathology, (2) disorder-specific couple intervention, and (3) couple therapy addressing relationship problems that are stressors on an individual with a vulnerability toward psychopathology. After we describe these three modalities of couple intervention, we explore how a transdiagnostic approach can be integrated with them in couple interventions that address individuals' vulnerabilities across diverse disorders.

Partner-Assisted Therapy for Individual Psychopathology

Partners' social support for each other has been found to be among the best resources they have in coping with life stressors (Cutrona, 1996). Consequently, partner-assisted therapy for individual psychopathology engages a symptomatic individual's significant other in a supportive role as the individual participates in standard interventions for the presenting disorder(s). Both the partner and the symptomatic individual receive psychoeducation regarding the disorder and its treatment, and then the partner serves supportive roles as the individual engages in components of the treatment. For example, after a couple learns about symptoms, causes, and treatment for social anxiety, the partner and symptomatic individual both take part in interoceptive exercises to increase the individual's tolerance of anxiety symptoms, which also may increase the partner's empathy for the person's anxiety experiences. Both members also are taught about tracking and counteracting negative cognitions, including the symptomatic individual's negative expectancies about their functioning when they meet a new person. The partner could play a supportive role in the individual's construction of an exposure hierarchy involving social interactions. Finally, the partner would accompany the individual during exposure exercises, providing encouragement and occasional mild coaching in combating negative thoughts and tolerating emotional discomfort rather than avoiding the situations. Partner-assisted therapies have been developed and evaluated empirically for a number of DSM disorders, such as depression, obsessive–compulsive disorder, and anorexia nervosa (Abramowitz et al., 2013; Baucom et al., 2020; Bulik, Baucom, Kirby, & Pisetsky, 2011).

Therapists need to be cautious in setting up this supportive role for a partner because there is some risk of creating unbalanced therapeutic alliances with the couple and reinforcing the members' skewed views of their roles (e.g., "Cheryl is psychologically healthy, but Robert is not"). When both members present with forms of psychopathology, this can be less of an issue; when one member presents with multiple DSM diagnoses and the other is basically symptom free, the issue becomes a sensitive one. Therapists also must be prepared for couples from cultural backgrounds that stigmatize mental illness, addressing their concerns about the meanings of symptoms.

Disorder–Specific Couple Interventions

When assessment indicates that particular interaction patterns between partners tend to elicit or maintain symptoms of an individual's disorder, interventions can alter those patterns. The patterns are not assumed to be expressions of unhappiness and conflict in the relationship. In fact, they often occur due to a positive bond in which a symptomatic member views their partner as a source of support and the partner's actions are intended to be helpful. In contrast to partner-assisted interventions for one member of the couple, disorder-specific interventions commonly focus on contributions that both members make to their interaction pattern. For example, when a depressed individual has low motivation and inertia, they may express helplessness to a partner and seek the partner's help with tasks, and the partner may respond by taking over the tasks. Although the partner's assistance is based on a desire to reduce the person's distress, after repeatedly helping, the partner may become frustrated. When those negative feelings become apparent to the depressed person, it may reinforce that person's depressive negative cognitions ("My partner is sick of me!"). In addition, when the partner takes responsibility for tasks, the depressed person misses opportunities to learn that they are competent and benefit from the depression-reducing effects of behavioral activation.

Because these couple interactions accommodate and maintain depression symptoms, dyadic interventions are designed to modify them. Interventions include psychoeducation for both members regarding couple processes that can unintentionally maintain or worsen an individual's symptoms, combined with guided behavior changes. An example of guided behavior change would be the partner reminding the depressed individual that efforts to accomplish even portions of tasks will be therapeutic, and the depressed person's role of thanking the partner for expressing confidence.

This type of couple intervention is labeled disorder-specific because the interventions target particular patterns specific to a disorder. The above example focuses on couple patterns that influence symptoms of inertia and helplessness that are common in depressive disorders. In contrast, individuals with panic disorder live in fear of symptoms of intense emotional arousal ("It's like I'm falling apart and going crazy!") and avoid situations in which they anticipate experiencing those symptoms. Commonly a partner also is intimidated by the individual's intense panic attacks and accommodates to the symptoms by helping the person avoid feared situations. Thus, treatment protocols have been developed to address particular dynamics of specific disorders (or classes of disorders), such as depressive disorders, anxiety disorders, posttraumatic stress disorder, alcohol use disorder, and eating disorders (Baucom et al., 2020; Chambless, 2012; McCrady et al., 2023; Monson & Fredman, 2012).

At this point, the reader may be thinking that, at least from our examples of disorder-specific couple interventions, the couple patterns that are targeted for depression and panic disorder have much in common. Even though symptoms associated with the two disorders are different (a panic attack feels quite different from a depressive episode), both disorders involve the three major domains of a transdiagnostic model. Both individuals experience *intense emotions* that are distressing and seem uncontrollable, both experience *negative cognitions* about their symptoms (e.g., self-criticism, helplessness, hopelessness regarding improvement, and dependence on the partner), and both have developed *behavioral coping responses* intended to avoid or escape from the distress. We will return to this point when we discuss the potential for transdiagnostic couple interventions for various presenting complaints.

Couple Therapy for Relationship Problems Eliciting or Exacerbating Psychopathology

Whereas partner-assisted and disorder-specific couple interventions involve collaboration between members of a couple and are most likely to be effective when both partners are satisfied with their relationship, couple therapy is also appropriate when relationship distress and negative couple interactions are creating stress that triggers an individual's vulnerability to experience psychopathology (Baucom et al., 1998, 2020; Epstein & Baucom, 2002). Based on this diathesis-stress model of psychopathology, an individual will remain at risk of experiencing symptoms as long as the relationship continues to expose the individual to stressors. Transdiagnostic models of psychopathology identify current life stressors as interacting with individuals' vulnerabilities (genetic factors and early life traumas) to elicit current symptoms (Eaton et al., 2015). Research consistently linking relationship conflict and distress with diverse forms of psychopathology suggests that interventions that improve the overall quality of couple interactions should help reduce members' symptoms. Consequently, therapies such as cognitive-behavioral couple therapy (CBCT) have been used with couples in which one or both members present with diagnoses such as depression, anxiety, and substance abuse (Baucom et al., 2020; O'Farrell & Fals-Stewart, 2006; Whisman et al., 2023). The couple therapy includes CBCT components (e.g., skills for communication and problem solving, emotion regulation, and modification of cognitions that influence relationship distress and conflict), although the skills are applied in particular with the couple's coping with psychopathology symptoms. It also includes psychoeducation regarding disorders the couple is experiencing and couple patterns such as accommodation that influence symptoms.

The application of general CBCT methods to couples experiencing psychopathology (which also applies to use of other couple therapy models) also takes psychopathology problems into account by addressing relational risk factors that have been identified in research. Chambless (2012) describes the use of psychoeducation with a distressed couple regarding a member's chronic obsessive–compulsive disorder and posttraumatic stress disorder, partly to counteract her partner's belief that she could "get over" her symptoms simply by trying harder, and partly to increase the couple's awareness of how the partner's accommodation to the individual's obsessive–compulsive disorder "checking" rituals reinforced that symptom. Expressive and empathic listening skills facilitated the partners' mutual empathy and emotional support for each other's experiences with the psychopathology, as well as reducing critical remarks and nonverbal behavior that conveyed hostility. Improved communication also helped improve the individual's emotion regulation (anger management) associated with her posttraumatic stress disorder. These interventions overlap with those in a disorder-specific approach but are designed to address how partners' dissatisfaction with each other fuels negative interactions that exacerbate an individual's symptoms. Whereas a therapist can count on mutual good will and collaboration when suggesting disorder-specific changes in the patterns of a happy couple, couples who present with chronic negative cognitions and emotional responses and behavior toward each other need couple therapy that focuses on reducing those negative patterns.

Psychopathology-Related Targets of General Couple Therapy

As we have described, general couple therapy is intended to improve a number of problematic aspects of distressed couple relationships that affect symptomatic individuals adversely, regardless of their particular disorder(s). Interventions for those common characteristics of distressed relationships are not tailored to improving specific individual disorders, but rather to reducing overall distress and conflict. Therapists assess how much each negative characteristic occurs in a couple and devotes an appropriate amount of session time to each of them. These general treatment targets (Chapter 1) are as follows:

- **Mutual negative behavior between partners.** Studies of communication in couples with a depressed partner have indicated that both members have a tendency for reciprocal negative behavior, such as both members criticizing the other person (Whisman et al., 2023). Florin, Nostadt, Reck, Franzen, and Jenkins (1992) found that both depressed individuals and their partners scored higher on a measure of EE than members of couples without depression. This finding does not indicate that symptomatic individuals are responsible for their psychopathology, but rather that interventions are needed to interrupt negative dyadic cycles in their relationship. Nevertheless, it is crucial that therapists be vigilant for evidence of cases in which an individual's psychopathology symptoms result from a partner's psychologically and physically abusive behavior and in which any negative behavior on the individual's part is a response to the victimization. Rehman, Gollan, and Mortimer (2008) critiqued interpersonal models of depression such as Beach, Sandeen, and O'Leary's (1990) model regarding negative interactions in a couple relationship that maintain or worsen symptoms because they do not identify the initial cause of a member's depression. However, models such as that of Beach et al. are consistent with transdiagnostic models of psychopathology that propose an interaction between predisposing vulnerabilities based on the individual's genetic and early life trauma factors and the individual's current life stressors that include aversive and unsupportive experiences with a significant other (Eaton et al., 2015).

- **A deficit in collaborative couple problem solving.** Chapters 1 and 4 describe deficits in collaborative problem solving and coping with life stressors that many distressed couples exhibit when they enter therapy. Many couples have never had opportunities in their lives to learn how to evaluate a problem systematically and generate potential solutions. Such deficits are relevant for couples in which one or both members experience psychopathology symptoms. Problem-solving deficits have been found to be especially problematic in couples experiencing depression. The psychopathology symptoms themselves not only are a stressor on both members of the couple, but also the symptoms interfere with partners engaging in effective problem solving that could reduce factors contributing to an individual's disorder. For example, the rumination that is common in generalized anxiety disorder, depressive disorders, and other forms of psychopathology interferes with logical thinking to generate potential solutions. Similarly, cognitive and behavioral avoidance strategies that symptomatic individuals commonly use to reduce their aversive emotional symptoms interfere with problem solving that requires thinking about a problem and possible solutions. Furthermore, couples experiencing depression have been found to exhibit more negative communication (e.g., verbal aggression) and less positive communication (e.g., self-disclosure) than distressed couples without depression (Rehman et al., 2008). Consequently, therapists need to assess a couple's problem-solving skills *and* how they apply them specifically to psychopathology within their relationship.

• **A deficit in partners' social support for each other.** Earlier, we noted the importance of social support in couples as a resource that protects individuals from the development or maintenance of psychopathology. This is a core concept in Beach et al.'s (1990) couple discord model of depression (see also Whisman et al., 2023). The Beach et al. treatment combines enhancement of social support with reduction of stressful couple interactions. Research has demonstrated that depressed individuals are not only the recipients of aversive behavior and low social support from their partners, but also exhibit problematic behavior toward their partners, such as excessive self-derogatory statements, reassurance-seeking, criticism of their partner, and withdrawal (Whisman et al., 2023). The depressed individual also provides limited social support for the partner, due to a tendency to be self-focused. Similar negative dyadic patterns can occur with other forms of psychopathology, such as anxiety disorders. For example, the partner of an individual who exhibits symptoms associated with generalized anxiety disorder may become frustrated with unsuccessful attempts to reassure the person that their excessive worries are unfounded and may communicate those negative feelings. In turn, the anxious individual may respond with additional worry regarding the couple's relationship and fail to provide social support for the partner. Across diverse disorders, a couple's negative patterns maintain the individual's psychopathology symptoms and mutual low satisfaction with the relationship.

• **Overall negative sentiment that partners have for each other.** Weiss's (1980) concept of sentiment override captures global cognitions and emotion that an individual develops for a partner, which can bias the individual's perception and behavioral responses to the partner's current actions. When a member of a couple has developed global negative sentiment toward a partner, therapeutic interventions that "chip away" at the negative view can reduce global negative EE toward the partner.

• **Partners' selective attention to negative aspects of each other's behavior, while overlooking positive actions.** This "negative tracking" (Jacobson & Margolin, 1979) may be influenced by negative sentiment override, but it also reflects a general tendency for people to attend to aspects of their environment that may pose threats to fulfillment of their needs.

• **Partners' negative attributions regarding intentions underlying each other's displeasing behavior.** Couple therapists must explore the content of this bias in each member's inferences regarding causes of the other's negative actions; for example, how much the person believes the partner's behavior was due to selfish motivation, not valuing or loving the person, a desire to control the person, or a reflection of compromised functioning due to psychopathology. The degree to which the partner's displeasing behavior is attributed to factors under the partner's control is relevant. On the one hand, when an individual's psychopathology-related negative actions are interpreted as intentional, it may elicit more anger and criticism of the individual. On the other hand, when those negative actions are viewed as caused by psychopathology and are assumed to be relatively uncontrollable, the partner may be more likely to be forgiving, although a sense of hopelessness may lead them to withdraw. When symptomatic and nonsymptomatic members of a couple attribute their negative interactions to negative characteristics of the other person, it can reduce cohesion for both of them (Whisman et al., 2023).

• **Negative emotion co-regulation between members of the couple.** In their emotion-focused model of intimate relationships and couple therapy, Greenberg and Goldman (2008) emphasize that the major sources of people's motivation in life, including their motives for becoming involved in close relationships, are based on the goals of experiencing positive emotions and avoiding negative emotions. Individuals are attracted to partners who help them regulate their emotions, increasing opportunities to experience pleasure and moderating unpleasant emotions. Unlike young children who rely heavily on parents or other caretakers to soothe their distressed feelings, adults normally have developed self-soothing strategies, but it is still normal for members of an adult relationship to help regulate each other's emotions. In a well-functioning relationship, messages of affection and validation from a partner contribute to one's self-esteem and positive affect. Furthermore, closeness, a sense of security, and nurturing actions in the relationship help soothe an individual who is experiencing stressors. In contrast, when a relationship breaks down, partners interact in ways that reduce each person's positive emotions and amplify negative emotional experiences. Studies have indicated that individuals whose partners do not provide intimacy and validation are more likely to be depressed. Distressed partners are linked emotionally but in negative ways. Greenberg and Goldman (2008) describe how emotion-focused couple therapy is designed to repair breakdowns in couples' mutual affect regulation. However, they emphasize that therapy also enhances each individual's capacity to self-soothe because many individuals enter close relationships with deficits in those coping skills. Thus, therapy involves maintaining a balance between dyadic regulation and self-regulation of emotion. CBCT also includes intervention goals that are focused on partners' mutual influences on each other's emotional experiences.

CLINICAL ASSESSMENT AND TREATMENT PLANNING

Assessment and treatment planning for couple interventions regarding psychopathology are based on empirically supported interventions for particular disorders; evidence of core transdiagnostic factors shared by individuals presenting with symptoms of diverse diagnoses; knowledge regarding links between couple relationship patterns and psychopathology; and knowledge of specific roles a partner can play in reducing an individual's symptoms. We begin with guidelines for screening appropriate cases for couple interventions and assessments that aid in designing a treatment plan to match each couple's needs.

Screening and Assessment for Psychopathology

Therapists can identify potential cases for couple interventions regarding individual psychopathology in a few ways:

- A couple contacts a therapist seeking assistance because of the distress in their relationship. As the therapist conducts an assessment, it becomes clear that psychopathology symptoms of one or both members is one of the factors contributing to their relationship problems.

- The couple initially identifies psychopathology symptoms as a source of conflict and distress, sometimes identifying a specific disorder and sometimes just describing symptoms they have not linked to a formal disorder (e.g., "He worries about everything! It's hard to have any fun with him").

- Couple therapists often receive referrals from other mental health practitioners who are treating a member of a couple for one or more disorders in individual therapy and have determined that couple therapy would help address influences between relationship problems and the member's symptoms.

When couples present with both relationship problems and individual psychopathology, it often is difficult to identify a causal direction between the two. Taking detailed histories of the individuals and the couple's relationship may clarify the degree to which a member's symptoms predated relationship problems or vice versa. To some degree, by the time a couple reaches a therapist's office, the two types of problems often have become so entwined that the treatment plan must address both reduction of relationship processes that contribute to symptoms and reduction of symptoms that influence relationship quality.

Individual Initial Phone Inquiry Regarding Couple Therapy

The therapist asks why the caller is seeking couple therapy, when the issues in the relationship seemed to develop, whether the person's partner also is motivated for therapy, and whether the partners currently are engaged in any therapy. As described in Chapter 5, safety concerns preclude in-depth questioning of the caller when it is unclear whether they have adequate privacy during the call. In addition, at this point the therapist only learns about one member's view of the presenting problems. Nevertheless, in some cases some relevant information is revealed about the presence of psychopathology symptoms and relationship issues.

The Couple's Initial Joint Assessment Session

The therapist collects a variety of types of information covered in Chapter 3, including a history of the relationship, with a timeline of when presenting issues arose and how the couple attempted to deal with them. The therapist can give the couple an assessment worksheet (Handout 10.1; available on the book's web page at *www.guilford.com/epstein-materials*) that includes questions about an individual's physical, emotional, cognitive and behavioral symptoms; situations in which they tend to occur; how the individual thinks, feels, and behaves when experiencing symptoms; prior treatments and effectiveness; couple communication about the symptoms; effects on the relationship; partner accommodations to symptoms; and ways the couple collaborate to cope with the symptoms. This handout serves the dual purpose of structuring the interview regarding an individual's symptoms and increasing the couple's attunement to effects they have on the two partners and relationship.

Given the CBCT attention to stressors the couple has experienced involving characteristics of the individuals, the dyad, and their environment, the joint interview is an opportunity to learn about any psychopathology symptoms that have affected the partners and their relationship. The therapist can inquire about how an individual has attempted to cope with their own symptoms, and how the partner tends to respond. On the one hand, the couple may describe how a partner accommodates to an individual's symptoms out of caring (and perhaps emotional overinvolvement) and how the symptomatic individual responds to the accommodating behavior. On the other hand, the therapist may obtain evidence of a partner's EE, in terms of either the partner describing frustration or the symptomatic individual reporting perceived criticism from the partner. If the couple reveals that a member's psychopathology has been severe and a significant stressor on the relationship, it is important to determine what treatment(s) the individual currently is receiving and whether the individual is willing to grant the couple therapist written permission to communicate with any involved professionals. Some forms of psychopathology (e.g., substance abuse, eating disorders, severe depression) require individual therapy to be the primary intervention, even though couple interventions also can be helpful in reducing relationship stresses and providing support for a symptomatic individual's engagement in treatment. Alternatively, if the relationship history and description of current relationship functioning reveal any past and ongoing partner aggression, including victimization of a symptomatic member, the therapist needs to consider whether couple therapy is appropriate (Chapter 5).

Partners' Completion of Questionnaires

Prior to or after the initial joint interview, the therapist can ask the members of the couple to complete measures of individual psychopathology, such as the Difficulties in Emotion Regulation Scale (DERS), Beck Depression Inventory–II (BDI-II), Beck Anxiety Inventory (BAI), and Generalized Anxiety Disorder–7 scale (GAD-7), as well as overall relationship satisfaction (see Chapter 3). Information from those instruments serves as a guide for in-depth inquiry into symptoms during each member's individual interview.

Individual Interview with Each Partner

The individual interviews cover the content described in Chapter 3 regarding the person's family of origin and other significant relationships (including prior couple relationships); social, educational, and employment history; any trauma experiences (such as discrimination, abuse, and significant attachment injuries) and their residual effects; physical health and current health behavior patterns; any prior or current substance use; history of and current psychopathology and treatments; level of satisfaction with the couple relationship and motivation to work on improving problems; past and current partner aggression in the relationship; and personal goals for entering couple therapy. Again, for individuals presenting with significant psychopathology symptoms, it is important to gain permission to share information with any individual treatment providers. Screening for suicidal risk also is important, as couple therapy often is stressful and might exacerbate risk of self-harm.

Sometimes a member of a couple reveals to a couple therapist psychopathology symptoms that are significantly interfering with daily functioning, but the individual has not been evaluated formally and is not in individual treatment. The therapist must determine whether to propose that the individual seek evaluation and potential treatment in order to begin couple therapy. Couple therapists with background in individual assessment of psychopathology may schedule an additional session with the person to conduct more thorough assessment. Otherwise, it is essential to have connections with local expert diagnosticians to whom clients can be referred. Given our emphasis on balancing traditional diagnosis with a transdiagnostic approach to psychopathology, thorough assessment of individual functioning is needed to determine the types and severity of symptoms and the degrees to which they can be treated in a couple context.

DECISIONS REGARDING THE APPROPRIATENESS OF COUPLE INTERVENTIONS

Because there are three approaches to using a couple context for treating individuals' psychopathology symptoms, the choice to do so can involve affirmative responses to any of the following questions:

1. Is there a mutually supportive relationship between partners, such that a member is motivated to learn about the other's psychopathology experiences and participate in sessions and homework exercises to facilitate the person's progress in treatment for symptoms? If so, partner-assisted interventions are appropriate. In partner-assisted interventions, the format is primarily individual therapy for the symptomatic individual, with the partner playing a supportive role. If the person is receiving individual therapy from another clinician, the couple therapist's role would be providing adjunctive interventions in collaboration with the primary clinician.

2. Is there evidence that the partner's behavior toward the individual elicits symptoms (e.g., critical remarks elicit self-criticism in a depressed person) or reinforces them through accommodation (e.g., the partner cooperates with avoidance behavior of an individual who experiences panic symptoms in public settings)? If so, disorder-specific couple interventions are appropriate. In a transdiagnostic approach, it is important for the clinician to evaluate, across diagnoses, how much a partner's actions influence an individual's symptoms. For example, when a partner suggests that an individual used to be stronger than their current anxiety, depression, and alcohol abuse symptoms indicate, it may increase the individual's tendency to catastrophize about all of those symptoms. It also is important to identify whether counterproductive partner actions are unintentional, based on caring feelings, versus reflections of unhappiness with the symptomatic individual. This distinction may not be clear initially, so the decision of whether couple therapy is needed in addition to interventions to modify well-intentioned but problematic partner behavior may require further inquiry.

3. Do stressful interactions between partners, regarding any aspect of their relationship (e.g., differences in desired degree of intimacy, conflicts regarding finances) trigger an individual's vulnerability to experiencing forms of psychopathology, eliciting emotion-regulation problems, interfering with executive cognitive functions such as the ability to devise solutions to problems, and contributing to negative behavioral coping patterns such as impulsive aggression or substance use?

If so, couple therapy designed to reduce aspects of stressful couple interactions may reduce psychopathology symptoms in the short run and help protect against relapse. In order to minimize ethical issues regarding dual relationships, it is most appropriate for the therapist to focus on the couple therapy while the symptomatic member is treated separately by an individual therapist. However, the couple therapist can collaborate with the individual therapy protocol by guiding the couple in using partner-assisted and disorder-specific interventions when appropriate.

In all three cases, couple interventions might be sufficient to alleviate an individual's symptoms. The existence of psychopathology symptoms in both members of a couple would not rule out couple-based interventions as long as each person is capable of providing support to the other and is motivated to change couple interaction patterns that elicit or maintain either person's symptoms.

Contraindications for Couple-Based Interventions

Contraindications for joint couple sessions include:

• Ongoing psychological and/or physical partner aggression that places either or both members of the couple at risk for physical and psychological harm, including psychopathology.

• Severe psychopathology symptoms in either partner that could interfere with collaboration in couple therapy.

• Ongoing substance use by either member of the couple that interferes with the ability to engage in couple therapy and that may exacerbate other psychopathology symptoms. Meyers, Smith, Serna, and Belon (2013) provide guidelines for clinicians in decision making about using input from significant others to engage treatment-resistant substance-abusing individuals into therapy.

• Evidence of lack of commitment to the couple relationship by either partner.

GOAL SETTING AND SOCIALIZATION TO TREATMENT

Goal setting that includes a significant focus on the psychopathology symptoms of one or both partners flows more readily when both members initially identify symptoms as a concern and reason for seeking assistance than when the therapist's assessment uncovers the psychopathology. Even then, establishing shared treatment goals and a positive therapeutic alliance with both members likely depends on each member's perception of the problem. When a symptomatic partner has been in individual therapy and is referred to the couple therapist by that clinician, a goal becomes identifying the degree to which couple dynamics are eliciting or maintaining the person's symptoms, the symptoms are stressors on the relationship, or both. In order to establish collaborative goals, the couple therapist needs to avoid participating in any blaming in which symptomatic and nonsymptomatic partners may be engaging. In cases in which the couple is self-referred and identifies psychopathology as a presenting problem, the therapist needs to identify each member's perception of the problem. Sometimes a symptomatic individual considers their stressful relationship as a major reason for their symptoms and pursues couple therapy rather than individual treatment. Alternatively, a partner of a symptomatic individual may seek couple therapy due to personal distress and frustration with the impact the person's symptoms have on their daily life. Therapists can minimize partners' blaming by emphasizing how symptoms are stressful for both members and how tension in the relationship has negative effects on both people. Therapy can therefore focus on reducing an individual's symptoms, decreasing negative couple interactions, and enhancing positive qualities of the relationship.

Because an individual's symptoms often are only one of a number of concerns that couples present for therapy, the goal setting should reflect all of those issues. In some cases, a couple may not even consider psychological symptoms a high priority, so the therapist should explore with them the degree to which a member's symptoms influence daily life (the impact may be minor) but also how symptoms may influence the couple's ability to manage the other issues they identified as significant (they may have underestimated that). For example, both members may see that a severely depressed individual's inertia led to unemployment and contributed to the couple's financial distress, and therefore reducing the depression should be a high priority goal. In contrast, the chronic low mood of a moderately depressed member of a couple may have reduced the partners' intimacy in a fairly subtle way that they failed to notice. In that case, the couple's stated goal of increasing intimacy would be a high priority, but as the therapist guides the clients in exploring factors that reduced their intimacy, it may become clear that reducing the individual's depression may be helpful to the relationship as well.

Socializing the couple to a dyadic approach to individuals' symptoms, and to a CBCT model that takes transdiagnostic factors into account specifically, involves psychoeducation about effective treatments for psychological problems, as well as the importance of a mutually supportive relationship for partners' emotional well-being. It also includes an overview of how structured interventions such as improving expressive and listening skills and regulating one's emotions can lead to partners feeling better understood, respected, and part of a team that can solve problems together. The therapist provides an overview of CBCT methods, including identification and modification of distressing thoughts, improvement of abilities to moderate negative emotional responses, facilitation of positive couple interactions, and routine homework to improve partners' experiences with each other in daily life. Then, the therapist can describe how couple-based methods are used to reduce individuals' psychological symptoms, at times in combination with individual therapy for the symptomatic person. It is emphasized that the treatment uses interventions that are helpful to individuals who have been diagnosed with a wide variety of psychological disorders such as depression and anxiety and some interventions tailored to specific disorders.

The therapist can elaborate with examples; for example, that individuals experiencing major depressive disorder and those experiencing panic disorder all tend to experience negative thoughts about themselves and benefit from interventions that help them think more reasonably. However, we also know that the types of negative thoughts associated with depression and panic tend to be different and require attention to the specific relevant content, even though the same types of cognitive restructuring methods are used. Similarly, individuals diagnosed with major depressive disorder and those diagnosed with panic disorder both exhibit reduced activities in the outside world and benefit from interventions designed to reengage them in such activities. However, the factors contributing to their low activity levels differ in some important ways. Whereas depressed individuals' activity level is impeded by symptoms of inertia, low energy, and hopeless thoughts about improving their lives, individuals with panic engage in limited activity as a result of avoiding situations in which they predict they will experience highly aversive and debilitating emotional and physical symptoms. Consequently, the behavioral activation interventions that were designed for depressed individuals and the exposure experiences designed to counteract avoidance by individuals with a history of panic differ, even though both involve counteracting the individual anticipating aversive experiences. For clients presenting with comorbid disorders (and their partners), therapists can emphasize how the transdiagnostic model can make understanding their difficulties and planning effective treatment simpler because common factors contribute to different disorders and can be reduced through similar types of treatment.

The therapist then can describe the differences among partner-assisted interventions, disorder-specific interventions, and couple therapy that addresses broader relational issues. The therapist also can discuss the degrees to which the assessment of this couple has suggested how much each of the three approaches seems to fit their needs. Because the three approaches are not mutually exclusive, the treatment plan may include components of one, two, or all three. Thus, regardless of whether a couple's relationship is happy overall or conflictual, providing both members with psychoeducation and engaging a partner in assisting a symptomatic individual in carrying out interventions can facilitate the individual's improvement. Similarly, whether a couple is happy or distressed, the assessment may indicate that the partner's responses to the individual's symptoms unwittingly accommodate or reinforce them, so changes in the partner's behavior would facilitate improvement. For distressed couples, couple therapy designed to reduce stressful conflict can be combined with partner-assisted and disorder-specific interventions to facilitate their effectiveness. Reducing relationship distress can make it easier for members of the couple to work together on partner-assisted and disorder-specific interventions. In turn, successful experiences of collaborating on those interventions can help partners develop more positive thoughts and emotions about each other.

In order to identify psychopathology symptoms in a couple and the members' responses to them, the therapist should review with the couple:

- any diagnoses that have been identified for either member prior to entering couple therapy, whether or not they were reasons for seeking the therapy.

- the cognitive, affective, and behavioral symptoms experienced by each member that are distressing to that person and/or to the person's partner, regardless of formal diagnoses.

- situations in which the symptoms are more likely to occur, as well as those in which they tend to be absent.

- each member's cognitions about an individual's symptoms (e.g., attributions regarding causes of the symptoms, perceptions of frequency and intensity of symptoms, expectancies regarding the potential for improvement, the degree to which the members believe they can tolerate an individual's symptoms).

- the ways in which each member tries to cope with an individual's symptoms (e.g., avoiding situations that trigger symptoms, trying to discourage a partner from venting emotional distress) and the degrees to which those coping responses affect the symptoms, as well as the partners' satisfaction with their relationship.

Because couple-based interventions rely on some good will and collaboration between partners, the therapist should inquire about the couple's history of solving life problems together. In order to minimize portraying a couple as unbalanced, with a poorly functioning symptomatic member and a well-functioning partner, the therapist can describe how any couple faces a variety of challenges together (e.g., finances, raising children, assisting extended family members, physical and psychological health issues), and their ability to work as a team is important. Psychological symptoms pose challenges for both the individual and the person's partner, so teamwork is essential for facing those challenges together and reducing them. Therefore, the therapist is interested to learn about other challenges the couple has faced and how they dealt with them. What approaches seemed to work best, and which ones were less effective?

This inquiry identifies positive and negative forms of individual coping and dyadic coping the couple has engaged in regarding problems they faced, including psychopathology symptoms. Both partner-assisted and disorder-specific couple-based interventions involve dyadic coping, so information about the couple's past coping will help in setting goals for this treatment.

Goal Setting and Procedures for Partner-Assisted Therapy

Enlisting a partner to support and assist a symptomatic individual's engagement in cognitive-behavioral interventions that target the person's symptoms begins with psychoeducation for the couple regarding factors contributing to the presenting problem(s), procedures used to treat them, and the advantages of having the partner participate. For individuals who enter couple therapy and who were previously diagnosed with comorbid disorders (which is often the case), psychoeducation about transdiagnostic characteristics can reduce the couple's distress about needing to cope with multiple problems. The interventions they learn to use can be applied to symptoms of more than one diagnosis. For example, a partner who learned to encourage a depressed individual in an empathic manner to engage in behavioral activation exercises can be guided in encouraging the individual to carry out *in vivo* exposure activities to counteract avoidance associated with panic disorder. The exercises differ somewhat for the two disorders, but the process is similar. Furthermore, the partner can learn to assist the individual in tracking and counteracting negative cognitions that have contributed to the behavioral inertia associated with depression (e.g., "I just don't have the energy to do anything") and with the avoidance associated with the anxiety disorder (e.g., "If I go to the store down the street, I'll have another panic attack and fall apart"). The negative expectancies (catastrophizing) are different, but the process and its negative effects on the person's emotions and behavior are similar.

In regard to the core foci of a Uniform Protocol, interventions that enlist the cooperation of a symptomatic person's partner target the three core vulnerabilities shared by individuals experiencing numerous disorders:

- A high level of negative affect in response to diverse life experiences
- A tendency to think about their emotional experiences negatively, which intensifies the aversive experience
- Engaging in counterproductive ways of trying to avoid or suppress their negative emotional responses

Regarding the individual's pervasive negative affect, psychoeducation for the couple about the components of emotion (thoughts, physical sensations, subjective feelings, behavioral manifestations) and how to track situations that trigger particular emotional responses allows the partners to work together in understanding and being less intimidated by the individual's emotions. The couple is taught the skill of nonjudgmental mindful awareness of emotions, a relatively detached perspective. In addition, after the couple is taught emotion-regulation techniques (see Chapter 4), the partner can provide encouragement and some coaching as needed as the individual practices them in daily life. In turn, the partner can use those techniques to manage their own emotional distress regarding the individual's symptoms. The couple can be sensitized to ways in which they co-regulate each other's emotions and can plan strategies to soothe each other rather than amplify each other's negative emotions.

The tendency to think about one's emotional experiences negatively can be addressed by teaching the couple about links between cognitions and emotional and behavioral responses and guiding them in tracking their automatic thoughts associated with various experiences, including interactions with each other (see Chapter 4). The Unified Protocol model focuses on two types of misappraisals in symptomatic individuals' cognitions: an overestimate that negative events will occur, and an exaggerated view of how severe the negative consequences of the event will be (Barlow et al., 2018). In our dyadic approach, instances in which each member's cognitions involve those negative appraisals are identified and treated. The therapist coaches the couple in tracking their own cognitions as well as supporting each other in that process.

For example, when a partner observes a symptomatic individual reacting to making a mistake by expressing self-criticism ("I'm so emotionally out of it that I can't do anything right!"), the partner can gently comment: "As we've discussed before, you criticize yourself when you don't perform as well as you think you should. What would be a more fair and less harsh way of thinking about the mistake you just made?" In addition, the partner might reduce irritation with the individual's negativity by noticing their own negative automatic thoughts, such as "I'm sick of my partner's self-criticism! It's hard to feel empathy for people who just feel sorry for themselves." Upon this self-reflection, the partner could challenge the negative thoughts; for example, "It's natural that I'm frustrated by my partner's negativity, but it's my partner's habit based on perfectionism. My venting my frustration just adds to the tension. What I can do is provide feedback about challenging one's perfectionism and focusing on what to do next after making a mistake. I'll also use self-soothing exercises myself to stay calm rather than getting angry and venting." The self-regulation not only helps one assist one's partner in carrying out interventions to modify negative cognitions; it also reduces negative reactions to the partner that reinforce the partner's upsetting cognitions.

Regarding a symptomatic individual's counterproductive strategies for avoiding or escaping from distressing emotional experiences, the therapist can provide psychoeducation for the couple on how those coping styles may be tempting but will have negative consequences (e.g., the individual never develops confidence in their ability to tolerate and overcome aversive symptoms; avoidance patterns constrict the couple's life together). Next, the therapist can coach the couple in working together to change counterproductive coping strategies, substituting new responses that can increase tolerance for discomfort and enhance their pleasurable experiences in daily life. For example, both members can repeatedly practice interoceptive exposure exercises in which psychopathology symptoms are simulated and become less threatening through desensitization, and the partner can accompany the symptomatic individual in working through a hierarchy of *in vivo* exposure experiences.

Although these exposure interventions are more often associated with treatment for anxiety disorders, they also are relevant for individuals who experience other distressing symptoms, such as those of depression. Commonly, depressed individuals who have experienced symptoms such as low mood, fatigue, inertia, and hopelessness regarding one's ability to carry out even mundane tasks avoid engaging in various activities, anticipating that they will be paralyzed by symptoms. Furthermore, an individual who has been feeling better for a while commonly is fearful that any symptoms may lead to a "slippery slope" and a relapse into dysfunction. This hyperalertness to their subjective experiences is similar to anxiety sensitivity in individuals with anxiety disorders. Interventions involving behavioral activation are designed not only to increase the individual's pleasant experiences; they also are exposure experiences that reduce negative cognitions about one's ability to tolerate unpleasant symptoms and carry out activities. Engaging both members of the couple in behavioral activation exercises can create pleasant shared activities, reduce joint avoidance patterns, and reduce their helpless and hopeless cognitions about the individual's symptoms. A hierarchy of joint activities can be constructed, based on the anticipated difficulty they pose for the symptomatic individual, and the therapist can help motivate the couple through encouragement and positive feedback as they report successes.

Goal Setting and Procedures for Disorder-Specific Couple Interventions

As we noted previously, disorder-specific interventions target couple interaction patterns that contribute to the occurrence and maintenance of an individual's symptoms. To date, disorder-specific couple treatment protocols have been developed for disorders such as posttraumatic stress disorder (Monson & Fredman, 2012), substance abuse (O'Farrell & Fals-Stewart, 2006), and obsessive–compulsive disorder (Abramowitz et al., 2013). Because each couple-based protocol is intended to be used with one specific disorder, clinicians who work with clients experiencing comorbid disorders need to learn a number of treatments and figure out how to integrate or sequence them. In this chapter, we focus on interventions with comorbid disorders that primarily involve anxiety and depression.

Our approach integrates existing treatments that focus on modifying particular couple interaction patterns associated with specific diagnoses and a Unified Protocol model of transdiagnostic treatment that addresses factors common to diverse disorders. Thus, a partner's way of accommodating to an individual's symptoms of depression (e.g., stepping in to complete tasks when the depressed individual exhibits inertia) may differ from ways of accommodating to symptoms of social anxiety (e.g., staying home rather than attending social gatherings together), but the function of the partner's accommodation is similar. Across disorders, the accommodation is motivated partly by the partner's caring and desire to protect the individual from emotional pain, partly by the partner's expectancy that the individual actually cannot function adequately in such situations, and partly by fear that failing to accommodate will elicit anger and relationship conflict from the symptomatic individual. Thus, we use the term *disorder-specific interventions* within an overall Unified Protocol framework to be consistent with descriptions in the field of partner behaviors that may be well intentioned but are counterproductive. When therapists understand the common elements across disorders, they can use similar interventions to address the accommodation process. Consistent with a Unified Protocol approach, therapists can reduce a partner's accommodation to and reinforcement of the individual's negative cognitions regarding distressing symptoms (e.g., that they are intolerable) by encouraging the partner to redefine helping as supporting the individual in exposure and tolerance of uncomfortable symptoms.

In spite of the common processes that couple therapists who apply the Unified Protocol framework can address across diverse disorders, the dynamics involved in a partner's accommodation may differ in some ways from one disorder to another that are relevant to treatment planning.

For example, "collaborating" with an individual's desire to avoid situations that may trigger symptoms may have different implications for the couple's life together, depending on the consequences of exacerbated symptoms and avoidance. Thus, when a partner accommodates to avoidance of social situations by an individual with social anxiety, the partner may lose opportunities to have their own social needs met, but the conditions at home may be tranquil for the most part and the partner may have independent social outlets. As a result, the costs of accommodation may be insufficient to motivate either member of the couple to try to change the status quo unless the therapist sensitizes them to the drawbacks of that pattern and addresses the partner's fear that challenging the other person's avoidance would disrupt the peace at home. In contrast, when a partner accommodates to a depressed individual's failure to engage in most activities (including couple interactions), the partner misses out on opportunities for enjoyment both inside and outside the home, and the chronic inactivity maintains or even worsens the individual's depression. Consequently, conditions at home are unpleasant for both people, so the costs of accommodation are more pervasive, and the therapist can focus motivational interviewing on partners' visions of what a happier life would look like for them individually and as a couple.

As we noted previously, research on EE indicates that a partner's negative sentiment toward a symptomatic individual can exacerbate symptoms. That negative sentiment can be a core aspect of overall relationship distress that is a major stressor in the individual's life (Baucom et al., 2020), although some partners may be upset about an individual's symptoms but have positive feelings toward the person otherwise. In either case, when the emotional distress of a symptomatic individual triggers negative emotion in the partner, it can result in mutual escalation of distress. Consequently, couple interventions that focus on reducing the partner's reactivity may be an important component of the treatment plan.

The distinction between global versus symptom-specific negative sentiment toward a symptomatic partner can have implications for treatment planning. Global negative sentiment regarding other aspects of the couple's relationship suggests a need for couple therapy, whereas symptom-specific negative feelings more likely call for interventions to help the partner develop better ways of coping with the other's stressful symptoms. Furthermore, the aspect of EE regarding a partner's emotional overinvolvement with a symptomatic individual's life may reflect caring, but it still can contribute to counterproductive overprotective accommodation. The couple therapist's job is to help both members see that expressing caring for a distressed partner is a strength of a relationship, but overprotecting the partner from facing and overcoming life challenges reduces the partner's opportunities to develop self-confidence and tolerate discomfort.

Given that an individual's symptoms are stressors for both members of the couple, interventions to reduce a partner's accommodation to the person's symptoms can be viewed within a dyadic coping model. Some forms of emotion-focused supportive dyadic coping (e.g., engaging the individual in distracting activities) and delegated dyadic coping (e.g., taking over some of the individual's tasks to reduce stress) may accommodate and reinforce the individual's counterproductive way of coping with symptoms. Some other forms of coping by a partner that tend to be counterproductive are hostile dyadic coping (e.g., blaming the individual for their psychological problems) and ambivalent dyadic coping (providing some support but communicating that doing so is a burden) because these tactics can exacerbate the individual's negative self-concept. In contrast, a combination of emotion-focused supportive dyadic coping that conveys affection and common dyadic coping (e.g., engaging in exposure exercises together) can facilitate improvement. These strategies can be used in a transdiagnostic manner.

Thus, goal setting that addresses couple interaction patterns influencing the occurrence of psychopathology symptoms combines a transdiagnostic model that identifies common patterns regardless of specific diagnoses and knowledge of variations in couple patterns that are associated with particular disorders. The Unified Protocol approach reduces the complexities of carrying out a set of couple treatment protocols for comorbid disorders, while knowledge of variations associated with different disorders helps tailor the details of the transdiagnostic interventions. For example, reducing negative cognitions is a core component of the Unified Protocol approach in individual and couple treatment modalities across diverse disorders. However, cognitive interventions for the common belief among individuals with generalized anxiety that worry serves a positive function in staving off problems can differ somewhat from interventions for the overly self-focused expectancies of individuals with social anxiety that others are scrutinizing them and evaluating them negatively. It is important for therapists to be aware of that difference in cognitive themes, but common cognitive restructuring interventions (e.g., behavioral experiments to test negative expectancies) can be used with both issues.

Goal Setting for Couple Therapy Addressing Relationship Factors That Elicit Psychopathology Symptoms

Although general couple therapy may be needed to assist some couples in reducing conflict and unhappiness associated with a member's psychopathology symptoms (e.g., by improving their communication and problem-solving skills, as well as joint emotion regulation), the treatment plan focuses even more on couple therapy when the assessment indicates that the couple's issues extend beyond psychopathology. As described by Epstein and Baucom (2002), sources of "primary distress" commonly involve conflicts over differences between partners' needs, preferences, personal styles, and life goals, and the couple's engagement in counterproductive attempts to resolve those differences creates "secondary distress" (i.e., their coping patterns make things worse). For example, a couple may experience primary distress because one member has a stronger desire than the other for autonomy and pursuit of individual interests, but their conflict and unhappiness have intensified due to a pursue–withdraw pattern they developed in response to their different needs, resulting in secondary distress.

Both forms of distress may be stressors that trigger or exacerbate a member's vulnerability to experience psychopathology symptoms. Consistent with the Unified Protocol model, an individual with a vulnerability toward insecurity and anxiety due to a mix of biological factors and prior traumatic life experiences may perceive a threat in a partner's desire for autonomy, eliciting anxiety symptoms. Furthermore, if the individual experiences negative cognitions about the anxiety symptoms (e.g., "This is awful! I can't stand it if my partner wants to be without me!"), those thoughts may contribute to pursuing the partner, seeking reassurance, or criticizing the partner as not caring about their relationship. The partner may also become upset (especially if the partner also has difficulty with negative cognitions and poor emotion regulation). The partner may contribute to an escalation of the pursue–withdraw pattern, perhaps through threatening comments (e.g., "Leave me alone! I can't stand much more of this!"). This secondary distress for both partners is likely to exacerbate the individual's symptoms. From a dyadic coping perspective, this couple's negative coping pattern is backfiring for both of them.

In the above example, the source of the couple's conflict and primary distress (a difference in the members' needs for connection versus autonomy) was related to the symptomatic individual's personal vulnerabilities, as was the source of their secondary distress (the pursue–withdraw pattern). However, in other cases the source of primary distress may be less relevant for eliciting symptoms in a vulnerable individual than the form and intensity of the couple's negative responses to the relationship conflict. For example, a couple's chronic arguments over parenting techniques may in itself have little bearing on an individual's tendency to experience anxiety, depression, and urges to engage in alcohol abuse, but the negative interactions that occur between the members during arguments may be crucial. The person's partner may make denigrating remarks that attack the individual's self-esteem and may engage in hostile withdrawal from the individual, responses that are highly relevant to the individual's underlying vulnerabilities and therefore trigger symptoms. In order to devise an appropriate treatment plan, therapists need to explore the degrees to which the stress on a symptomatic member of a couple is associated with sources of primary distress (areas of difference between partners) or to negative ways the couple interacts in response to their issues.

In applying a Unified Protocol model to assessment and treatment planning, couple therapists need to examine vulnerabilities in the three areas of emotional overreactivity, negative cognitions, and counterproductive ways of coping with distressing experiences on the parts of both members. Those vulnerabilities may differ from one couple to another, so treatment planning must take into account individual differences. Nevertheless, if therapists structure their assessment and identification of appropriate interventions within those three core domains, they should be able to devise treatment plans that address a variety of clients' symptoms in a manner that is clear to the couple and counteracts their hopelessness regarding their perception that they have many problems. CBCT interventions can be used to substitute constructive communication and problem solving for negative behavioral interactions, regulation of negative emotion for mutual escalation of emotional upset, and flexible thinking for unrealistic cognitions about symptoms and each other. Those interventions can reduce relationship problems as a major source of stress on individuals with diverse and comorbid psychopathology symptoms.

The evidence that relationship conflict and distress are risk factors for development and maintenance of various forms of psychopathology indicates that treatment of the overall relationship is essential when the couple has unresolved issues. In that sense, couple therapy is a transdiagnostic intervention that applies to couples with diverse psychopathology symptoms. Nevertheless, a complete treatment plan also will include components of partner-assisted interventions and disorder-specific or Unified Protocol interventions that are designed to foster couple collaboration and change interaction patterns such as accommodation that influence a member's symptoms. Improving a couple's ability to collaborate on strategies to reduce a member's psychopathology symptoms has potential to improve the members' overall cognitions, emotions and behavior toward each other.

PLANNING TREATMENT

Couple-based interventions for forms of psychopathology emphasize the involvement of a symptomatic individual's partner in ways that facilitate the effectiveness of empirically supported individual therapy protocols, typically with a CBT focus. The published programs apply one or a combination of partner-assisted, disorder-specific, and couple therapy approaches (Baucom et al., 2020), which are tailored to the individual therapy protocol for each disorder. To date, there has been relatively little application of a transdiagnostic Unified Protocol model in couple-based treatments for diverse and comorbid disorders. This section describes such a couple-based application of a Unified Protocol model.

A Unified Protocol Treatment Model Tailored to a Couple-Based Intervention

Figure 10.2 identifies how each component of Barlow et al.'s Unified Protocol can be conducted conjointly, targeting both partners' cognitions, emotional responses, and behavior, with an emphasis on influences between partners. The figure describes ways in which components of the Unified Protocol can be carried out with partner-assisted, disorder-specific, and couple therapy approaches. Partner-assisted and disorder-specific interventions are relevant for all couples, regardless of level of relationship satisfaction, whereas couple therapy is used with couples who are experiencing conflict and dissatisfaction. Following this description of the transdiagnostic Unified Protocol approach, we describe CBCT interventions for emotions, cognitions, and behavior that can be used to address its components in partner-assisted, disorder-specific, and couple therapy modes.

Transdiagnostic CBCT Couple-Based Interventions

This section describes CBCT interventions therapists can use with couples presenting with various symptoms, including those diagnosed with comorbid disorders. For detailed treatment of protocols focused on specific disorders (e.g., obsessive–compulsive disorder, posttraumatic stress disorder, major depressive disorder), readers should consult publications such as those cited in this chapter.

The following presents separate sections on interventions for modifying difficulties with emotion regulation, negative cognition, and counterproductive behavioral patterns of coping with symptoms within the couple. We begin with interventions for emotion regulation, followed by interventions for negative cognition, and finally interventions for behavioral responses, to be consistent with the Unified Protocol conception of individuals with a variety of disorders experiencing emotion dysregulation, negative thinking about those symptoms, and counterproductive coping with the symptoms. In clinical practice, however, therapists integrate the interventions for those three major domains. In addition, we note how the three domains are used in partner-assisted, disorder-specific, and couple therapy modalities. The degree to which the treatment plan includes partner-assisted, disorder-specific, and couple therapy interventions depends on the therapist's appraisal of how much the interventions need to focus on:

- couple teamwork in treating an individual's symptoms
- modification of couple patterns that maintain the symptoms
- reduction of stressful conflict and dissatisfaction in the overall couple relationship that elicit or exacerbate symptoms in a vulnerable individual

Interventions for Emotion Dysregulation

Because emotional distress commonly dominates the daily experiences of individuals with psychopathology and their partners, it is important to reduce emotion dysregulation not only on the part of a symptomatic member, but also on the part of the partner as needed. Furthermore, because members of a couple commonly "co-regulate" each other's emotions (Greenberg & Goldman, 2008), therapists often need to intervene with the couple's dyadic emotional process; that is, it is

Session 1: Functional Assessment and Introduction to Treatment

Information is collected about an individual's symptoms, any formal diagnoses, conditions in which they occur, and how both members think about those symptoms, respond emotionally to them, and attempt to cope with them, especially using avoidance or escape strategies. The therapist's focus is on whatever symptoms an individual experiences, regardless of diagnoses. The therapist provides a rationale and an overview of treatment components designed to reduce an individual's symptoms and emphasizes how the partner can be a major resource in the treatment. Although interventions will vary somewhat depending on the individual's symptoms (e.g., behavioral activation to reduce depression; a hierarchy of exposure exercises to reduce anxiety), they focus on emotional distress, cognitions regarding symptoms, and strategies used to avoid or escape symptoms. The therapist notes evidence of ways in which the individual's symptoms affect both members and the quality of their relationship, emphasizing benefits that the individual's improvement will have for the couple. The therapist identifies degrees to which partner-assisted, disorder-specific, and couple therapy approaches are appropriate and provides a rationale for the treatment plan. Standard CBCT interventions such as communication training used with discordant couples also are included whenever there is evidence of communication difficulties that could interfere with partner-assisted or disorder-specific couple interventions.

Module 1: Setting Goals and Maintaining Motivation

This module focuses on maximizing both partners' motivation to invest time and energy into the interventions, guiding them in setting concrete goals for overcoming an individual's symptoms and any links with relationship problems, and planning manageable steps toward achieving each goal. For generally satisfied couples who are low in conflict, the therapist can focus on goals for partner-assisted interventions. The supportive role of the partner in helping the individual carry out CBT interventions is clarified. Each person's role in carrying out interventions that target core transdiagnostic components (emotional distress, cognitions regarding symptoms, and counterproductive coping) is described. Each individual's thoughts and emotions regarding the partner playing that supportive role are explored in order to minimize labeling a symptomatic individual as "the dysfunctional" member and to maximize their collaboration. For satisfied couples in which a partner's accommodation responses maintain the other's symptoms, the therapist points out patterns in a nonblaming manner and emphasizes collaboration in eliminating couple patterns that are counterproductive. Finally, for couples in which distress and conflict elicit or exacerbate symptoms, psychoeducation includes a diathesis-stress model and enlists the couple in setting a goal of improving their relationship to reduce stress for both members.

Module 2: Understanding Emotions

The couple receives psychoeducation about emotions: their components, functions, internal and external triggers, ways members influence each other's emotions, and constructive and problematic ways that symptomatic individuals and their partners cope with aversive emotions. This psychoeducation facilitates a partner's empathy for the emotional experiences of a symptomatic individual and supports the rationale for collaborating on interventions to down-regulate excessive negative affect and up-regulate positive emotional experiences such as pleasure from behavior activation. Partners who become aware that they engage in actions that accommodate the other person's attempts to avoid negative affect can become motivated to support the individual's increased acceptance and tolerance of unpleasant emotions. For discordant couples, understanding how members "fuel" each other's upset helps motivate them to engage in dyadic CBCT interventions to regulate negative moods and communicate constructively.

(continued)

FIGURE 10.2. Conjoint couple interventions applying the Unified Protocol (UP) for Transdiagnostic Treatment of Emotional Disorders.

Module 3: Mindful Emotion Awareness

The couple is taught about a nonjudgmental approach to observing their own and each other's emotional experiences rather than evaluating particular emotions as undesirable and avoiding them. They are taught and practice exercises for mindful emotion awareness during sessions. The psychoeducation and focus on noticing emotional responses can contribute to partner-assisted interventions in which a partner encourages a symptomatic individual to attend nonjudgmentally to emotional experiences and value them as indicators that triggering events have significant meaning to the individual. The symptomatic individual supports the partner's own emotional self-exploration to identify significant meanings; for example, a partner's anger was triggered by frustration that their attempts to make the symptomatic person feel better have been ineffective. Thus, it may become clear that a partner's fear that an individual's possible panic attack will disrupt daily life may motivate the partner to help the individual avoid threatening situations. Regarding couple therapy for discordant relationships, mindful awareness can contribute to members noticing cues that anger is building, so they can take actions to forestall escalation.

Module 4: Cognitive Flexibility

Traditional CBT interventions are used to increase both partners' awareness of their cognitions about a member's cognitive, affective, and behavioral psychopathology symptoms (e.g., excessive worry, lethargy) and how those interpretations influence how each member copes with the symptoms. Psychoeducation covers automatic thoughts, cognitive distortions (e.g., catastrophizing), and approaches to considering more constructive ways of thinking about each other's responses. Although some negative cognitions may be relatively specific to a type of disorder (e.g., danger themes especially common in anxiety disorders, themes regarding loss and hopelessness prevalent in depressive disorders), there are transdiagnostic cognitive themes. For example, across diagnoses individuals tend to be hypervigilant for distressing symptoms and catastrophize about negative outcomes (e.g., that any symptoms of depression signify a "slippery slope" in which functioning will deteriorate). Partners are guided in exploring their own cognitions, as well as inquiring about each other's in a respectful manner, with a goal of supporting each other in testing the validity of upsetting thoughts. This process also is used to attune a partner to their cognitions that lead them to engage in accommodating behavior. Finally, these interventions are used to improve dissatisfied members' abilities to counteract cognitions that fuel their negative emotional and behavioral responses to each other.

Module 5: Countering Emotional Behaviors

The couple is taught about the behavioral responses individuals and their partners use to try to control their own and each other's distressing emotions and the negative consequences of some strategies. Partner-accommodating behaviors to reduce an individual's symptoms are targeted, including exploration of some benefits that the nonsymptomatic partner also may have gotten from those strategies (e.g., relief when the individual temporarily stops complaining about emotional distress). The couple is guided in experimenting with "alternative actions" that produce more positive results. This is applied within a partner-assisted approach and a disorder-specific approach, but is also relevant for discordant couples. For example, a partner may cooperate with a socially anxious individual's desire for the couple to avoid social gatherings but is also resentful of missed socializing with friends, which contributes to unhappiness with the relationship.

Module 6: Understanding and Confronting Physical Sensations

The couple is guided through *interoceptive exposure,* which simulates an individual's distressing symptoms. The goals are the symptomatic individual's increased awareness and tolerance of unpleasant

(continued)

FIGURE 10.2. *(continued)*

symptoms, as well as greater empathy on the part of a partner. Interoceptive exposure prepares the couple to collaborate on partner-assisted interventions. It also is applied within a disorder-specific approach, as exposure experiences counteract couple interactions that accommodate an individual's avoidance of distressing symptoms. With regard to couple therapy for discordant relationships, a partner's increased empathy for an individual's uncomfortable symptoms can reduce the partner's criticism and negative affect, which has been a stressor for a vulnerable symptomatic individual. The partner's participation in interoceptive exposure also can contribute to the symptomatic individual's ability to form a more positive view of the partner.

Module 7: Emotion Exposures

The couple receives psychoeducation about the importance of staying in situations that elicit strong emotions rather than avoiding or escaping them. The clinician guides the couple in constructing a hierarchy of challenging exposure situations and using repeated exposures to increase tolerance for more challenging levels. The partner's role as a support and coach, as well as the importance of eliminating accommodation behavior, is detailed. This is another component of partner-assisted treatment and also contributes to disorder-specific couple intervention as it counteracts a partner's accommodating behaviors. For discordant couples, it is helpful for increasing positive collaborations between partners and positive attributions regarding each other's good intentions in working to solve problems that affect both people.

Module 8: Recognizing Accomplishments and Looking to the Future

The couple is guided in reviewing gains, especially through teamwork, toward treatment goals. Areas for future work and improvement are noted, and strategies are planned for relapse prevention—for example, periodic couple meetings to assess functioning and any signs that additional practice of interventions is needed, scheduling a "booster session" with their therapist.

FIGURE 10.2. *(continued)*

more than two parallel interventions for the individuals. Throughout this process, the inclusion of both members of the couple validates the distress experienced by a nonsymptomatic partner and balances the intervention rather than focusing on an identified patient.

However, it is crucial for therapists and their clients to acknowledge and accept the ubiquity of distressing experiences in people's lives and to help clients accept the idea that living a full life involves experiencing a full range of emotions rather than trying one's best to avoid all unpleasant feelings or to aid loved ones in such avoidance (Leahy, 2019). In a CBCT approach, therapists convey to clients that it is normal to experience negative as well as positive emotions, and that one's emotional responses are important reflections of one's personal needs, preferences, and life goals (see Chapter 1). Becoming aware that a partner's actions led to anger is a cue to self-exploration about the meaning that one has attached to the partner's actions and implications for seeking changes. The problem is not the individual's experience of anger, but rather the intensity of the anger and how it is expressed toward the partner (see Chapter 5 on partner aggression). The goal of couple-based interventions is to maximize awareness of emotions, identify their significance, increase partners' ability to regulate their intensity, and facilitate the couple's skills for sharing them. Therapists also need to be attuned to the cultural beliefs and traditions of some couples that do not support any direct expression of strong emotions, so interventions will not detract from a positive therapeutic alliance and effectiveness of therapy. In Chapter 11, we discuss cultural adaptations of a model such as CBCT that emphasizes recognition and communication about emotion.

If the assessment of a couple indicates that a member's psychopathology symptoms have been elicited or worsened by the couple's intense emotional responses to other issues in the relationship, interventions to reduce both partners' negative emotional responses that are part of global relationship stress can reduce negative effects on the symptomatic individual. Thus, couple therapy is used to reduce the impact of emotion dysregulation regarding relationship problems on individual functioning. However, if the assessment indicates that the couple has a mutually satisfying relationship overall, but a nonsymptomatic partner experiences some emotion dysregulation specifically due to difficulty coping with the other person's symptoms, interventions for both members' emotional responses can facilitate partner-assisted and disorder-specific couple approaches.

As described earlier in this chapter, intervention regarding the couple's emotions associated with psychopathology typically begins with psychoeducation regarding the role of emotion in various forms of psychological distress and disorders, as well as in unhappiness with one's relationship. Information is presented not only about the physiological, cognitive, subjective feelings, and behavioral components of each individual's emotions, but also about co-regulation processes that can occur rapidly and can turn a calm discussion into a tense argument. The therapist then probes for both partners' emotions associated with an individual's psychopathology symptoms. For example, the emotional experiences of an individual who presents with moderate depression symptoms are explored by tracking situations that trigger them and the degree to which the individual appraises them as overwhelming and uncontrollable. The therapist simultaneously explores the other partner's emotional experiences when the individual exhibits depression symptoms; for example, anxiety associated with an expectancy that "my partner's depression will engulf us and turn our daily life into gloom and doom!" In turn, the intensity of the depressed individual's emotion may be intensified by the partner's negative emotion. The therapist's goal is to increase the couple's awareness of each person's emotional process, as well as the dyadic co-regulation process.

The psychoeducation process is extended by coaching the couple in differentiating various emotions that they experience and tracking emotional experiences in various life situations, including couple interactions. The therapist surveys the range of distressing emotional symptoms an individual experiences, including those that are responses to the other person's emotions. Members of a couple can be introduced to keeping logs of their emotional experiences, including apps that they can download on their phones. In particular, the therapist gives the couple in-the-moment feedback regarding instances of co-regulation during their interactions within therapy sessions. The therapist also guides the couple in noticing their automatic thoughts that are associated with particular emotions, such as anxiety regarding perceived danger, sadness or depression regarding perceived losses, and anger regarding perceived injustices. This leads to interventions to modify unrealistic or inaccurate negative cognitions that fuel negative emotions.

Although the insight provided by psychoeducation is an important step in improving a couple's emotion regulation, couples typically also need guidance in developing their abilities to regulate negative emotions individually and as a dyad as they occur. Therefore, the therapist then introduces a variety of emotion-regulation strategies (see Chapter 4) and collaborates with the couple to identify particular methods they can try for their personal emotional responses, as well as those they can use to reduce escalation of negative emotion between them. It is emphasized that some emotion-regulation methods may be more palatable and work better for one member than for the other. Furthermore, the most relevant strategies may differ based on the types of emotional symptoms each person experiences. For example, an individual's depressed moods may be counteracted best by behavioral activation exercises, whereas another person's physical anxiety symptoms may respond best to muscle relaxation and mindfulness exercises. An individual's participation in partner-assisted interventions for a symptomatic person's emotion-regulation problems is more likely to occur if the individual knows and accepts the methods that are most effective for that person. In cases in which symptomatic and nonsymptomatic members escalate each other's negative emotions, a disorder-specific approach can be used that focuses on reducing the nonsymptomatic partner's negative reactions (e.g., expressed irritation) that exacerbate the other's symptoms. When couples include two members with significant psychopathology symptoms, the emphasis is on contributions that both people can make to reducing negative emotion within their relationship.

As emphasized in the Unified Protocol model, problems that both members of a couple experience with an individual's emotional distress are due not only to difficulties in regulating negative affect, but also to poor tolerance of emotional and physical distress. In fact, excessive focus in therapy on a goal of reducing one's own or a partner's emotional distress can convey a message to the couple that negative feelings are dangerous and unacceptable, and exercises designed to reduce arousal may become avoidance strategies. Therefore, psychoeducation and emotion-regulation interventions also should emphasize that stress and emotional discomfort are inevitable in life, and developing acceptance and tolerance of those experiences is a significant strength. Linehan's (2015) book *DBT Skills Training Handouts and Worksheets* includes a variety of interventions to improve individuals' distress tolerance, which can be used in couple therapy as well. Partner-assisted and disorder-specific couple therapy protocols for a variety of disorders include psychoeducation regarding the importance of reducing the avoidance of symptoms and the situations that elicit them, as well as interventions that repeatedly expose clients to them. The ways that individuals experience distressing symptoms vary across presenting problems (e.g., uncomfortable feelings associated with depressed moods, fear of panic symptoms, urges to drink alcohol). However, the more the individual and partner come to accept and tolerate discomfort, the less likely they are to try to avoid or escape the situation. Behavioral interventions that focus on reducing individual and dyadic avoidance that are described below are integrated with emotion-regulation interventions. Furthermore, behavioral interventions that improve partners' abilities to express emotions and thoughts to each other and convey empathy and support for each other can help reduce partners' concerns about experiencing emotions.

Interventions to Modify Cognition

Cognitive-behavioral conceptualizations include identification of the specific predominant content of cognitions that differentiate one disorder from another. For example, social anxiety tends to involve expectancies that other people will scrutinize and negatively evaluate the individual; depressive disorders involve cognitions of loss, self-criticism, and hopelessness; panic disorder involves negative expectancies of severe and dangerous anxiety symptoms, as well as hypervigilance for bodily cues of emotional arousal (anxiety sensitivity); eating disorders involve perfectionistic thinking and distorted body image; and alcohol abuse commonly involves expectancies regarding the positive effects of drinking on emotional distress and sociability. The negative cognitions in all disorders involve individuals' standards, assumptions, attributions, expectancies, and selective perceptions, but their content has some disorder-specific themes.

Although the Unified Protocol model also recognizes some specificity in cognitions associated with particular types of symptoms, it also emphasizes negative and distorted cognitions that are consistent across disorders. In particular, transdiagnostic cognitions have themes that one's emotional symptoms are reflections of being defective and weak, are intolerable, make it impossible to function adequately in life, and need to be avoided or escaped. For couple therapists working with psychopathology, both disorder-specific and transdiagnostic negative cognitions are targets of treatment.

In couple-based treatment, interventions for the cognitions of a symptomatic individual are similar to those used in individual therapy, although they are carried out in the dyadic context. For example, common "cognitive restructuring" methods used in individual cognitive therapy (J. S. Beck, 2021; Leahy, 2017; Leahy et al., 2012), such as exploring exceptions to an individual's selective negative perception of her ability to complete tasks, exploration of advantages and disadvantages of perfectionism, or psychoeducation regarding particular cognitive distortions such as catastrophizing, are used conjointly with the couple. In addition to transdiagnostic cognitions (e.g., that emotional distress is intolerable), the therapist draws the couple's attention to cognitions that are especially associated with particular symptoms (e.g., intense concern about being evaluated by other people associated with social anxiety). In partner-assisted interventions, the partner is engaged in reminding the symptomatic individual to use cognitive interventions during daily life and praising the individual for even small successes.

However, intervention with the partner's own cognitions is important too, particularly when the therapist identifies ways in which the partner's responses to the symptomatic individual worsen the problem. In disorder-specific couple intervention, the partner may have cognitions that are similar to those of the symptomatic individual (e.g., that the person cannot tolerate distressing symptoms; that emotions are signs of weakness). In such cases, the members of the couple reinforce each other's negative thinking. The partner may have additional negative cognitions (e.g., that the person's self-criticism is unattractive self-pity) that result in negative emotion toward the individual and may lead the partner to behave negatively.

Psychoeducation can increase both members' knowledge about psychopathology symptoms and both the individual's intrapsychic factors (e.g., cognitive distortions) and couple patterns (e.g., accommodation behavior by a caring partner) that must be altered to produce improvement. Furthermore, psychoeducation regarding forms of dyadic coping can emphasize the advantages of teamwork to manage and reduce the impact of symptoms on both members. Similar to the process of externalizing the problem in narrative therapy (Freedman & Combs, 2023; White & Epston, 1990), orienting the couple toward collaborating to overcome a shared problem of psychopathology symptoms, rather than viewing it as belonging solely to the symptomatic individual and each other as adversaries, is a fundamental cognitive shift.

CBCT interventions can help partners resolve differences in life goals, preferences, and personal standards. When conflict is due to partners having rigid or extreme personal standards for the qualities that their relationship "should" have, making negative attributions about each other's motives, selectively attending to each other's displeasing actions, and overlooking positives, the cognitive interventions described in Chapter 4 are used.

Interventions to Modify Behavior Associated with Psychopathology Symptoms

The Unified Protocol approach to psychopathology emphasizes modifying counterproductive actions that individuals take to avoid or escape aversive symptoms. Across disorders these actions commonly involve restricting one's activity in daily life, and behavioral interventions are designed to activate and expose the individual to situations they find intimidating. The behavioral interventions draw from established individual therapy methods such as those in cognitive-behavioral therapies (Dobson, & Dozois, 2019; J. S. Beck, 2021; Leahy, 2017). They are incorporated into partner-assisted and disorder-specific couple approaches by building couple collaboration and teamwork in managing psychopathology symptoms. For example, Monson and Fredman's (2012, 2023) conjoint couple protocol for posttraumatic stress disorder addresses forms of partner accommodation to a symptomatic individual, involving ways of avoiding conditions that could upset the person, such as avoiding public places that trigger posttraumatic stress disorder symptoms. Behavioral interventions used to reduce avoidance by the symptomatic individual and couple include communication and problem-solving skills training, a hierarchy of *in vivo* exposures to avoided situations, and interventions to increase safety within the relationship by reducing any partner aggression. Increasing joint pleasant activities also reduces stress within the relationship.

Because dyadic accommodation patterns are motivated by both members' concerns about exposing the individual to distressing symptoms, it is important for the therapist to provide rationales for behavioral interventions that unbalance the status quo and likely will be uncomfortable. It is important that the therapist explore a partner's discomfort with procedures that initially may increase the other person's symptoms, or fear of the symptoms, and discuss the short-term and long-term pros and cons of making changes. Otherwise, the partner's reluctance to change the status quo may be as much a barrier to carrying out interventions as the symptomatic individual's fear of emotional pain.

Similarly, individual and couple behavioral responses to depressive symptoms commonly involve low-level activity, especially regarding situations and tasks that the individual (and often the partner) believe are too taxing and upsetting for the person. Both the Unified Protocol model and couple treatment protocols specifically designed for depression focus on partner assistance with cognitive-behavioral individual therapy interventions that counteract avoidance and inactivity. Interventions emphasize working through a hierarchy of behavioral activation exercises, with a goal of increasing experiences of mastery, self-efficacy, and pleasure. When the therapist identifies ways in which a partner accommodates the individual's avoidance and inactivity, the therapist intervenes to reduce the partner's cognitions that support the accommodation. Thus, the partner of a depressed person may hold an assumption that the individual is fragile and an expectancy that the individual will be damaged if exposed to stressors, as well as a personal standard that a loving partner protects the other person from pain. The goal of cognitive interventions is to prepare the partner to play a therapeutic role in supporting and encouraging the depressed individual to engage in activities that will reduce inertia, increase self-efficacy, and add to mood-enhancing experiences. The therapist also can emphasize that the shared behavior activation exercises can enhance both members' enjoyment of the relationship.

When the therapist identifies broad negative couple behavioral interaction patterns regarding issues other than psychopathology that act as stressors on an individual who is vulnerable to experiencing symptoms, common CBCT behavioral interventions (Chapter 4) are used in a transdiagnostic manner to reduce the aversive interactions and increase positive interactions. This approach is consistent with an interpersonal model of psychopathology (Beach et al., 1990; Whisman et al., 2023) that focuses on a high level of aversive interaction between partners. Their exchanges include expressions of negative cognition and emotion on the part of a symptomatic individual and a low level of support between partners, both of which contribute to relationship distress and symptoms. Behavioral interventions focus on reducing EE and increasing intimacy, cohesion, constructive communication and problem solving, and mutual social support (including partner dependability and positive dyadic coping with stressors).

TROUBLESHOOTING PROBLEMS IN COUPLE THERAPY FOR PSYCHOPATHOLOGY

In this section, we describe problems that can arise in couple-based interventions for psychopathology and some guidelines for addressing them. Because these issues have been identified in other chapters or previously in this chapter, they are described concisely here.

Severe Psychopathology and Partner Aggression

Chapter 2 discussed severe psychopathology as one of the possible exclusion factors for conducting couple therapy. This is not because couple dynamics are less influential in the individual's functioning, but rather because of the degree to which severe symptoms interfere with the individual's capacity to participate in and benefit from couple interventions.

- Partner-assisted and disorder-specific couple interventions still may be productive in many cases with severe symptoms, as a partner's guidance and support may make it easier for an individual to carry out procedures to improve emotion regulation, negative cognitions regarding oneself and one's symptoms, and counterproductive ways of coping with emotional distress (Mueser & Gingerich, 2006).

- Chapter 5 emphasizes that couple-based treatments are contraindicated when there is evidence of severe aggression perpetrated by one or both members of the couple, especially resulting in physical injury. Psychopathology can be a risk factor for perpetrating aggression, and in turn, aggression victimization has been found to be a risk for mental health problems. Consequently, before considering couple interventions for psychopathology, therapists should screen for partner aggression and make referrals for individual therapy focused on treatment of aggressive behavior as needed, as a prerequisite for couple therapy. Evidence that a member of a couple has been victimized also should lead to safety planning and referrals to protective community resources.

- Although substance abuse is among the range of disorders that have been treated in a couple context, severe use can interfere with an individual's ability to participate in couple interventions in ways similar to other forms of severe psychopathology. Again, the clinician can evaluate whether partner-assisted and disorder-specific interventions can support the individual in carrying out standard substance abuse interventions (McCrady et al., 2023; O'Farrell & Fals-Stewart, 2006), or whether individual therapy for the symptomatic member must be a prerequisite for any conjoint treatment.

Environmental Stressors Influencing Psychopathology

Consistent with our contextual approach to understanding and treating individual and relational problems within couples, comprehensive case conceptualization and treatment planning must take into account stressors within the couple's physical and interpersonal environment (e.g., job demands, parenting stressors, discrimination based on minority group characteristics such as race, ethnicity, age, gender identity, sexual orientation, and disabilities).

• In some cases, the negative effects of environmental stressors on individual and couple functioning can interfere with couple-based treatment unless they are identified and targeted for intervention. Because research has indicated that a variety of life stressors can elicit or maintain psychopathology symptoms in vulnerable people (Barlow et al., 2018), the therapist needs to interview the couple and both individuals to identify stressors that are affecting them and ways that the members have attempted to cope with them, both individually and as a dyad. The interviews with the couple and individual partners described in Chapter 3 include questions regarding stressors and coping responses.

• In order to devise appropriate couple-based interventions, the therapist needs to identify which individual and dyadic coping strategies a couple has been using to deal with stressors affecting either or both of them, as well as their effectiveness or lack thereof. The assessment should explore circumstances in which specific stressful experiences elicited or exacerbated a partner's symptoms. The therapist can guide the couple in devising plans to use positive dyadic coping strategies to buffer the negative effects of stressors and to use the resources available to them (e.g., sources of social support) to reduce stressors.

Sociocultural Factors Influencing the Experience and Expression of Psychopathology

As described in Chapter 11, cultural beliefs and traditions are other contextual factors that influence couple and family relationships. People's conceptions of causes, meanings, and appropriate treatment of psychopathology often are influenced by their cultural backgrounds, potentially leading to a gap between their expectations of therapy and a therapist's case conceptualization and treatment plan.

• Therefore, therapists should inquire about individuals' beliefs regarding the causes of their own or a partner's symptoms (e.g., as manifestations of internal moral conflict, personal weakness, genetic factors, damage from life traumas, severe unhappiness with one's life, overwhelmed ability to cope with current life stressors). The therapist also can ask about each person's culturally based beliefs about the stigma associated with mental illness, as well as knowledge and assumptions about treatments that may help (e.g., individual or couple therapy, medication, changes in diet and lifestyle, some form of penance). The therapist needs to demonstrate empathy for individuals whose cultural background involves shame for a symptomatic person and their family, and also needs to convey optimism that treatment has the potential to alleviate symptoms and build individual and family strengths.

• In order to foster a positive therapeutic alliance with the couple, it is important for the therapist to describe their conceptualization of factors contributing to the psychopathology symptoms the couple has presented, as well as the therapist's treatment methods, and to show interest in hearing about the clients' thoughts and emotions regarding therapy. The therapist also should interview partners about past experiences within their culture with interventions for symptoms and convey optimism that the present treatment can help.

• While showing respect for clients' cultural backgrounds, the therapist can provide psycho-education regarding causes and effective treatments for psychopathology, including the advantages of collaborative couple approaches.

KEY POINTS

• Psychopathology traditionally has been thought of and treated as a characteristic of individuals, but links have been found between forms of psychopathology and problems in the functioning of individuals' significant relationships.

• Three forms of couple-based interventions for psychopathology are (1) partner-assisted interventions, (2) disorder-specific protocols, and (3) traditional couple therapy designed to reduce the interpersonal sources of stress affecting an individual's symptoms.

• A symptomatic individual's partner also has cognitive, affective, and behavioral responses to the individual's symptoms, and the two members mutually influence each other's coping with psychopathology in problematic or constructive ways.

• Research indicating the high comorbidity of DSM disorders in presenting problems has led to development of transdiagnostic models of psychopathology and its treatment.

• The three core transdiagnostic domains of client vulnerability are (1) severe, persistent, and poorly regulated negative emotional responses, (2) distorted and inappropriate negative thinking about one's emotional and related symptoms, and (3) counterproductive ways of attempting to cope with one's negative symptoms, such as avoidance.

• Although CBCT therapists still need to be familiar with the client characteristics associated with particular disorders (e.g., in social anxiety, preoccupation with being evaluated negatively by others), a transdiagnostic approach can help in treatment planning for clients with diverse and often comorbid psychopathology symptoms.

CHAPTER 11

Intercultural Couples

Intercultural couple relationships have received increasing attention in the last two decades in both the research and the clinical literature and in diverse societies such as the United States, which has been shaped by waves of immigration. Similar to Killian (2015), we define intercultural couples as those in which partners identify with different nationalities, ethnicities, races, and/or religions "who may possess quite different beliefs, assumptions, and values as a result of their socialization in different sociocultural spaces" (p. 514). Within intercultural, interracial, and interfaith couples, one or both partners may not be part of the dominant culture, race, or religion in the country or region in which the couple resides. Furthermore, one or both members may be immigrants from another country, who have faced significant adjustments and challenges from the dominant culture. Thus, one or both partners may belong to a minority group in terms of ethnicity, race, and/or religion and experience varying levels of discrimination and challenges outside their relationship, which influence them individually as well as their relationship. In this chapter, we describe ways in which being a minority where one lives is an important contextual factor to consider in couple assessment and treatment.

WHAT IS CULTURE?

According to the Merriam-Webster online dictionary (*www.merriam-webster.com*), *culture* is defined at a broad level as "the customary beliefs, social forms, and material traits of a racial, religious, or social group." Despite its wide use in social science literature, this definition can create an illusion that a particular culture is a set of homogeneous, clearly identifiable characteristics shared by all of its members and that individual members passively incorporate those characteristics through the socialization process (Falconier et al., 2016; Markus, 2004). This view contributes to the notion that the characteristics of a culture do not change over time, leading to stereotyped descriptions of differences among cultural groups, when in fact large changes within cultural groups commonly occur over time (Markus, 2004; Varnum & Grossmann, 2017).

In reality, the characteristics of cultures (such as South Asian, Jewish, Black, Latine, Spanish, and Muslim) exhibit ongoing transformation as their members adapt to changes in their environment that can vary from gradual to abrupt (Varnum & Grossman, 2017). An example of a recent abrupt change that has influenced cultures around the world has been the COVID-19 pandemic that markedly changed people's experiences of work, education, and social interaction (Varnum & Grossmann, 2021). Thus, culture is far from being a system with clearly delineated boundaries and permanent elements, but rather is fluid and dynamic. Cultural contexts shape individuals' beliefs, emotions, and behaviors, but individuals also interpret and act out culture idiosyncratically. Individuals experience and perform culture in a variety of ways. The ways individuals cook and eat, dance, work, parent children, express affection, communicate, and deal with stresses and losses are performed within cultural frameworks and scripts, but with each person's and family's idiosyncratic versions.

On the one hand, individuals reinforce broadly shared practices, values, and worldviews of their culture(s), but on the other hand they also introduce variation. One specific example is chefs who develop fusion forms of cuisine that integrate a traditional cultural style with aspects of other cuisines. Those variations are introduced through identification with the characteristics of other cultural groups, the effects of a dominant cultural system on immigrants' traditions (and vice versa), generational shifts in preferences (as in music), contextual demands (such as phasing out of certain types of jobs due to technological advances), and individuals' social location. As regards social location, the intersection of various identities based on one's age, gender identity, sexual orientation, socioeconomic status, and race (among other elements of one's identity) has a major influence on how one perceives, experiences, and performs culture. Based on the intersection of such social identities, members of the same cultural group will inevitably have different understandings and definitions of their culture. Consequently, it is important that therapists avoid making potentially stereotyped assumptions about their clients' culture(s), constantly examine their work for implicit bias. and actively seek to learn about clients' personal views and definitions of the culture(s) with which they identify. In couple therapy, therapist curiosity must extend to degrees to which partners share each other's views and definitions of their cultures.

In addition to understanding clients' idiosyncratic views of their cultures of identification, couple therapists need to explore whether and to what extent each member views themself as belonging to more than one cultural group (e.g., Jewish and Latine, Muslim and Asian, Black and Caribbean). These observations apply to any couple, but they are especially relevant when treating intercultural relationships, given the greater potential for differences between partners.

When inquiring about cultures with which partners identify, couple therapists may find that it is not easy for all clients to describe the elements of those cultures. People vary in their awareness of aspects of culture that shape their worldviews, interpretation of interactions with other people, emotional responses, and behaviors (Ting-Toomey & Oetzel, 2001). People constantly interpret the world and perform aspects of culture, but not necessarily in a conscious way. Although children commonly are taught some aspects of their heritage culture explicitly in their families of origin, schools, and religious institutions, they internalize other aspects of culture implicitly through observational learning, without a word being spoken. In addition, people often are not required to think explicitly about and define culturally linked roles (e.g., parent, spouse, child) while they are engaged in them. It is often during contacts with other cultures that elements of one's own become more salient. For many people, it is when they become involved in a romantic relationship with a member of different cultural groups that they become aware of characteristics of the cultures that have shaped their own life experiences. As we discuss in the assessment section of this chapter, therapists' inquiries may assist partners in identifying and reflecting on the elements of their cultures.

TRENDS TOWARD INCREASED INTERCULTURAL COUPLES

Waves of migration around the world have resulted in increased cultural diversity in many countries (United Nations, 2015), creating the potential for the formation of intercultural relationships. The passage of statutes legalizing such relationships has significantly transformed that potential into more intercultural couples. In the United States, for example, since the Supreme Court's decision in the case of *Loving v. Virginia* in 1967, which legalized interracial marriage, interracial coupling has steadily increased and a gradual shift toward acceptance of such unions has taken place. According to the Pew Research Center's report (2017a) on intermarriages, these marriages grew from 3% in 1967 to 17% in 2015, with 1 of every 10 married people reporting a spouse of a different race or ethnicity. However, groups differ significantly in their tendency to marry outside their race or ethnicity. The Pew Research Center report indicated that among U.S. newlyweds in 2015, 29% of Asians, 27% of Latines, 18% of Blacks, and 11% of Whites intermarried. The largest percentage of intermarried couples included a Latine individual and a White spouse (42%), followed by an Asian person and a White individual (12%). The report also indicated that the number of intermarried individuals is even higher for second-generation immigrants. In 2015, 39% of U.S.-born newlywed Latines and 46% of U.S.-born newlywed Asians intermarried.

Similarly, the number of interfaith couples has risen. Since 2010, in the United States 39% of people have married a person from a different religious group, compared to only 19% of those who got married before 1960 (Pew Research Center, 2015). The most frequent interfaith marriage is between Christians and individuals with no religious affiliation. Similar to married couples, 45% of cohabiting couples are also interfaith. Nonetheless, the rate of partnering with someone outside one's religious group is not the same across different religious groups. For example, in the United States 42% of married Jewish people have a non-Jewish spouse, and 61% of those who have married since 2010 have non-Jewish partners, with a higher concentration among younger couples (Pew Research Center, 2021c). By contrast, only 9% of Hindus, 18% of Mormons, and 21% Muslims in the United States are married or are living with a partner with a different religion (Pew Research Center, 2015). Therapists should consider these differences in interfaith combinations in order to understand the social context that exists when an individual partners with someone of a different faith or no faith, concerning levels of acceptance or criticism they may receive from their religious group.

Because young people born in the United States have been choosing to marry partners of a different race or ethnicity, and interfaith coupling also is more common in younger generations, it is reasonable to expect the upward trend in intermarriage to continue. As a result, couple therapists are increasingly likely to find themselves treating intercultural, interracial, and interfaith couples. Thus, it is important for couple therapists to understand the strengths of intercultural partnerships as well as risk factors they may face in order to assist them.

RACIAL, ETHNIC, AND RELIGIOUS DISCRIMINATION EXPERIENCED BY INTERCULTURAL COUPLES

Despite the upward trend in interethnic, interracial, and interfaith unions, partners in such relationships in the United States still often face discrimination, either individually or as a couple. At the individual level, a partner who is part of a minority population is already likely to encounter prejudice and even violence. For example, African Americans continue to report experiences of discrimination when interacting with the police (50%), applying for jobs (56%), and at work (57%) regarding being paid equally or considered for promotion (Robert Wood Johnson Foundation, 2017a). A recent study on the deaths due to police violence in the United States from 1980 through 2019 found that police have killed Black people at a rate three to five times higher than White people (Sharara, GBD 2019 Police Violence US Subnational Collaborators, & Wool, 2021). Cases such as the murder of George Floyd by an officer in Minneapolis and the hate crime murder of Ahmaud Arbery in suburban Georgia have increased public attention to widespread racism toward Black individuals and couples across people and institutions in the United States.

Similarly, Asians, Latines, and Native Americans continue to experience discrimination. A Pew Research Center report (2021b) indicated that 8 in 10 Asian Americans thought violence against them was increasing, and 3 in 10 reported that they were afraid of receiving threats or being attacked physically. They attributed the increase in violence toward them to their being viewed as responsible for the outbreak of the COVID-19 pandemic. However, 73% of Asian Americans shared that they had experienced discrimination due to their race or ethnicity before the pandemic (Pew Research Center, 2021a). At the end of 2019, almost 1 in 10 Latine individuals in the United States reported experiencing discrimination by being treated unfairly, called offensive names, criticized for speaking Spanish in public, or told to go back to their "home country" (Pew Research Center, 2020). More than one in three Native Americans report having personally experienced racial or ethnic slurs, and one in four say they have received offensive comments about their race or ethnicity. Thirty-eight percent report that they or a family member has suffered from violence, and 34% have been harassed nonsexually or have received verbal threats (Robert Wood Johnson Foundation, 2017b).

Regarding religion, non-Christian groups and atheists tend to experience discrimination in the United States (Scheitle & Ecklund, 2020). Muslims have experienced a rise in assaults in recent years, surpassing the levels of victimization following the September 11, 2001, terrorist attack. The Pew Research Center (2017b) survey found that 75% of Muslims believe that there is "a lot" of discrimination against them in the United States, and 50% conclude that discrimination, racism, and prejudice have made it more difficult to be a Muslim in the United States. Both Muslims and Jewish individuals are at greater risk for discrimination and hate crimes than Christian individuals, but Muslims tend to experience more harassment and unfair treatment by the police than any other religious group (Scheitle & Ecklund, 2020). Furthermore, individuals who identify publicly as nonreligious experience more interpersonal hostility and discrimination, harassment, or violence than Christian people (Scheitle & Ecklund, 2020).

Minority groups' perceptions of discrimination based on race, country of origin, and religion seem to be consistent with the general public's perception of discrimination toward minorities. According to the Pew Research Center Report (2021a), 80% of the general population think Black people face discrimination, and 76% and 70% think the same about Latines and Asians, respectively. In terms of religion, 78% reported that Muslims face some or a lot of discrimination, and 68% reported the same for Jews. Furthermore, 39% believed Muslims face "a lot" of discrimination, compared to 14% who believed Jews face that severe level.

Individuals in intercultural groups often face prejudice, discrimination, inequities, and even violence, not only because of their minoritized race, ethnicity, and/or religion but also because of their gender identity, sexual orientation, disability, and other social identities. This is a frequent situation among same-sex couples who are more likely to marry interethnically or interracially than opposite-sex couples; 28% of men in same-sex marriages versus 16% in opposite-sex marriages are intermarried, and 20% of women in same-sex marriages are intermarried, versus 16% those in opposite-sex marriages (Pew Research Center, 2021d). In such cases minority stress is greatly exacerbated, severely affecting their individual mental health and their couple and family relationships.

Besides bias and discrimination based on ethnicity, race, religion, gender identity, sexual orientation, and other minoritized social identities, partners in intercultural couples may experience discrimination and a lack of safety due to the interethnic, interracial, or interfaith nature of their relationship. Pittman, Kamp Dush, Pratt, and Wong (2023) found that in spite of the legalization of intermarriages and the increasing rate of intercultural unions, interracial couples continue to experience discrimination and stigma in contemporary America. Skinner and Hudac (2017) found a tendency for individuals to report disgust when observing interracial couples and to view them in a dehumanized way. As already noted, interracial couples' experiences of discrimination are exacerbated by minority stress related to their other minority social identities. For example, studies found that interracial couples in which one of the partners is Black report more discrimination than those without a Black partner (Midy, 2018; Yancey, 2007).

The chronic stress resulting from the everyday experiences of being subjected to rejection, inequalities, discrimination, and stereotypes/stigma, as well as the individual's tendency to internalize negative self-images, has been referred to as minority stress (Meyer, 2003). Partners in intercultural couples each have to cope with their own minority stress as members of racial, ethnic, religious, or other minority groups, but also due to people's prejudice against intercultural relationships themselves. A substantial body of research has found that minority stress negatively affects individuals' psychological and physical health. For example, a meta-analysis of 134 studies (Pascoe & Richman, 2009) found that perceived discrimination has a negative impact on individuals' physical health and mental health (e.g., depression, low-self-esteem, traumatic stress symptoms). Minority stress also affects the quality of couple relationships. As one example, Pittman et al. (2023) found that members of Black–White interracial couples reported significantly more discrimination toward their relationships and perceived stress than White couples, as well as greater depression symptoms and poorer self-rated overall health. Foeman and Nance (2002) found that Black members of Black–White interracial couples tended to perceive that their White partners were unaware of the level of discrimination they face in society, and thus they feel they are facing the minority stress alone. Therapists working with intercultural couples need to be aware of and understand the context of chronic discrimination within which their clients live and the effects of minority stress on each partner's psychological well-being as well as their relationship.

A COGNITIVE–BEHAVIORAL VIEW
OF INTERCULTURAL COUPLE FUNCTIONING

A cognitive-behavioral framework is helpful in understanding the functioning and potential challenges experienced by intercultural couples, due to its emphasis on learning processes through which individuals' ways of thinking, experiencing emotions, and behaving with other people are shaped beginning in childhood. Furthermore, a cognitive-behavioral model is helpful for understanding how intercultural couples cope with stressors originating both inside their relationship (e.g., differences between partners' culturally based standards for relations with extended family) and outside the relationship (e.g., others' discrimination against intercultural couples). Ways in which members of a couple appraise the meaning and dangers associated with such stressors, as well as the strategies they use to cope with them individually and as a dyad, involve cognition, emotional responses, and behavioral patterns.

Due to the great diversity of people's cultural socialization experiences, especially when one considers the intersection of each person's multiple cultures, we emphasize culturally shaped cognition, emotion, and behavioral patterns broadly in this chapter rather than those patterns that may be experienced by an individual with a particular cultural background. Therapists must avoid applying generalized assumptions about people who share a culture broadly and who in fact may experience diverse versions of that culture. In the assessment section of this chapter, we propose questions that can help reveal each partner's culturally based cognitions, experiences of emotion, and behavioral patterns, some of which are very common among members of a culture, and some of which are idiosyncratic to the individual.

Culture and Relationship Cognition

Having been socialized within a cultural context leads an individual to carry out various roles and traditions based on cultural beliefs. Those beliefs include assumptions about the normal characteristics of people and their relationships (e.g., types of parenting that lead to healthy child development, how one communicates with significant others via explicit messages or contextual cues) and standards about the characteristics individuals and relationships should have (e.g., gender roles, ways of demonstrating respect for each other). At times, individuals are aware of the cultural beliefs guiding their behavior toward a partner, but at other times they are not necessarily thinking explicitly about those beliefs. For example, an intercultural couple's different styles of parenting their children are likely to have been influenced by their cultural backgrounds, but at any moment they may not be cognizant of the particular beliefs that underlie their attempts to shape their children's behavior, or of each other's beliefs that contribute to their parenting conflict. Similarly, individuals' personal standards for an intimate couple relationship (e.g., appropriate gender roles, communication styles, emotional expression, ways of demonstrating caring and being intimate, relationships with and obligations to extended family and friends, relationship boundaries) that were developed within their cultural background often operate implicitly; they seem natural and normal to each person. In addition, personal standards for how one should relate to the outside world, including as a member of a minority group (e.g., how to deal with discrimination and injustice, how to engage with social institutions such as schools, health care agencies) may seem intuitive and natural to each person based on the ways they were socialized.

When one's partner behaves in ways that are inconsistent with one's cultural beliefs, however, one is led to make some conscious judgments about the partner and their actions. As discussed in Chapter 1, selective attention to partner actions that violate one's cultural beliefs may contribute to a global negative view of the partner and elicit negative emotions. The individual may explicitly evaluate the partner's behavior negatively, in relation to their own personal standard, which they may realize is culturally based, but not necessarily. Furthermore, the individual may make attributions about *why* the partner has behaved that way. For example, if a partner's actions violate one's standards about appropriate gender roles or about constructive ways of communicating when in conflict, it is natural to consider possible causes, such as a lack of caring or respect. Individuals may be more likely to make negative attributions when they are not aware that their partner's actions are based on beliefs that are normative within the partner's culture. Some cultural differences may be relatively minor and nonthreatening (e.g., differences in traditional food preferences), whereas others may involve significant differences in core values and worldviews (e.g., individualistic vs. collectivist orientations, what constitutes respectful behavior; Bustamante et al., 2011). Because it is natural to consider one's own standards as normal, the danger arises that a partner's different ways will be interpreted as inappropriate and abnormal. When members of a couple with different cultural backgrounds fail to normalize, accept, and negotiate diverse standards and personal styles, they are at risk of becoming polarized, increasingly thinking of the gaps between them as unmanageable and non-negotiable.

Culture and Couple Behavioral Interactions

Interpersonal behavior patterns that individuals learn beginning early in life in interactions with family members, various significant others, and media portrayals of relationships include communication styles, actions that convey caring for a partner and commitment to the relationship, and problem-solving and coping styles, among others. Although some behavior interaction differences can be identified across cultures, substantial diversity also exists within each culture, so a detailed assessment of each intercultural couple is needed to identify possible sources of conflict. Furthermore, individuals develop behavioral patterns through interacting with a specific partner over time and through mutual influences on each other. Although members of any couple are likely to have some different relational backgrounds due to the idiosyncratic qualities of their families of origin and other learning contexts, differences between members of intercultural couples tend to be greater. On the one hand, adapting to such differences can be a challenge, as when one member of a couple grew up in a culture that emphasized indirect contextual communication, whereas the other member was raised in a culture that emphasized explicit verbal messages. On the other hand, diversity can be a valuable resource if partners learn ways of interacting from each other's culture that enrich their relationship. For example, perhaps one member of a couple comes from a background that emphasizes collectivist values in which one prioritizes the needs of one's family and community over one's personal needs, whereas the other member grew up in a cultural context that emphasized individual achievement and autonomy. Rather than developing polarized perceptions of the two cultures, the partners may focus on the strengths that each framework offers and may attempt to interact in ways that balance family bonds and self-actualization.

Culture and Emotional Experience

Cultural contexts also shape individuals' emotional experiences, including within their intimate relationships. Some cultural influences involve the effects of cognition on emotions. For example, an individual who was raised with strong collectivistic family-oriented values but has been unable to help an extended family member financially may experience strong guilt or even shame, whereas their partner who was raised with more individualistic values may experience less personal distress about the family member's plight. Furthermore, cultural socialization influences forms of emotional expression that individuals consider acceptable or normal, versus inappropriate and troubling. For example, cultures vary in norms for overt verbal and nonverbal expressions of affection, such as hugging and kissing, especially in public. Similarly, expressing emotional distress (e.g., sorrow, anxiety, anger) verbally or nonverbally may be welcomed, tolerated, or discouraged in various cultures.

Research suggests that "cultural practices and beliefs provide meanings to emotions (e.g., which emotions are good, bad, useful, or familiar), leading to cultural differences in how emotions are interpreted, expressed, and regulated" (Yoo & Miyamoto, 2018, p. 1). A well-known distinction is that people in Western cultures tend to exhibit greater emotional expressivity than those in East Asian cultures (Mauss & Butler, 2010; Rychlowska et al., 2015). Western cultures tend to prioritize each individual's well-being and unique emotional states, and therefore, understanding one's emotions and communicating about them to others are viewed as healthy assertion and protection of one's independent self (Yoo & Miyamoto, 2018). In the collectivistic orientation shared by a variety of East Asian cultures, a person prioritizes family and other social relationships over individual needs. Overt expression of the individual's emotions is not expected, due to the risk of disrupting interpersonal relationships and group harmony. Others would be likely to attribute expression of one's strong positive or negative emotions about events as being due to selfish motivation, in which the individual prioritized their personal needs over those of the group. Furthermore, because of these cultural variations in values attached to expression of emotions, some emotion-regulation strategies that couple therapists might consider introducing may have different effects depending on the cultural background of the client. For example, emotion suppression has been found to exacerbate negative emotional states in individuals from Western cultures (Gross & John, 2003), but it has been reported to reduce negative emotion experience and expression in Asian women (Butler, Lee, & Gross, 2007). As we emphasize throughout this book, examples such as this are offered only as illustrations of group diversity, and it is important not to overgeneralize and stereotype emotional patterns of cultural groups that likely have significant diversity within them.

There also is cultural variation in the intensity of emotions that individuals experience and in the way emotional states are interpreted as desirable or negatively undesirable. For example, cultural differences have been found in what individuals consider ideal emotional states. Tsai, Knutson, and Fung (2006) found that Americans (taking into account cultural diversity within the United States) value high-arousal positive emotions such as excitement more than East Asians do, whereas East Asians prefer low-arousal positive emotions such as calmness. In Western cultures, negative emotions are more likely to be considered undesirable and are linked to negative psychological outcomes (Goetz, Spencer-Rodgers, & Peng, 2008). As a result, a common goal of psychotherapy in Western cultures is to decrease clients' negative affect. By contrast, East Asians (e.g., Koreans, Chinese) view negative emotional states such as sadness and guilt as more desirable and positive emotions as less desirable, when compared to European Americans (e.g., An, Ji, Marks, & Zhang, 2017; Bastian., Kuppens, De Roover, & Diener, 2014; Sims et al., 2015). In East Asian cultures, negative emotions are seen as necessary forms of motivation for personal growth (Miyamoto, Ma, & Petermann, 2014). Given these differences, it is not surprising that East Asians tend to report more negative feelings and less positive emotions in relation to Western individuals (e.g., Ng, 2002). Therapists must therefore be cautious in assuming their Asian clients' emotional expressions reflect lower overall satisfaction with life. East Asians also are less likely than Western individuals to expend effort toward reducing negative emotions and increasing positive ones (Yoo & Miyamoto, 2018). When developing treatment goals, therapists whose cultural backgrounds are different from those of one or both members of a client couple need to be aware of ways in which their assumptions about partners' emotional experiences and expression may be inaccurate. They also need to explore whether members of an intercultural couple experience and evaluate positive and negative emotional states differently and whether or not partners empathize with and validate each other's approaches to emotion.

Religiosity is another cultural factor that has been found to influence individuals' experiences and coping with emotions. For example, Vishkin and colleagues (e.g., Vishkin, Bloom, Schwartz, Solak, & Tamir, 2019; Vishkin, Bloom, & Tamir, 2019) examined whether emotion-regulation strategies mediated the association between religiosity and life satisfaction in samples of American Catholics, Israeli Jews, and Turkish Muslims. They found that the overall association between greater religiosity and life satisfaction is mediated by emotion regulation and that more religious individuals are more likely to use cognitive reappraisal (finding positive meaning in negative life experiences) to regulate their distress and experience satisfaction. In contrast, the coping strategy of expressive suppression (concealing the overt expression of one's emotions) did not mediate the positive link between religiosity and life satisfaction. Such culturally based meaning making associated with religiosity should be part of the assessment and possible intervention with intercultural couples' emotional experiences.

Differences in expression of emotions also may be related to broader cultural differences in low-context versus high-context communication styles (Gudykunst et al., 1996). Low-context communication emphasizes verbal content that directly conveys the speaker's message (e.g., "You are very important to me, and I feel lonely when we are apart for a long time"), whereas high-context communication relies on the listener noticing contextual cues when interpreting the speaker's words (e.g., an individual arrives home late from work, and the partner says, "You must have been very busy today," and offers a cup of tea). Although high-context communication tends to be associated more with relatively collectivistic cultures and low-context communication with relatively individualistic cultures, it is more realistic to avoid dichotomizing communication styles (or cultures) and to examine the degrees to which the members of an intercultural couple exhibit them. Furthermore, members of some couples reach mutual acceptance of cultural differences in their standards for ways of expressing love and caring (e.g., "I would prefer my partner to hug me and verbalize love, but I know I'm loved from the ways my partner takes care of me in daily life"), whereas others experience emotional distress from such differences.

CULTURAL DIFFERENCES: A STRENGTH OR RISK FACTOR?

Even though partners in all couples have to handle differences in various areas, intercultural couples have the potential to face a larger number of them. Coming from dissimilar cultural backgrounds, partners may need to manage discrepancies in multiple aspects of their life together, such as collectivistic versus individualistic beliefs regarding family relationships, roles within the couple, communication styles, language, emotional expression, sexual life and intimacy, food and music preferences, standards regarding parenting roles, religious beliefs and participation, significance attached to major life transitions and events (e.g., weddings, birth of a child, retirement, deaths), management of finances, relationship with the community, and responses to discrimination and oppression. Bustamante et al.'s (2011) study identified dissimilarity in child-rearing practices, time orientation, gender role expectations, and relationships with the extended family as major areas of partners' cultural differences. However, as Killian (2015) points out, these differences can be stressors on a relationship or opportunities.

For several decades, differences in intercultural couples were seen primarily as a source of stress and conflict, and therefore posed a major threat to relationship stability. Findings from studies that took this deficit perspective found support for the principle of homogamy in which partners' similarity is a critical factor for relationship satisfaction and success (e.g., Rosenblatt & Stewart, 2004). This empirical literature on intercultural relationships emphasized challenges from differences in communication styles (e.g., Waldman & Rubalcava, 2005), parenting (e.g., Romano, 2001), and cultural values (Garcia, 2006), as well as religious beliefs and practices, language, and so on. Higher rates and severity of interpartner violence in interracial couples have been attributed to the stressors that such couples face (e.g., Fusco, 2010). Because members of an intercultural relationship commonly differ on several characteristics simultaneously, it is important for clinicians to identify which characteristics are the main sources of stress in order to design an appropriate treatment plan for each couple.

In contrast to that deficit model, based on the work of Celia Falicov (1995), some scholars have adopted a more strength-based conceptualization of intercultural couples that focuses on the benefits such unions can bring to the two individuals, their relationship, and any children they may have. Potential benefits include greater cultural literacy and sensitivity, tolerance of diversity, and enhanced ability to adapt and accommodate (e.g., Crippen, 2011; Troy, Lewis-Smith, & Laurenceau, 2006; Singh, Killian, Bhugun, & Tseng, 2020; Singla, 2015). This strength-based model has emphasized how intercultural relationships can be transformative opportunities for all family members and increase partners' relationship satisfaction. Furthermore, qualitative studies (e.g., Seshadri & Knudson-Martin, 2013) produced evidence that it is actually discrimination and disapproval from other people that affect intercultural relationships negatively rather than the partners' cultural dissimilarities.

Even though some issues that intercultural couples face (e.g., conflict over parenting styles, relations with extended family) are similar to those experienced by couples from the same cultural background (Poulsen, 2003), therapists should be mindful of the unique challenges intercultural couples experience. Sometimes these couples seek assistance explicitly for cultural factors contributing to their relationship distress. However, in some instances, they have not identified how cultural dissimilarities influence their areas of conflict—for example, how culturally based standards regarding ways to express love influence dissatisfaction with their emotional bond. A strength-based approach to therapy can help these couples turn cultural dissimilarities into opportunities for growth, connection, and a positive couple relationship identity.

A STRENGTH-BASED VIEW OF INTERCULTURAL RELATIONSHIPS

In well-functioning intercultural relationships, partners are aware of their cultural differences and view them as a strength of their relationship, or at least a challenge that can be overcome and lead to growth. For many couples, these differences were the source of attraction to each other in the first place, as partners identified characteristics in each other that they admired and enjoyed. Regardless of whether the differences were apparent and attractive from the beginning or whether they surfaced over time, satisfied intercultural couples have managed them successfully, with appreciation for each other's background.

Killian (2015) described three configurations of couples that manage their differences successfully: integrated, coexisting, and singularly assimilated, although an intercultural couple may exhibit a blend of these characteristics. Members of *integrated* couples honor and appreciate the characteristics of each other's culture and intentionally integrate them into their own lives. Partners have been curious and respectful about each other's cultural background, and they have been able to evaluate their own cultural background critically, identifying both strengths and limitations. They value their differences, seeing opportunities to incorporate what they view as the best aspects of each culture into their life together. For example, a couple may follow one partner's collectivistic cultural values in maintaining close relations with extended family while emphasizing the other's individualistic cultural values in supporting each other's career development. They also may combine elements of both partners' cultures in some areas of couple and family life, such as incorporating ethnic foods, clothing, music, and rituals (e.g., styles of celebrating weddings, births) from both cultures. These couples may not have had models of couples who were successful in integrating each other's culture, so they may have experimented, through a process of trial and error. Integrated couples commonly need to develop strategies for managing pressure from their family, friends, and community to retain aspects of their culture of origin (Killian, 2015).

In contrast to the integrated couple, in the *coexisting* form each member identifies completely with their own heritage culture's values, traditions, communication style, and beliefs. This type of relationship functions well as long as the partners feel mutual respect for, interest in, and understanding of each other's culture. They consider their cultural differences as positive and enriching for their relationship, even though they have not adopted aspects of each other's culture. Each partner shares with the family some elements of their personal culture, such as food preferences, music, and holiday traditions. It is common to see this structure in interfaith couples, in which each partner may decide to maintain their spiritual belief system, rituals, and/or organizational affiliations. Each member may support the other's religious background by participating in celebrations of holidays significant to the other person. These couples likely need to negotiate some areas of their life together, particularly in relation to children (e.g., the role that religion plays in their upbringing, what values they are taught; Killian, 2015).

In a *singularly assimilated* couple, one partner is more assimilated to the other's culture. This process functions well when the assimilated partner has freely agreed to this accommodation, without any direct or subtle coercion based on a power differential between partners (e.g., due to financial dependence). Similar to the coexisting structure, this configuration often is found among couples whose partners have different religious backgrounds and one partner decides to convert to the other's faith. It also is found among couples in which one partner is an immigrant and the other is a member of the dominant local culture. Regardless of the reasons for one person assimilating to the other's culture, the relationship tends to be functional when the assimilated partner has freely agreed to this conversion, has not been coerced through a power differential between the partners (e.g., financial dependence, access to citizenship/legal immigration status), and has positive feelings about it (Killian, 2015).

This description of three intercultural relationship configurations likely underestimates the complexities of the decisions members of a couple face. Partners may be searching for ways to integrate multiple cultural differences simultaneously (e.g., dissimilar religious parenting traditions, cultural communication styles, and expectations regarding gender roles).

Furthermore, intercultural couples often include one or both members who are immigrants and are faced with the stresses associated with acculturation to the dominant culture as well as coping with the cultural differences between the partners. Therapists who work with intercultural couples need to be sensitive to such multiple struggles that their clients are experiencing and should help partners explore those stresses in a mutually supportive way.

Over time, the intercultural couple configurations described by Killian (2015) may shift for a couple due to changing circumstances. For example, the birth of a child may motivate a couple who had a predominantly coexisting structure (essentially leading parallel cultural lives) toward more of an integrated configuration, based on their desire to avoid creating pressure on their child to choose between the parents' beliefs, traditions, and the like.

In all three configurations described by Killian (2015), but particularly the integrated and coexisting structures, partners tend to consider their cultural differences positive aspects of their relationship. In successful relationships, they are open to addressing differences without imposing their own worldview on the other person. Partners in these unions have been found to value learning about other cultures, and they believe that being in an intercultural relationship provides opportunities for personal growth (Bustamante et al., 2011). However, partners also seek cultural similarities with each other, particularly regarding core values such as appropriate ways of treating other people (Bustamante et al., 2011). They tend to have strong communication skills for conveying their preferences and values to each other, as well as problem-solving skills for negotiation and compromise. They also are purposeful about defining a "we" relational identity as they present themselves to their families and communities. They may need to be intentional in building a network of friends, family members, and community organizations (e.g., schools, religious organizations) who support the multicultural identity they developed.

In successful intercultural couples, the partners support each other in dealing with discrimination from the outside world, whether it is directed toward the relationship or just one member. When one partner is a member of a dominant group (e.g., racial majority) and the other is part of a minority group, the member of the dominant group understands the minority stress that their partner experiences, ranging from microaggressions to violence, and the couple has developed strong dyadic coping skills.

SOURCES OF STRUGGLE IN INTERCULTURAL COUPLES

Intercultural couples that seek therapy typically experience two types of challenges: (1) managing cultural differences between partners in particular areas of their relationship and/or (2) responding effectively to discrimination toward individual partners and/or the intercultural nature of their relationship, as well as lack of support from their families, friends and their community. The following sections describe those challenges and the types of conflict and stress involved.

Difficulties in Managing Cultural Differences between Partners

Intercultural couples face the challenge of finding ways to manage the different cultural beliefs and traditions they bring to their relationship. As we described earlier, some couples resolve these differences by intentionally or implicitly negotiating them and either creating an integrated combination of their backgrounds or deciding to allow their different beliefs and traditions to coexist (e.g., each partner is responsible for organizing the couple's celebration of particular holidays).

However, even members of these culturally sensitive and inclusive couples may sometimes exhibit biases toward each other's beliefs and traditions that can create tension. For example, if one partner's background emphasizes high-context communication and the other's background favors low-context communication, they may find themselves critical of the other's communication style. Couple therapists can foster a safe setting in which partners can verbalize their cultural biases without fear that their discomfort with unfamiliar cultural ways will be judged harshly by either their partner or the therapist.

Couple therapists may encounter couples who have successfully navigated some cultural differences but need assistance with other areas or with addressing new areas of cultural difference that have arisen at various points of developmental change (e.g., becoming parents, having elderly parents move in with them). It is common for intercultural, interracial, and interfaith couples to feel challenged by differences in their beliefs and traditions in some areas even after many years of being together (Biever, Bobele, & North, 1998; Bustamante et al., 2011; Daneshpour, 2003; Negy & Snyder, 2000; Seshadri & Knudson-Martin, 2013; Tubbs & Rosenblatt, 2003).

Furthermore, some intercultural couples with an *unresolved* relationship structure may have sought therapy due to significant conflict in multiple areas of their relationship, as they have not been able to integrate their cultural characteristics or live harmoniously through acceptance of coexistence (Seshadri & Knudson-Martin, 2013). These couples may experience a sense of hopelessness and helplessness about their potential to find a way to live together happily, associated with negative emotions (anxiety, depression, anger). It is important that their couple therapist encourage the couple to reframe their situation as a significant challenge rather than a crisis.

Some topics a therapist can explore with a couple to explore their experiences with navigating cultural differences are as follows:

• To what degree have members experienced difficulties in navigating cultural differences between them (with examples of these difficulties)?

• If one or both members of the couple are immigrants, to what degree have they had to deal with stresses related to immigration (e.g., adjusting to living in an unfamiliar host culture, limited language fluency with the host culture, missing family and friends they left behind, discrimination by individuals and agencies such as health care services and social service agencies)? If one partner is from the host culture and the other is not, how have they have managed those differences?

• To what degree is a member of an intercultural couple dealing simultaneously with individual stress from belonging to one or more minority groups (based on race, country of origin, gender identity, sexual orientation, or religion) and stress from being part of an intercultural relationship?

• What individual and dyadic coping styles have the partners used to manage their cultural differences, and how effective have they been?

Responding Effectively to Discrimination

Intercultural couples commonly must cope with discrimination toward the individual partners and/or the intercultural nature of their relationship itself. The sources of discrimination may include school personnel, health care professionals, employers, staff in stores, and strangers on the street. A partner who assimilated to the other's values and practices may have to deal with discrimination from members of their own culture(s), who may view the person as disloyal (Daneshpour, 2003).

Lack of support from various sources within their community, as well as from people close to them, including their families and friends, is an ongoing source of stress (Seshadri & Knudson-Martin, 2013; Tubbs & Rosenblatt, 2003). Consequently, assessment of each couple should include an inquiry about specific discrimination experiences, as well as ways they have coped with discrimination and the sources of support they have had available.

THERAPIST SOCIOCULTURAL ATTUNEMENT AND HUMILITY

In order to work with intercultural couples, therapists need to be aware of their own level of prejudice and bias against interethnic, interracial, and/or interfaith couples, as well as about each of the cultural identities that partners present in therapy. They should examine their social location and understand forms of privilege they may have taken for granted based on being members of dominant groups, which members of their intercultural couple clients may not share. It is important to understand the sociocultural and political contexts affecting the lives of the minority clients with whom they work. As we noted in Chapter 2, therapist awareness and critical examination of one's potential bias against other cultural groups are necessary first steps toward developing cultural sensitivity and reducing implicit bias. Therapists can keep a journal of reflections about their ongoing reactions to cultural material within and outside therapy sessions, potential effects on their clinical work, and strategies to maximize multipartiality. For example, a therapist may realize a tendency to consider one partner's perspective more than the other's due to identifying more with the former's culture.

Therapists should educate themselves about the cultures of the clients they work with and the socioeconomic-political contexts in which such cultures have developed and exist (Knudson-Martin, McDowell, & Bermudez, 2020). They should also educate themselves about potential differences and issues between the cultures of members of intercultural couples. Furthermore, therapists treating intercultural couples need to convey the importance of partners being sensitive and supportive of each other's cultural beliefs and traditions. At times, this exploration may uncover instances in which societal oppressor–oppressed dynamics have been replicated within a couple's relationship in terms of power inequities between partners.

SCREENING AND ASSESSMENT

This section focuses on ways therapists can tailor assessment methods used in a cognitive-behavioral approach to couple therapy with intercultural couples. We begin with screening for the cultural backgrounds of the partners and ways in which they have taken their cultural differences into account. In addition, we screen for forms of discrimination the clients have experienced based on their individual cultural identities and being members of an intercultural relationship. We then describe methods to assess partners' cognitions, emotional responses, and behavioral patterns associated with their cultural backgrounds and differences.

Screening for Intercultural Couple Status

A demographic questionnaire or interview protocol (see Figure 3.2 in Chapter 3) will show whether the couple is intercultural, interfaith, interracial, or the like. It is important to include questions that identify how each member of the couple defines themself in terms of gender, sexual orientation, race, ethnicity/country of origin, religion, or any other reference group. In addition, when one or both may be from an immigrant family, the questionnaire should ask about whether individuals are first- or second-generation immigrants. When working with first-generation immigrants, the therapist should learn about the individual's country of birth and immigration status, the reasons for immigrating, the length of time they have lived in their current country of residence, whether other family members immigrated with them or they were reunited in the host country, the existing family network in the host country, whether there currently are family members living with them, the degree of connection they have with local communities from their countries, their communication with family members in their country of origin, and whether they provide financial support to those members. The therapist must be sensitive to the possibility that some undocumented immigrants will be concerned about divulging information about their status.

Similarly, when working with interfaith couples, therapists should not only inquire about their religious affiliation and/or spiritual beliefs, but also about the importance of beliefs and practices in the individual's life. Therapists also should ask about the frequency and type of religious practices that partners have adopted individually and/or together and how they have managed differences in their religious beliefs and practices. Finally, it is important to inquire about any instances in which religious differences have been a source of stress and conflict between an individual and their partner's family and religious community.

Screening for the Role of Cultural Characteristics

When assessment of presenting problems includes a screening questionnaire such as the Relationship Issues Survey (RIS; Epstein & Werlinich, 1999) and an interview with the couple (Chapter 3), one should inquire if and how conflicts are related to partners' individual cultural characteristics and couple differences. Couple conflict on any of the RIS topics (e.g., communication, intimacy, conflict management, recreation, emotional expression, parenting, relationship with extended family, division of household labor, gender roles, spirituality, values) may be influenced by cultural differences.

Sometimes couples spontaneously reveal whether their struggles are related to their being an intercultural relationship. If they do not, the therapist can ask in an open-ended manner about factors affecting a particular issue they have identified in their relationship. For example, an individual may describe couple conflict based on their own mother's frequent criticism of their partner's parenting style. When the therapist asks about the source of the criticism, the individual may reveal that it is based on cultural differences between the beliefs that the mother and partner hold regarding listening empathically to children's feelings. The therapist also may learn that the individual feels caught in the middle of the conflict between mother and partner, which leads to couple conflict.

Even when partners may believe that a presenting problem is unrelated to cultural differences, their ways of viewing the problem and addressing it may be shaped by their cultural backgrounds. For example, an intercultural couple may come to therapy because one member engaged in infidelity, and they share a view that the individual's violation of their explicit vow of monogamy is a problem, but they may not see their cultural differences as playing a role in their conflict. However, further exploration by the therapist may reveal that the betrayed partner's religious beliefs include strong condemnation of infidelity as a shameful major sin, in contrast to the perpetrator's more secular belief that it is an insensitive way of treating one's partner that requires restitution and rebuilding of trust. Thus, deeper mutual understanding is needed between partners of cultural factors contributing to their conflict. Those differences in core beliefs can therefore be taken into account during therapy.

The therapist should avoid inquiring about possible challenges and conflicts the couple has experienced in a manner that suggests the therapist assumes that intercultural couples inevitably have problems. One way to introduce an inquiry would be to state the following:

"Couples with different cultural backgrounds [add specific forms of culture for this couple, such as religion, ethnicity, etc.] commonly find that the diversity in their backgrounds enriches their life together. Sometimes those differences can be challenging. I would like to hear about what living with your differences has been like for you as a couple."

Assessment of Discrimination Experiences and Coping

Some intercultural couples directly describe discrimination experiences they have had stemming from their being a minority individual and/or a member of an intercultural couple. They also may describe a lack of support for their cultural characteristics from their extended families, friends, neighbors, religious organizations, schools, workplaces, and community health and social service agencies. However, other couples may not describe issues regarding discrimination and limited support as a major presenting concern, or may not even mention them. Therapists can interview intercultural couples about possible discrimination experiences, as well as about who they can turn to for support, and groups/places from whom they do not perceive support. It also is important to inquire about the degree to which members of a couple believe it is appropriate to seek or accept help from others when they experience such problems (Holzapfel, Randall, Tao, & Iida, 2018). Therapists may begin this screening by administering the widely used 9-item Everyday Discrimination Scale (EDS; Forman, Williams, & Jackson, 1997) that has demonstrated strong reliability and construct validity in diverse cultural groups (e.g., Clark, Coleman, & Novak, 2004; Gonzales et al., 2016). Respondents indicate the extent to which they experience discrimination based on their specific identity (e.g., culture, religion, race). The EDS items have stems such as "Are you treated with less courtesy than other people?"; "Do people act as if they are better than you?"; "Are you called names or insulted?"; and "Do people act as if you are dishonest?" with an identifier added that tailors it to the respondent's specific cultural group, such as "based on being African American" or "because of your race." Clinicians and researchers have used various response scales that assess the frequency with which individuals perceive each type of discrimination, such as from 1 = never to 4 = often, or from 1 = never to 6 = almost every day. The EDS is easy to administer and provides a view of each individual's experiences. It is available online on Dr. David Williams's website (*scholar.harvard.edu/davidrwilliams/node/32397*).

Therapists also can ask members of a couple to complete the EDS in relation to discrimination that they perceive regarding the intercultural nature of their relationship; this scale identifies whether that type of discrimination is another stressor that the partners experience. Based on the partners' responses to open-ended interview questions or their responses to the EDS, the therapist then can expand the assessment of discrimination with topics described in Figure 11.1.

ASSESSMENT OF PARTNERS' CULTURAL IDENTITIES AND MANAGEMENT OF COUPLE DIFFERENCES

A number of assessment methods can be helpful in understanding partners' cultural identities, which often include multiple aspects (e.g., country of origin, ethnicity, race, religious affiliation, gender, sexual orientation), and the way the couple manages their differences. Our experience is that couples feel most comfortable with the personal therapeutic relationship conveyed during interviews, in which the therapist raises topics and asks follow-up questions tailored to partners' responses about their identities and experiences.

The following are topics regarding discrimination experiences that can be explored in both joint couple assessment interviews and individual partner interviews:

- Ask each member of the couple about details regarding discrimination incidents they have experienced, large or small, based on either their own personal minority status (race, ethnicity, cultural background, religion, gender, sexual orientation, etc.) or their being part of an intercultural couple. Inquire about who behaved in a discriminatory way toward them; and in what setting (e.g., neighbors, staff in stores, school personnel, personnel in social service agencies, health care professionals, people at their job). What did the individuals say and do?

- Inquire about the effects that such a discrimination experience tends to have on the individual (e.g., emotional responses such as sadness, anxiety, anger, shame; cognitive responses such as self-criticism, desire for retribution; behavioral responses such as withdrawal from situations such as work, school, stores, or arguing with perpetrators). Also ask about effects on the couple relationship, such as spillover effects in which anger about discrimination leads to arguing with one's partner about neutral topics.

- Inquire about ways they cope individually and as a couple with discrimination experiences (see Chapter 3 regarding assessment of coping styles). For example, the therapist can ask, "You have said that people in stores sometimes act as if you are dishonest. When that has happened, how do you think and feel about it? How do you cope with an experience like that as an individual?" Follow up as needed with questions to identify any emotion-focused and problem-focused strategies they tend to use.

- Ask about dyadic coping strategies the couple use, in which they collaborate to deal with discrimination stresses (communicating to each other about an experience; empathic listening; joint problem solving). Inquire about the effectiveness of the couple's coping strategies in terms of individual and relationship well-being.

- Evaluate how effective the communication is between the partners regarding stressful discrimination experiences. In addition to any difficulties a couple may face even if they share the same primary language, probe for any challenges a couple experiences if they have different language backgrounds (e.g., misunderstandings due to inability to understand the nuances of words and different cultural communications styles). If the therapist has the same primary language as one member but not the other, the potential imbalance in communication this can create in therapy sessions should be discussed, and any ways of facilitating clear, balanced communication (e.g., adding a co-therapist who is fluent in the other language) should be considered.

- Identify how much support each member of the couple experienced individually and as part of an intercultural relationship from family, friends, neighbors (including members of their own country of origin), religious organizations, social service agencies, health care providers, employers, and school personnel. To what degree have they sought support from those sources, have their efforts been rebuffed, and if so, how did they respond? Explore both members' views on the appropriateness of asking for or receiving help, from either one's partner or outsiders.

FIGURE 11.1. Interview topics regarding discrimination experiences.

Individual Interview with Each Partner

The standard initial individual assessment interview with each partner (Figure 3.2) is an opportunity to gather information regarding cultural background and the current role of culture in the person's life. The personal history questions include an inquiry about where the individual was born and how the person was socialized. For immigrants, it also includes questions about the circumstances associated with moving from one country to another, as well as ways in which the individual still has contact with their heritage culture. The therapist also asks about the cultural make-up of the individual's friendships and prior romantic relationships.

Couple Interview

The initial couple assessment interview (Figure 3.1 in Chapter 3) also includes an inquiry into cultural factors, including those that may have contributed to the partners' attraction to each other and decision to form a committed relationship. Cultural factors in various decisions the couple made regarding their life together (e.g., whether to have a religious marriage ceremony, what if any cultural organizations they are affiliated with, what cultural beliefs and traditions they will teach their children) are explored. The therapist asks whether any cultural differences between them have been challenging, and if so, how they managed any conflicts.

Relationship History

In addition to gathering information regarding the overall history of the couple's relationship, which is covered in detail in Chapter 3, the therapist asks about how differences in the partners' cultural backgrounds have influenced their life together. How have they shared their backgrounds and cultural identities with each other? How much did they express interest in learning about each other's background? What aspects of the other's culture did they find attractive and as potential sources of making them a good match, and what characteristics, if any, led them to be concerned about compatibility?

The therapist can then ask the couple how they initially approached their cultural differences. To what extent did they explicitly discuss the differences and how they believed they could harness them as strengths for their relationship? What memories do they have of early experiences of confronting a cultural difference between them (e.g., realizing that they have different styles of communication when they are upset about someone's behavior)? What strategies did they adopt for coping with differences (e.g., listening to each other's preferences and negotiating ways of integrating them; avoiding in-depth discussions), and how well did each strategy work? To what extent did they integrate their cultural traditions versus each maintaining their own or one partner primarily adopting the other's? What advantages and strengths have they experienced from sharing aspects of each partner's culture?

With regard to the couple's relationships with other people, the therapist can inquire when and how they told their families of origin, extended family members, and friends about their relationship. If they hid it, did they differ in their desires to do so? To what degree did their families and others immediately embrace the intercultural nature of their relationship? To what extent were there any negative responses from significant others, and how did others' reactions affect the couple's relationship? Has either member of the couple felt torn between pressure to adopt or support their partner's culture and pressure to adhere to cultural traditions of their own family of origin? If so, how have such conflicts affected those relationships?

The relationship history interview then tracks cultural influences on the development of the couple's relationship. The therapist asks about processes such as increased involvement with each other and potentially a decision for marriage or a similar formal commitment, decisions regarding having children, levels of involvement with each person's family of origin, and choices of what cultural traditions to adopt jointly. The therapist also asks the couple to give examples of times when they felt they best handled their cultural differences (and what strategies seemed to work best) and times when they struggled more. In addition, what challenges have they faced individually or jointly from the world around them, such as discrimination? What strategies did they use to cope, and how effective were those strategies? What kinds of support have they experienced for their intercultural relationship from various sources, such as families, friends, neighbors, community organizations, schools, and religious organizations?

Another generic line of inquiry that can be revealing regarding each partner's subjective experience of the quality of their intercultural relationship can begin with a question such as "All in all, how have your experiences in your couple relationship over the time you have been together compared with the dreams you had for your life together?" The therapist can follow up with questions about goals that each person currently has for the future of their relationship, including changes they would prefer.

Cultural Genogram

We propose using a cultural genogram to identify the racial, ethnic/cultural, and religious composition of each partner's family of origin, as well as the partners' and couple's current cultural identifications. It is conducted via an interview with the couple, but it has a clear structure as the therapist asks about particular details regarding the members of each partner's family of origin across at least three generations. The version that we recommend is an integration of the cultural genogram described by Hardy and Laszloffy (1995) for therapists in training and the spiritual ecogram developed by Hodge (2005) for understanding family-of-origin influences on the spiritual aspects of an individual's, couple's, or family's life. The therapist constructs a diagram of a family tree with information on the generations of each partner's family (McGoldrick et al., 2020). It indicates the name, age, gender identity, and relationships (e.g., parent–child) of all family members, including those who have passed away. It also indicates closeness/distance and conflict in relationships, as well as information about each family member's race, ethnicity/country of origin, and religious/spiritual orientation, indicated with colors and symbols. The genogram also includes immigration information, specifically when individuals left their countries of birth and the countries they migrated to.

Following Hardy and Laszloffy's (1995) suggestions, the therapist can also ask about issues of pride and shame in the cultures of families of origin. For example, one partner may describe the pride they share with their family of origin's culture regarding their strong work ethic. Another partner may take pride in the parenting practices of their culture and may express a strong desire to continue those traditions when raising their own children. In contrast to pride, a partner may express shame about a cultural tradition in their family of origin, such as rigid gender roles.

The pictorial representation of both partners' families of origin and their couple relationship in a single diagram allows the therapist and couple to observe:

- members' races, countries of origin, religious/spiritual orientations, and migration patterns (diversity of demographic characteristics).
- the quality of family relationships (e.g., distant, close, cutoff) among family members who were/are racial, ethnic, and/or religious minorities.
- the presence of interracial/interethnic/interfaith relationships in either partner's family of origin and the family's acceptance or rejection of such unions.
- the couple's current cultural identity in the context of the racial, ethnic, and spiritual identity of each partner's family of origin.

It may require more than one session to complete a cultural genogram, and sometimes partners need to gather information from their families of origin between sessions. Cultural genograms can also be used during treatment. For example, if a couple has sought therapy to resolve differences in parenting beliefs and strategies, the therapist may return them to examining their cultural genogram and differences in parenting practices in relation to family cultural backgrounds. This may help partners understand each other's perspective and appreciate the strengths that each person's cultural identity can bring to parenting.

Assessment of Cognition in Intercultural Couple Relationships

The methods used to assess intercultural partners' cognitions regarding their relationship are consistent with the generic cognitive-behavioral procedures detailed in Chapter 3. The types of cognition involved in intercultural relationships include cultural *assumptions* about individual and relationship functioning (e.g., about normal ways of experiencing emotions; parenting strategies that shape positive child behavior), cultural *standards* about appropriate behavior (e.g., regarding gender roles, ways of demonstrating care for one's partner), *attributions* about the causes of behavior one observes in one's partner (e.g., attributing a partner's desire to pursue independent achievements to selfishness), *expectancies* (e.g., predicting that the partner's interpretation of one's messages will be influenced significantly by contextual cues, not only one's words), and *selective perception* (e.g., paying close attention to the ways in which a partner responds to preferences expressed by one's parents). The following are procedures for identifying the types of cognition that are contributing to an intercultural couple's conflict and dissatisfaction with their relationship.

Assessment of Culturally Based Assumptions Contributing to Couple Conflict and Distress

As described in Chapter 1, couples may experience conflict and unhappiness when they view events in life through different lenses based on different assumptions about natural and normal characteristics of individuals and relationships. Cultural beliefs can contribute to partners' different assumptions. For example, partners may differ in the degree to which they hold cultural beliefs that disagreements between them are signs of dysfunction and are dangerous to their bond. If members of a couple do not mention concerns about the meaning and consequences of conflict and the expression of anger between them, the therapist questions them about the meanings they attach to the conflict and anger directly, for example:

"You mentioned that the two of you sometimes argue about your different child-rearing approaches. To what extent does each of you believe that disagreements like that are natural in any couple with children, or are you concerned that it is harmful to your relationship?"

Similarly, the therapist can initiate a discussion with an intercultural couple regarding their assumptions about the pros and cons of raising children in a multicultural family, as well as their assumptions about adopting a bicultural life themselves. Is it healthy and an opportunity for personal growth? Is it likely to confuse children and lead to psychological problems? Is it disloyal to one's culture? We find that interviews in which the therapist uses follow-up probes to uncover partners' culturally based assumptions provide rich details about their beliefs.

Assessment of Culturally Based Standards Contributing to Couple Conflict and Distress

Because conflict and distress often result from differences between partners' standards for the characteristics they believe individuals and couple relationships should have, therapists need to listen for partners' spontaneous expressions of those beliefs during the individual and couple assessment interviews. When clients fail to voice standards on their own, the therapist can probe for them. For example, a couple may present with conflict about the involvement of extended family members in decisions regarding the treatment of their children's health conditions. One member of the couple may invite grandparents on both sides of the family to attend the children's medical appointments and help administer treatments at home. Because that partner's family is from a culture that holds older family members in high esteem and tends to involve them in decision making about family life, the partner may adhere to a standard that grandparents should be involved in the medical care of grandchildren. Therefore, the individual expresses gratitude to their own parents for their assistance and reacts negatively when the other partner's parents avoid such involvement, making an attribution that they do not care about their grandchildren's health. Furthermore, the other partner, who comes from a more individualist culture that places grandparents in a secondary role to parents, may hold a standard that the in-laws should avoid "butting in" regarding treatment of grandchildren. This partner may attribute the involvement of the other partner's parents to a lack of confidence in them as parents.

Another common example of a difference in partners' standards that often is not initially stated explicitly but becomes evident when a therapist interviews the couple and observes their interactions involves their beliefs about appropriate ways of communicating ideas and emotions. For example, when the cultural background of one member emphasizes high-context communication and the other's background focuses on low-context communication, conflict may surface when the therapist asks them a question such as "How do the two of you express your love and affection for each other." After a pause during which one individual has little eye contact with the therapist or partner, the other individual may state, "He does a lot of nice things for me, so I know he cares, but he almost never tells me that he loves me." When the therapist asks the other partner about his perceptions of how the two of them express love and caring, he may respond, "I grew up in a family in which people didn't express their feelings through a lot of words or hugs and kisses, but everyone took good care of each other. I like it when she tells me she loves me, but it also feels awkward."

Similarly, when a therapist asks a couple how they manage situations in which they disagree, they may respond that they are able to either find a compromise or "agree to disagree," as long as their discussion occurs in private. However, with other people present, one partner may be comfortable expressing disagreement, whereas the other finds it embarrassing and experiences a loss of face. The therapist's exploration of each partner's standards regarding public displays of conflict may reveal that the former individual was raised in a culture that encourages independent thinking and considers overt disagreement (as long as it is polite) to be a reflection of self-esteem. The other individual may describe being raised in a more collectivist culture that emphasizes interpersonal harmony and saving face. The couple's contrasting reactions to public displays of disagreement are consistent with their cultural backgrounds, and the therapist can engage them in collaborating on devising ways to bridge their difference.

In addition to challenges that naturally occur when two partners have different cultural assumptions and standards regarding ways of conducting their life together, stress is likely to increase if one or both partners hold standards that are nonaffirming of their intercultural relationship. One or both members may hold a belief that was not acknowledged and expressed early in their relationship that their own cultural traditions are more appropriate and correct than the other's. Cognitions that lead partners to the conclusion that their cultural disagreements will be solved by choosing one culture over another can invalidate one person's worldview and cultural identity, interfering with a mutually satisfying relationship. For example, an interfaith couple may have difficulty deciding what religious traditions to emphasize when looking ahead to the birth of their first child. One or both partners may have an expectancy that attempts to integrate their religious beliefs will confuse the child, so they believe they need to choose one of their religions for raising their child. This thinking may tap into one or both partners' underlying beliefs that their personal religion is superior to that of the other, triggering conflictual discussions in which they perceive they are being invalidated by each other. The therapist's inquiry into each partner's cognitions in this area can contribute to a treatment plan that includes strategies for resolving their cultural beliefs in ways that are validating to both individuals.

Although clinical interviews are the primary method for identifying partners' culturally based standards for their relationship, therapists also can use a limited number of questionnaires that tap relationship standards. As described in Chapter 3, Epstein, Chen, and Beyder-Kamjou (2005) administered the Inventory of General Relationship Standards (IGRS; Epstein et al., 1990), which assesses standards that individuals hold regarding boundaries around the couple and between partners, partners' degrees of instrumental and expressive investment in their relationship, distribution of power between partners, and attainment of perfection in their relationship to samples of couples in the United States and mainland China. Overall, the standards were associated with level of relationship satisfaction in both cultures, with some differences between cultures in adherence to particular standards (e.g., U.S. couples more strongly endorsed maintaining clear boundaries around their relationship than Chinese couples did; Chinese couples more strongly believed that partners should share values than U.S. couples did). Measures such as the IGRS, the Inventory of Specific Relationship Standards (Baucom et al., 1996), and the Relationship Belief Inventory (RBI; Eidelson & Epstein, 1982) emphasize beliefs from a Western cultural perspective. Consequently, Hiew, Halford, van de Vijver, and Liu (2015) designed the Chinese–Western Intercultural Couple Standards Scale (CWICSS) to cover both Western relationship standards (regarding demonstrations of love, demonstrations of caring, intimacy expression, and intimacy responsiveness) and Chinese relationship standards (regarding relations with extended family, relational harmony, face, and gender roles) that are also prevalent in other collectivist cultures. Therapists can administer those scales as screening instruments, or they can become familiar with their contents to guide interviews regarding couples' standards.

Assessment of Culturally Based Attributions and Expectancies

As described throughout this book, individuals commonly make attributions involving inferences about the causes of others' actions, which can vary in their accuracy, and those attributions tend to be shaped by the individual's assumptions and standards. For example, in a scenario described earlier, a member of a couple attributes in-laws' reluctance to be involved with the medical care of grandchildren to a lack of caring on their part, based on the individual's cultural standard that grandparents' involvement is important. In turn, their partner whose cultural standard emphasizes a clear hierarchy in which grandparents have limited authority in childrearing attributes their in-laws' suggestions about medical care of grandchildren to a lack of respect for the couple's abilities. Sometimes the members of a couple explicitly voice their attributions (e.g., "My mother-in-law has a lot to say about how we should raise our children, because she thinks she's an expert and we are clueless!"). In other cases, the therapist can probe for attributions with questions such as "When your mother-in-law makes suggestions about childrearing, why do you think she does that?" After each partner's attributions about the causes of each other's actions, as well as those of significant others, are uncovered, the therapist can explore with the couple underlying assumptions and standards that influenced those inferences. With intercultural couples, this may lead to an exploration of partners' different cultural beliefs and traditions, and how an individual's behavior that is consistent with or violates them naturally leads one to make inferences about why the person would behave that way.

Individuals' culturally based assumptions and standards also can lead them to have *expectancies* about the likelihood of particular outcomes in their couple and family relationships, which they may reveal spontaneously during interviews or which may surface in response to therapist questions. For example, an individual whose background emphasizes collectivist cultural values for maintaining harmony and avoiding loss of face in relationships may have an expectancy that expressing frustration with their partner's attempts to maintain strong boundaries with extended family will insult the partner, and therefore may "sit on" those feelings and build resentment toward the partner over time. Although the person's partner who may have more individualistic cultural values might express irritation that the person "is secretive with me about feelings," the person's avoidance actually is convenient for the partner, who does not need to negotiate boundary issues. The therapist's role is to ask questions of each individual regarding their expectancies of what will occur between them if they take particular actions that are consistent or inconsistent with their own personal standards and those of their partner. Uncovering members' different culturally based cognitions during the assessment process is likely to increase their insight into each other's experiences in their relationship, but it also is likely to highlight some conflicts in their preferences that will need attention in the treatment plan.

Assessment of Culturally Based Selective Perception

As we described in Chapter 1, individuals' values, standards, and other core beliefs tend to influence what they notice or overlook in daily life. Consequently, the members of an intercultural couple may be attuned to different aspects of their behavioral interactions. A common example that we already noted is the difference between high-context and low-context communication, which differ in the degree to which a speaker relies on a listener interpreting verbal content-based contextual cues such as nonverbal behavior (e.g., saying "It really doesn't matter to me" while avoiding eye contact) or aspects of the situation (e.g., the presence of a third person who the listener is expected to understand is inhibiting the speaker from expressing true feelings). If one member's cultural background makes them highly attuned to contextual cues as a speaker or listener, whereas the other's background emphasizes unambiguous direct messages so that a listener can rely on verbal content, their perceptions of their communication may be quite different. The therapist's role is to ask questions about verbal content, nonverbal communication, and situational cues that each member of a couple considers important to notice. The therapist should portray such cultural differences as normal factors that seem to influence their communication and instances of conflict, and they should collaborate with the couple in attending to those differences in the treatment plan.

Assessment of Couple Behavioral Interaction Patterns

Therapists can assess culturally based couple behavioral interactions by observing their spontaneous interactions or asking partners to discuss with each other the conflict topics they have identified either on the Relationship Issues Survey (RIS) or during the initial couple interview. The therapist should attempt to obtain a sample of how the couple discusses issues within their relationship as well as external factors such as discrimination and lack of support from extended family. When the couple and therapist discuss their intercultural background during the relationship history interview, the therapist can ask the partners to talk together about their perceptions of the strengths of their intercultural life as well as how they have coped together with any challenges.

In addition to observing patterns in the couple's communication as they talk with each other in session, the therapist can ask them about any patterns they have noticed in daily life. A goal is to identify any aspects of the couple's interaction pattern (e.g., a demand–withdraw pattern; mutual escalation of criticism) that contributes to difficulties in their ability to manage cultural differences and stressors such as discrimination experiences. The therapist's awareness of the partners' different culturally based styles of communication will prevent the therapist from viewing some partners' behaviors as problematic or deviant when they are actually normative and acceptable in the person's culture. For example, an individual's hesitation or silence in response to the therapist's questions may reflect that person's cultural norms rather than difficulty with self-expression. Furthermore, some cultures may have gender-based communication differences, perhaps expecting women and men to behave differently (e.g., who talks first, who can talk about certain matters in public), whereas other cultures may not. It is important for a therapist to avoid taking for granted that any communication pattern is universal across cultures. The therapist should also be curious in asking members of each couple whether the behavior they have been exhibiting in sessions is common in their cultural background.

The therapist needs to determine what aspects of the couple's dyadic communication may be contributing to conflict and preventing them from coping effectively with challenges from inside or outside their relationship. The therapist should use the assessment methods described in Chapter 3 to focus on how each member of the couple copes with stressors and how the couple copes dyadically. To what extent are the partners' individual coping styles compatible? For example, some religions focus more than others on accepting circumstance as "fate" rather than attempting to take actions to change one's negative circumstances. Thus, partners who differ in this regard may have different coping responses.

The therapist should also assess the couple's joint behavioral problem-solving skills (Chapter 3) while considering each partner's cultural style that may contribute to differences. To tailor the assessment to an intercultural couple, the therapist could ask them to identify an unresolved challenge they are facing together that involves a cultural factor (such as a difference in religious affiliation) and to discuss possible solutions to it as the therapist observes them. The therapist observes the degrees to which the partners are able to reach consensus on the nature of the problem, brainstorm possible solutions without criticizing each other's ideas, and discuss the advantages and disadvantages of each possible solution. Based on those observations, the therapist probes for each partner's cultural beliefs and traditions that contribute to difficulties with any stage in joint problem solving.

Assessment of Emotion in Intercultural Relationships

Therapists need to be aware of cultural differences in how emotional states are interpreted, which emotional states are considered desirable, and how (and to what extent) emotions are expressed and regulated. The culturally sensitive assessment can begin with the therapist asking each partner during the initial couple interview and their individual interview:

- what emotions they experience regarding their presenting problems
- the meaning they attach to each type of emotion (e.g., whether they consider it a useful or dysfunctional experience)
- strategies they use to regulate (reduce or enhance) such emotions
- the effects they perceive their emotions are having on the quality of their own and their relationship's well-being

The therapist also needs to inquire about whether the partners' cultural differences in the experience and regulation of particular emotions (such as anger or joy) may be contributing to conflict and a sense of disconnection. For example, in addressing disagreements regarding preferred degrees of involvement with each other's family of origin, one member of a couple may be more comfortable expressing anger as a means of negotiating, whereas the other may consider overt expression of anger to be disrespectful and harmful to family relations. When partners have different primary languages, therapists should be on the lookout for potential misunderstandings during discussions of their differences regarding emotional experience.

Another important factor to keep in mind when assessing partners' emotional responses from a cultural perspective is that research has indicated that bilingual individuals prefer to express both positive and negative emotions in their first language rather than their secondary language. In addition, they exhibit stronger emotionality when communicating in their first language (Dylman & Bjärtå, 2019). Consequently, if members of an intercultural couple tend to speak with each other primarily in what is the first language of one member but the second language of the other member, the person communicating in their second language may be at a disadvantage in conveying their emotional experiences to their partner. In addition, if their therapist's first or only language matches that of one member of a couple but not the other member, the accuracy of the therapist's assessment of the two individuals' emotional experiences may be biased toward the partner with the same primary language. In order to track partners' emotional responses during sessions, probing for instances in which one person's actions elicit the other's emotions, the therapist must be attuned to nonverbal as well as verbal cues of both partners' emotional expression. The therapist's personal cultural experience with communication of emotions is likely to influence the ability to "decode" those cues. Although a therapist may have no practical solution to this lack of balance, it still is important to be aware of potential difficulties in understanding a partner's emotions and discuss with the couple strategies for the therapist to probe more with that individual for descriptions of subjective feelings during sessions.

GOAL SETTING AND SOCIALIZATION TO TREATMENT

Some intercultural couples seek therapy for problems they have been experiencing as a result of their intercultural status. In those cases, the therapist can collaborate with the partners in identifying goals such as managing differences between them or coping together with discrimination from outside sources. However, therapists must be cautious and avoid attributing all of a couple's difficulties to cultural factors, as some may be due to other sources such as partners' personal characteristics (e.g., rigidity, vulnerability to chronic depression) and other life stresses (e.g., job stress). Thus, the therapist conducts a comprehensive standard assessment covered in Chapter 3 to identify sources of distress and goals for change.

Some other intercultural couples may seek therapy for difficulties they have not conceptualized as being related to their cultural backgrounds. The therapist therefore needs to conduct an assessment that differentiates problems influenced by culture from those that are relatively independent of culture. In contrast to the couples who have clearly identified cultural factors as affecting them individually and/or as a couple, the therapist's introduction of possible cultural influences may catch these clients by surprise. They may initially be put off by the therapist's attribution of problems to their intercultural identity, perhaps even experiencing it as a microaggression, especially if the couple has been motivated to cope with their cultural differences by minimizing them. Therefore, it is important to present any suggestions regarding culture in the context of specific information that the couple provided. For example, a couple may report that their arguments about preferences regarding taking parenting advice from their parents seems to be associated with different types of relations and communication with their respective parents throughout their lives. The therapist can describe to the couple a broad definition of culture as beliefs and traditions that are a part of daily life associated with one's country of origin, religion, race, etc.—ways of being that are familiar and generally comfortable. One therefore tends to take them for granted until one interacts with people with different backgrounds and experiences. It also can be helpful to describe to clients how one works with diverse couples, with the goal of learning a lot about each person's life experiences, including those experiences influenced by culture. Alternatively, the therapist can discuss their cognitions, emotions, and behaviors with the couple without even mentioning the term *culture*, focusing on the ways the partners tend to manage any differences they experience. As with the couples who enter therapy identifying cultural factors in their presenting problems, the therapist can propose that the three of them survey a variety of factors from their backgrounds that might be relevant in their relationship, including some that involve culture and others that do not. With all couples, a primary goal is to help them work as a team to identify and change sources of conflict and distress, all in the interest of achieving a more satisfying relationship.

PLANNING TREATMENT

Intercultural couples have been thought to be at risk for failure due to deficiencies based on partners' differences. Some research has found that they had higher rates of dissolution than partners from similar cultural backgrounds. Consequently, interventions focused on remediating deficits have implicitly, or even explicitly, conveyed a potentially pessimistic message to clients regarding the quality and future of their relationships. In order to counteract potentially iatrogenic interventions, treatment plans for intercultural couples must take a strength-based approach in which cultural differences are seen as beneficial for their life together, even if the differences pose challenges such as partners needing sustained efforts to understand each other's perspectives. Therapists should draw partners' attention to the drawbacks associated with attempting to impose their own culture on the other person, rather than each person making their own decision about aspects of the other's culture they would like to adopt. The therapist can help partners understand each other's cultural cognitions, emotional responses, and behavioral patterns through discussions of each other's background. Those discussions can be facilitated by using cultural genograms and coaching the couple in expressive and empathic listening skills.

Overall, the treatment plan we suggest draws on generic CBCT interventions but applies them to modifying behavioral patterns, cognitions, and emotional responses involved in partners' conflict and distress about their different cultural characteristics. Therefore, in the following sections we describe interventions focused on cognition, behavior, and emotional responses. CBCT methods described in Chapter 4 are used, with examples focused on reducing the sources of conflict and unhappiness in intercultural relationships.

Interventions to Modify Cognitions

In a CBCT approach, behavior change is facilitated by intervening simultaneously or beforehand with clients' cognitions and emotional responses that influence individuals' behavior. Here we describe a number of interventions for cognition that are especially relevant when working with intercultural couples.

Modifying Negative Attributions Regarding Cultural Differences

Members of an intercultural couple are more likely to be upset if they attach negative meanings to their differences or to how the other person responds to those differences. As we describe in Chapter 4, couple therapists commonly guide individuals in examining the validity of such negative inferences and in considering more positive ways of interpreting particular experiences, thereby broadening the clients' negative views. This process emphasizes taking an objective view of causes of events, based on logic and evidence. If the analysis suggests that a person's negative attribution about a partner's behavior is accurate (e.g., that a partner indeed intended to ignore the individual's desire to attend a religious event), the focus is on addressing how the couple is managing their differences (e.g., regarding the role that religion plays in their lives). However, if logic and evidence suggest that the partner's upsetting behavior (e.g., their failure to plan to attend the religious event together) was due to a more benign cause (e.g., the partner was distracted by stress at their job), the focus may shift to the couple making more use of expressive and listening skills in order to "stay on the same page" regarding their priorities and plans.

As another example, an individual whose background emphasizes high-context communication may feel hurt when their partner's parents fail to call them to extend good wishes during a major holiday that is part of the individual's culture. When the individual's partner comments that the individual seems to be in a bad mood, and the individual replies, "I guess they forgot about the holiday because they don't celebrate it," the partner responds, "Yeah, that's probably it." The individual then becomes more upset that the partner did not "get" the underlying message that the parents seemed insensitive to important cultural aspects of the individual's life. Thus, the individual made a negative attribution that the partner's response was due to a lack of caring. At this point, the therapist can begin by asking the individual questions to uncover the negative attribution, which otherwise would have remained unstated, so the couple can consider it together. The therapist also intervenes quickly if the partner responds defensively (e.g., "That's not true! I care about your cultural traditions a lot. I think you are being unfair to my parents"). The therapist should propose that the couple avoid debating this issue and think about communication differences between them and their families of origin that can be challenging. The therapist then initiates a discussion of the advantages of both a high-context and a low-context approach to communication, asking the partners to think about ways in which having the choice between the two approaches in various situations may actually be a strength of their intercultural relationship. The discussion can then expand to consider how each person can help their partner and in-laws learn about the goals of the communication style that is unfamiliar to them.

In a CBCT approach, the therapist may take the lead in suggesting more positive meanings for events or may coach the clients in generating alternative attributions themselves. An advantage of the latter approach is that it more directly develops the clients' skills for examining and modifying their cognitions when the clinician is not present.

Modifying Assumptions and Standards That Contribute to Conflict

A therapist can identify the assumptions and standards intercultural partners hold about relationships that produce conflict, dissatisfaction, and distance, and can guide the couple in substituting more appropriate or realistic beliefs. Examples are an assumption that cultural differences between partners inevitably result in conflict and the demise of the relationship, and a standard that one's cultural beliefs and traditions are superior to those of one's partner.

As detailed in Chapter 4, interventions for rigid beliefs include listing and evaluating the advantages and disadvantages of living according to a belief; making a logical analysis of the degree to which the assumption or standard makes sense; examining past and present evidence that the belief is valid; and designing and implementing behavioral experiments to test their validity. Regarding polarized standards that one set of cultural beliefs and practices is better than the other, the therapist can guide the couple in examining the characteristics of each other's culture that contributed to their being attracted to each other, and in thinking of ways to integrate valuable aspects of their cultures to lead a rich life together. Any discussion of why following a particular aspect of one culture over the other may be advantageous should explicitly address the matter of advantages and disadvantages, without conveying the notion that one culture is better than another.

For example, a couple may report that they often misunderstand each other's preferences when trying to reach a decision about aspects of daily life, such as money management, child rearing, and relationships with extended family members. The therapist may identify that the cultural background of one member of the couple emphasizes low-context communication (meanings are conveyed primarily by explicit content of messages), whereas the other member's background emphasizes high-context communication (meanings are conveyed to a significant degree by contextual cues such as nonverbal behavior and what is left unsaid). It may become clear that the couple's misunderstandings are influenced by their different communication styles. Although each member may view their accustomed communication style as superior, the therapist can guide them in examining the advantages of each style and considering adoption of a hybrid way of reaching joint decisions. The discussion could take into account the advantages of low-context communication (e.g., partners' ability to discuss how closely their preferences align) and high-context communication (e.g., partners seek a desirable goal of avoiding loss of face when expressing disagreement with each other).

Strengthening Assumptions and Standards That Validate the Relationship

As we have noted, intercultural relationships have potential to provide richness to a couple's life together, but couples who have sought therapy may overlook those strengths as their attention has been drawn to their problems. A therapist can guide partners in identifying opportunities for personal growth and the pleasurable aspects of cultural diversity (e.g., warm holiday rituals, delicious cultural foods, and music—shared traditions that contribute to strong bonds with extended family and friends). The couple can generate a list of these positive characteristics and refer to them frequently as affirmations of the value of their relationship.

Enhancing the Couple's Perception of Themselves as a Dyad

Increasing an intercultural couple's bond can be facilitated by guiding them in shifting their perception of themselves primarily as two different individuals who need to coexist to a "we" dyad that is greater than the sum of its parts (Seshadri & Knudson-Martin, 2013). Their "we-ness" consists of shared goals, values, and enjoyable life experiences, including a feeling of connection from enjoying aspects of each person's heritage culture(s) together.

In addition, couples may selectively notice negative experiences in their intercultural relationship, such as microaggressions and incidents of major discrimination from other people. The therapist can help them counteract this negative view by reviewing the ways they have developed to cope as a team with discrimination, experiences of inequities and social injustice, and other life stresses. Their selective perception of negatives can be reduced by having them keep track of instances of positive dyadic coping, as evidence of the strength of their relationship.

Interventions to Modify Behavioral Patterns Regarding Culture

Teaching and Practicing Communication Skills

Given the importance of members of an intercultural couple understanding and respecting each other's cultural beliefs and traditions, teaching the couple communication skills for expressing thoughts and emotions and for listening empathically to the other person is a high priority. As we noted previously (Chapter 4), communication skills training concepts and procedures are largely based on Western ways of communicating, which emphasize open and direct sharing of thoughts and emotions. However, some clients enter therapy adhering to those Western beliefs and traditions, whereas others do not (e.g., those whose cultural beliefs emphasize relational harmony and saving face). Consequently, the therapist should provide psychoeducation regarding the concepts and traditions underlying CBCT communication skills. Then, the therapist can explore with the couple the extent to which that approach may differ from communication patterns in their cultural backgrounds, emphasize that it is crucial that they both be comfortable as they communicate with each other, and brainstorm ways of modifying expresser and listener guidelines to foster that comfort. For example, an individual who has been frustrated and irritated by a partner's sharing couple information with an extended family member might preface a description of those reactions with comments such as the following:

> "I know that you care about our relationship as much as I do, and you have been concerned about our financial situation as I have. I also know that you have always been close with your sister, and you respect her knowledge about many things. I think she is really smart, so it seems natural to you to discuss our finances with her. However, in my cultural background members of a couple keep most of their relationship issues just between the two of them, and it feels like a violation of our privacy when you tell your sister so much."

Thus, rather than using communication guidelines in a one-size-fits-all manner with all couples, the therapist explores styles that are familiar and comfortable with each person and explores with them how their cultural traditions can be taken into account without sacrificing the overall goal of increasing their understanding of each other's thoughts and emotions.

As is typical in communication skills training, the therapist has the couple begin with benign topics that are unlikely to elicit conflict for the couple or flashbacks to stressful experiences that they had individually or as a couple, based on their cultural identities. A key purpose is to increase mutual understanding of ways in which each person's cultural background shaped the way the person experiences the world and their couple and family relationships. For example, an individual related details of personal discrimination experiences at her job in which a supervisor treated her as incompetent in front of co-workers, and it was clear that the individual's racial minority identity played a role in the supervisor's bias. The client also described how the experience and her decision to seek another job were very stressful and harmful to her self-esteem. When the individual's partner used empathic listening skills well in the couple therapy session, conveying the partner's deep understanding and emotional support for the distress the individual had experienced, it helped strengthen their couple bond. It also motivated the individual's partner to reveal her own painful discrimination experiences, which the couple also had never discussed so openly before.

Strengthening the Couple's Dyadic Coping Processes

As a couple has engaged in expresser and empathic listener skills consistent with their cultural traditions regarding expression of thoughts and emotions, the therapist can guide them in discussing their stressful experiences with discrimination from outside the relationship, acculturation challenges, and lack of support from others. This process can help partners understand the specific forms of discrimination and other stressors that each person has experienced and the effects they have had on their individual well-being (e.g., anxiety symptoms, insomnia, lowered self-esteem). Each person can learn about cues they can look for that their partner currently is experiencing stress and could benefit from help, including subtle high-context communication cues common in some cultures. Experiencing mutual empathy and knowing that one has a close partner in facing those difficult experiences can help build a strong couple bond.

Through discussions of cultural traditions and preferences, the therapist can guide the couple in communicating about the types of support each person prefers from their partner. The therapist should be attuned to instances when an individual finds it difficult to understand how their partner from a different culture prefers a type of support that is atypical within the individual's own culture. In cases in which only one partner deals with discrimination, due to belonging to a minority group, additional discussion may be needed for the other person to understand and validate the discrimination experiences fully, especially regarding common microaggressions. Partners may also need to understand the history of oppression and/or persecution of certain religious, racial, and sexual and gender minority groups. This understanding will help them fully grasp the intergenerational impact of structural racism and cumulative trauma on their partner's emotional well-being (e.g., Hankerson et al., 2022).

The therapist can encourage the couple to consider forms of dyadic coping that address discrimination experienced primarily by one member or jointly as a couple. The couple can brainstorm ways of coping they can engage in together that will benefit them. For example, if a member of one person's extended family behaved in unwelcoming ways toward the person's partner during a holiday gathering, the couple might place a joint FaceTime call to that individual. They could explain that they consider family very important, but both felt put off by the individual's specific actions and want to have more positive experiences in the future. This form of dyadic coping not only supports the partner who experienced the discrimination; it also validates the individual who chose that person as a life partner.

Strengthening the Couple's Problem-Solving Skills

Dyadic coping can be enhanced by strengthening the couple's problem-solving skills, using the steps detailed in Chapter 4. During the process of introducing and practicing standard problem-solving steps, the therapist should check on possible cultural differences that may influence the couple's ability to collaborate. For example, partners from different backgrounds may define the characteristics of a problem differently. Thus, one member who grew up in an interfaith family may identify a neighbor's comments such as "Don't your kids get confused when you have Christmas decorations on your house and also light candles for Hannukah?" as a distressing microaggression, whereas the other member whose family all had the same religious affiliation and predominantly secular traditions may view the comments as innocent curiosity. The therapist needs to guide the couple in understanding each other's views of whether or not the neighbor's behavior constituted distressing discrimination, and if one member finds it stressful, how the other can collaborate in dyadic coping through joint problem solving. In the brainstorming solutions stage of problem solving, the therapist may need to guide the couple in resolving their different opinions regarding actions they believe would be appropriate responses to the neighbor's comments. For example, one partner from a cultural background that values expression of one's needs may favor having a direct discussion with the neighbor about the negative impact of the comments. The other partner whose background more strongly supports maintenance of harmony and avoidance of loss of face may prefer casually introducing the neighbor to their interfaith family life and how they and their children enjoy their respect for diversity the next time they and the neighbor are catching up with each other during a sidewalk chat. This gives the therapist an opportunity to coach the couple in collaborating to find solutions that support both members' cultural beliefs.

Helping the Couple Define Themselves as a Couple with Others

The therapist can introduce the idea that the way partners behave toward their extended families, friends, and larger community conveys important information to others regarding their identity as a couple (Seshadri & Knudson-Martin, 2013). The therapist can use specific terms when talking with others (e.g., "We are looking forward to celebrating the Lunar New Year together with our children"). It also may involve demonstrations of solidarity such as giving feedback to one's family member who made a discriminatory comment to one's partner. Participating in the cultural and religious activities of each other's families and social networks also can increase mutual support and strengthen the couple bond.

Enhancing the Couple's Behavioral Management of Their Cultural Differences

The therapist can guide the partners in identifying actions that have worked relatively well for them in managing their cultural differences, even if some improvement would be desirable. For example, a couple may have felt more mutual understanding and acceptance of each other's cultural backgrounds by teaching each other about their fond memories of traditions practiced in their families, visiting each other's family to participate in holiday celebrations or a traditional cultural meal, and discussing similarities between partners' core cultural values, strategies that many couples identify as effective (Bustamante et al., 2011).

If a couple is in an early stage of developing their relationship, they may need assistance with integrating their cultural backgrounds or building a "third' culture that is somewhat different from each person's traditions but sufficiently consistent with both their cultures that both people feel comfortable (Bustamante et al., 2011). They may find that certain key moments/events (e.g., their wedding, the birth of a child) provide opportunities for being creative and designing unique rituals of their own that contain elements that reflect both individuals' values. For example, creating roles for each person's family of origin in their wedding ceremony can reflect the couple's joint valuing of family bonds and the joining of their families. This can send strong messages to family, friends, and the community about the couple's cultural identity.

In tandem with strategies for finding common ground and some integration of their cultures, the therapist also can guide the couple in finding room for some individuality and separateness (Seshadri & Knudson-Martin, 2013). Each person should feel free to devote some time and energy to their heritage culture, without needing to be concerned that their partner will feel rejected. For example, a couple in which one member is Catholic and the other is Jewish may share holiday celebrations for both religions, but they may have decided to attend occasional church and synagogue services, respectively, primarily on their own.

Building Acceptance and Support from Significant Others

Understandably, members of an intercultural couple desire significant others to support their relationship from the beginning and demonstrate acceptance of their partner. However, that process may be gradual, which can be stressful for both the couple and the other people in their lives

(Seshadri & Knudson-Martin, 2013). The therapist can provide guidance to the couple in ways of giving each person's family members and others time and space to demonstrate acceptance of the other partner and their relationship, especially initially. This may require a shift toward more accepting cognitions, such as softening one's standard that "If my family members care about me, they'll be happy to learn that I found someone I love," combined with regulating one's anger when significant others communicate discomfort with the relationship and regulation of one's urges to behave negatively toward them. The therapist can coach the couple in devising dyadic coping strategies for accepting their anger toward others who respond negatively to their relationship. However, the partners need to regulate the intensity of their anger so that it does not take a toll on their personal well-being or result in them venting it toward the other people in counterproductive ways. For example, the therapist can coach the couple in problem solving regarding ways to talk with relatives and friends about their commitment to each other as a couple, and their desire for support from them. They also can devise plans for limiting exposure to people who exhibit limited acceptance of their relationship, with the option of increasing contact if and when the other people demonstrate a more positive response to them. In the meantime, the couple can engage in dyadic coping to reduce each other's emotional distress. They can do this by listening to each other's upset feelings empathically, discussing how they will face discrimination as a team and present their "we-ness" to the world, and focusing on pleasant joint activities to soothe their emotions.

Helping the Couple Build a Network of Support

The therapist can guide the couple in problem solving that focuses on developing a network of support for their intercultural relationship and minority members of the couple, from individuals and organizations (Seshadri & Knudson-Martin, 2013). This can include seeking out similar couples in the community, selectively spending time with friends and relatives who are supportive, and accessing community agencies that provide support services to intercultural couples and individuals who are experiencing minority, acculturation, and other forms of stress. For those whose cultural backgrounds discourage seeking help from outsiders rather than managing one's life stressors by oneself, cognitive interventions can introduce the concept of help-seeking as a continuum in which a strong, self-sufficient person is skilled at recruiting and using resources to solve problems.

Interventions to Modify Emotional Responses Regarding Culture

Psychoeducation Regarding Cultural Factors Affecting Emotion

The therapist can guide partners through psychoeducation and discussions of each other's cultural experiences to improve their understanding of each other's experiences of emotions. Discussions, with examples from the couple's daily life, can focus on how each person experiences and expresses various positive and negative emotions, and what cues and information each person can use to interpret the other's emotions. Partners may learn that certain styles of expressing emotions should be interpreted differently for each of them. For example, a Spanish-speaking Latine individual may use intense language to emphasize their emotional states, even when they are describing a relatively mild emotion to their partner, because such highly expressive descriptions of emotions are common in Spanish language usage. A partner from a culture that uses less emotionally expressive language may need to understand the difference in their Spanish-speaking partner's verbal expression of emotions. In a qualitative study of Latines with non-Latine partners, Seshadri and Kundson-Martin (2013) reported an example of a Latina female describing how "Latinos do things with passion and fire!" (p. 51), and that she needed to adjust her cultural style of emotional responses to conflict somewhat so that her husband would listen to her and not shut down as a way of coping with her intensity. In turn, her husband needed to learn that her external displays of emotion often were considerably more intense than her internal feelings. In contrast to issues arising from cultural traditions emphasizing intense emotional expression, individuals from cultures that emphasize relationship harmony may consistently inhibit external displays of their emotions, especially negative ones. This may result in their partners from more expressive cultural backgrounds underestimating the intensity of their feelings.

A therapist can help a couple adjust to their cultural difference in emotion expression through psychoeducation, discussions about experiences in their upbringing, and their current beliefs about appropriate communication of one's feelings to others. The therapist can engage them in setting a goal of improving their understanding of each other's experiences within their relationship. This understanding can be facilitated by both members making a commitment to tell each other explicitly about the type and intensity of their emotional states (e.g., using a 1 to 10 intensity scale) and to express interest in hearing about the other's feelings. The therapist can then coach the couple in practicing these adjustments in communication about their emotions.

Psychoeducation about Negative Emotions and Somatic Symptoms

When working with couples that include individuals whose cultural background involves expression of negative emotion through somatic symptoms (e.g., body aches, fatigue), a therapist can include information about that process in psychoeducation and discussions of partners' cultural experiences, to increase their understanding of each other's emotions. This information may be surprising to individuals whose backgrounds have not included exposure to somatization of emotions. A goal is increasing both partners' awareness of the possibility that symptoms of physical discomfort might sometimes reflect feelings that should be explored.

Cultural Differences in Comfort Expressing Affection and Love

Partners' different cultural backgrounds may result in differences in their comfort and verbal skill in expressing affection and love. An individual who is accustomed to explicit expression of affection may be frustrated at a partner's relative lack of such expression, even questioning whether the partner truly loves them. In turn, an individual who is unaccustomed to and uncomfortable with explicit expression of affection may feel even more uncomfortable when their partner criticizes and pressures them to be more expressive, and may feel embarrassed when the partner "gushes romantically at me." A therapist can address these differences by exploring each person's experiences regarding emotion in their family of origin during a joint couple session, with reference to a cultural genogram that was constructed during assessment of the couple. The therapist can emphasize that after interacting with significant others for many years in accordance with an emotional expression style, it would likely feel awkward and seem somewhat inappropriate to try to behave differently now with one's partner. This does not mean that either person's familiar style is right or wrong—just different. The goal is not to abandon the emotional expression style from one's background, but to increase one's understanding and acceptance of each other's style of processing and expressing emotions. The therapist notes that if members of a couple wish to try to adjust their styles of expressing emotions somewhat to make them more compatible, that is fine, but it is less important than becoming more comfortable with their differences and not interpreting them negatively.

Achieving increased acceptance may involve examining one's cognitions about the aspects of a partner's expressive style that one finds distressing. For example, an individual who strongly believes that a partner who rarely expresses affection could not possibly truly love them may need to hear more about their partner's strong emotional attachment and caring for them, along with the partner's disclosure of their lifelong pattern of keeping their feelings to themself. In addition, the individual may need guidance from the therapist in examining other evidence that their partner cares deeply. Further psychoeducation regarding different but normal styles that all express caring for a partner also may help shift an individual's beliefs.

TROUBLESHOOTING PROBLEMS IN COUPLE THERAPY WITH INTERCULTURAL COUPLES

It is natural and common for therapists to encounter some challenges when working with intercultural couples. The following are some issues that may arise and some suggestions of ways a therapist can respond to them.

Implicit Bias and an Unbalanced Therapeutic Alliance

A therapist may unconsciously promote one partner's cultural beliefs and practices over the other's because of stronger identification or understanding of the former's culture or because of bias and prejudice toward the latter's culture. This may not be clear to the therapist until cues arise, such as the couple arguing increasingly about their differences, or the partner whose culture the therapist has favored citing the therapist's comments to bolster their debates with the other partner. This imbalance in the therapeutic alliance must be addressed quickly if the therapy is to be helpful to the couple.

• Using interventions that we described in Chapter 2 for maintaining multipartiality and establishing a strong alliance with a couple, the therapist emphasizes the goal of making both partners feel understood and respected, describes the cues the therapist noticed that the partners were experiencing some lack of balance, encourages them to share any discomfort with therapist's behavior, and returns to a discussion of how the couple can share their cultural differences in a mutually enjoyable and enriching way.

• If a therapist becomes aware of personal bias in favor of one partner's culture, the therapist should plan some forms of "self of therapist" work to counteract the bias. The therapist may become aware of a need for further education about a culture that is unfamiliar and perhaps uncomfortable, and to seek professional peer supervision regarding self of therapist issues, including one's personal cultural history. Therapists should cultivate cultural humility (self-exploration and critique in the service of understanding and honoring other people's cultural beliefs, values, and traditions). They should beware of viewing their own ways of communicating and expressing emotions as normative across cultures. It may be easier for therapists to identify their own standards as culture-specific than to moderate their own ethnocentric ways of communicating, coping with problems, and conveying their emotions. Similarly, when treating interracial couples as well as racial minority couples, White therapists should be aware of their White privilege and should understand their clients' experiences of racial oppression and the implicit power dynamics in the therapeutic relationship. Their non-White clients may not initiate expression of their past experiences and their feelings about race, but therapists need to be attuned to the likelihood that such experiences and feelings exist.

Client Psychological Characteristics Impeding Cultural Integration

Sometimes conflict between partners regarding their cultural differences may reflect the psychological characteristics of one or both individuals that need attention. For example, an individual may exhibit difficulty integrating a partner's cultural characteristics into their own life that may reflect a broader inflexible cognitive style that permeates their negative responses to other life experiences. Sometimes differences in partners' levels of cognitive flexibility become evident during the therapist's initial couple assessment interview and interviews with the individuals, but sometimes it only becomes obvious when the therapist delves into the development of their intercultural relationship. Such rigidity may be linked to an underlying psychopathological condition (e.g., a personality disorder) or issues with family of origin such as members engaging in long-term "cutoffs" of others with whom they had conflicts. Those patterns may become clear during construction of the couple's joint cultural genogram.

- The therapist can begin by reviewing with the couple characteristics that attracted them to each other and drawing their attention to cultural factors that contributed to them being drawn to each other. The therapist can emphasize that every person is a mixture of characteristics, and any characteristic can have both advantages and disadvantages. Using knowledge from the assessment, the therapist can point to an example of "double-edged" characteristics. For example, Marcus emphasized that he was drawn to Sylvia's strong valuing of family, based on her collectivist cultural background, and he felt confident that they would form a close-knit nuclear family. However, as time went on, he was upset that she spent so much time interacting with her family of origin. He grew up in a culture in which independence and personal strength were valued, and Sylvia's level of involvement with her family led him to perceive her as unable to develop what he believed was healthy independence. The couple's therapist pointed out that Marcus seemed to enjoy Sylvia's collectivist values for their own nuclear family but was uncomfortable when she expressed them with her family of origin. Sylvia replied that all family relationships are very important to her, and Marcus seems to apply a double standard. The therapist noted that Marcus indeed valued Sylvia's family orientation when he viewed her as an excellent life partner, but the degree to which that characteristic led her to remain connected to her family of origin was uncomfortable for him, and Marcus agreed. The therapist guided the couple in discussing how a person's emotional ties to family members probably can exist on a continuum, and as an intercultural couple an important goal may be to explore ways in which they can balance connection and independence in their relations with their extended families. In this case, both partners were flexible enough to accept a need to negotiate ways to balance cultural values regarding connection versus independence. The therapist guided them in problem solving about shifts in relations with extended family that could satisfy both of them.

• If one or both partners exhibit persistent rigidity in response to the therapist encouraging a focus on positive aspects of cultural differences, as well as on cultural characteristics existing on continua that allow a balance between acceptance and negotiations for behavioral changes, a referral for individual therapy may be needed. Chapter 2 suggests procedures for minimizing negative reactions when introducing referrals.

• In this chapter, we have noted that within any group of people who share a culture, there likely is considerable variation in individuals' personal "versions" of cultural beliefs and traditions. Consequently, therapists might miss identifying an individual's mental health condition that needs treatment due to attributing the person's cognitive, emotional, and behavioral responses to normal cultural differences between partners. For example, a therapist might attribute a member's very strong venting of negative emotions to that person's cultural background, which encourages emotional expression, although in this case the individual's personal trauma history may play a significant role in an emotion-regulation problem. When a therapist suspects individual psychological issues, an additional interview with the individual to assess personal functioning is appropriate.

Microaggressions

Traditional literature on discrimination and minority stress has tended to emphasize severe forms of discrimination and trauma, but increased attention has been paid to microaggressions that can be more subtle but very harmful (Sue et al., 2007). In working with intercultural couples, therapists need to be on the lookout for microaggressions, not only from outsiders, but also by one partner toward the other.

• Upon noticing such interactions, the therapist needs to explore what the individual did or said and what the impact was on the recipient. If the recipient of what appears to the therapist to be a microaggression does not comment on it, the therapist can pause the interaction and explore the recipient's experience. The recipient may report an unpleasant response, but not necessarily, leaving the therapist with a judgment call about whether the incident should be explored. The process can be framed as a way the couple can strengthen their relationship by increasing understanding of each other's experiences, including the microaggressions they and others may enact without realizing it.

• Furthermore, therapists need to be attuned to gaps in their own cultural sensitivity that lead them to engage in microaggressions with clients. Explicitly taking responsibility for one's blind spots and the need for cultural sensitivity and validation of clients' identities can be a valuable model for one's clients.

• Discussions of microaggressions may lead a couple to describe instances committed by significant others such as in-laws. Because receiving feedback about perceived microaggressions is likely to be threatening and uncomfortable for perpetrators, the therapist can coach the couple in brainstorming ways of communicating with those individuals to produce positive change and to minimize the potential for escalating conflict.

• Some intercultural couples make good-faith efforts to build bridges with their families of origin, friends, and others who have engaged in discrimination toward them. Their efforts gradually pay off, with more supportive and validating responses from the other people. However, in some other cases, the couple receives unrelenting negativity, which creates persistent stress for them as individuals and as a couple. When a therapist becomes aware that a couple has given particular people time and opportunity to connect with them in positive ways but the others continue to be sources of stress, it is important to discuss with them individual and dyadic coping strategies to maintain their own well-being. This may include reducing or even eliminating further exposure to discrimination from those individuals, an option that can be painful and frightening when it involves significant others. An option that avoids creating complete "cutoffs" involves changing one's standards regarding the nature of particular relationships (i.e., continuing to interact to some degree but lowering one's expectations for the degree to which a relationship will meet one's needs). In such cases, it is important that the couple's choice of a coping pattern not take a toll on their individual and couple well-being. For example, the couple may decide to attend some family holiday celebrations but may limit conversations with particular members, but they also may rehearse concise, firm, yet non-aggressive responses they can use if someone makes a derogatory remark about a partner's culture.

KEY POINTS

• Most therapists will work with intercultural couples, and they need to be skilled with ways of connecting with them and helping them manage challenges from outside their relationship (discrimination) and within the relationship (e.g., managing differences).

• Attunement is crucial as therapists work with couples in which one or both partners have cultural beliefs and traditions different from those of the clinician.

• Therapists need to assess and factor into the treatment plan how culture shapes partners' cognitions regarding self and close relationships, ways of experiencing and expressing emotions, and patterns of behaving toward significant others.

• Treatment plans need to emphasize partners' understanding of each other's cultural framework and accepting their differences.

• Assessment and treatment planning should examine the positive and negative consequences of forming an integrated, coexisting, or singularly assimilated intercultural relationship.

• Therapists should focus on the ways cultural differences can be sources of challenges and stress, yet also be enriching sources of strength and personal growth.

CHAPTER 12

Conclusions and Future Directions

Our central goal in this book has been to describe a cognitive-behavioral approach to the assessment and treatment of distressed couples that can be applied across a variety of presenting problems the clinician is likely to encounter in general practice. It is beyond the scope of this volume to survey the range of problems that tend to be covered in couple therapy handbooks (e.g., Lebow & Snyder, 2023) that apply numerous theoretical orientations, but the topics we have addressed are among the most common presenting problems identified in research surveys (Doss, Simpson, & Christensen, 2004; Miller, Yorgason, Sandberg, & White, 2003; Whisman, Dixon, & Johnson, 1997). Although our chapters focus on a smaller number of presenting problems, the concepts and methods they describe are readily applicable to other relationship issues. For example, CBCT can be used with couples experiencing challenges associated with loss and grief, chronic illnesses and disabilities, infertility, discernment issues regarding the future of the relationship, caretaking for family members, and alcohol and substance use. Although we addressed co-parenting in nuclear families in Chapter 9, there are special parenting issues experienced by couples who are forming a stepfamily, such as coping with members' unresolved grief from losses of prior relationships through death or divorce and defining the roles nonbiological stepfamily relatives will have with each other (Papernow, 2023).

All of these presenting problems, as well as those we detailed in this book, require that the therapist acquire a solid background in the particular challenges and stressors that members of a couple likely will experience. For example, when working with infertility, therapists need to educate themselves about numerous issues, including intrusive infertility treatments that can be quite stressful, current sociopolitical factors that may influence access to treatments, ways of collaborating with a fertility counselor, available resources for the couple (e.g., support groups, reading materials), and gender differences in partners' coping with infertility stressors. The introduction to each chapter of this book includes a review of literature regarding the characteristics and incidence of the problem, risk factors for it, traditional treatments, and the relevance of our CBCT approach for treating it. We have cited literature that clinicians can consult to increase their knowledge of the topic. There are additional clinical resources (available on the book's web page at *www.guilford.com/epstein-materials*) regarding couple therapy presenting problems and their treatment besides those we covered in this book's chapters.

Furthermore, we have attempted to broaden the scope of couple therapy practice through our emphasis on sociocultural relevance, significant contextual factors such as stressors experienced by minoritized couples, and couple interventions for problems in individual functioning that apply a transdiagnostic model of psychopathology. All of the chapters focused on specific presenting problems apply the concepts and methods of a CBCT model, with an emphasis on developing and implementing treatment goals that target risk factors and that are tailored to each couple's characteristics. We have described a process through which a therapist strives to understand the inner worlds of the two partners as well as problematic interaction patterns, forms a strong therapeutic alliance with the couple, and collaborates with the clients to work toward their personal goals for their relationship.

Our clinical work also is informed by a common factors model that identifies client characteristics, therapist factors, and the therapist client relationship that are crucial influences on the effectiveness of couple therapy (Sprenkle, Davis, & Lebow, 2009). Development of strong therapeutic relationships depends on the therapist's ability to inquire about and empathize with each partner's subjective experiences of events within the couple relationship as well as broader contextual factors, both present and in the past. It is crucial to create an atmosphere in which each person can explore and share with their partner cognitions and emotions beyond those they initially describe, such as deep sadness and insecurity from a partner's past betrayal. Partners can develop hope for facing the challenges of life together when the therapist guides them in shifting initial complaints toward descriptions of longings for connection, safety, equity, and respect. In contrast to a stereotyped view of CBCT as rote teaching of various skills for modifying negative behavior, cognition, and emotional responses, the clinical practice of CBCT is a nuanced human connection between the therapist and couple, tapping past and current processes that have contributed to their presenting problems and broadening the couple's ways of addressing their concerns.

Even though we tried to be inclusive of many types of client populations, this book does not take an in-depth look at the specific issues present in the lives of particular populations such as LGBTQ+ couples, open relationships, specific intercultural/racial/faith couples, immigrant couples, couples with adoptive children, and those who have experienced traumas such as warfare or violent crime. We have briefly identified types of stress experienced by populations that are minoritized due to gender identity, ethnicity, race, sexual orientation, ability, religion, age, and so on, but clinicians who work with these clients need to learn as much as they can about their lives. Sources include readings such as those in the Additional Clinical Resources, professional workshops, and clinical supervision, as well as those demonstrating cultural humility that allows for learning from the clients themselves, with true nonjudgmental curiosity. Consistent with a common factors approach, the clinician needs to address self-of-the-therapist issues that may arise when working with diverse clients, including implicit biases one may hold about clients who are different from oneself. Because clients may be reluctant to give therapists feedback when they feel misunderstood or devalued, the clinician needs to communicate the idea that such feedback is highly valued. Furthermore, given the inherent power differential between therapists and their clients, it is therapists' responsibility to educate themselves about stressful factors in the lives of their clients, especially those who are minoritized and may not feel empowered to educate their therapist.

Cognitive-behavioral therapies, including CBCT, tend to place the therapist in a role of expert who teaches and guides clients toward positive changes, but success in developing a positive therapeutic alliance with clients also depends on meeting clients' expectations for the therapist's role, such as identifying the degree to which couples want their therapist to use their expertise to direct them toward change and the degree to which they value therapists who relate to them in a personal way. Therapists who fail to attend to differences in power and resources between the social locations of themselves and their clients, in terms of race, ethnicity, socioeconomic status, gender identity, sexual orientation, age, ability, religion, language ability, and other minoritized identities, are likely to carry implicit biases in their work and to have difficulty establishing strong therapeutic alliances. Although the therapist has valuable knowledge and skills, the clients are the experts on their personal life experiences, as well as their goals for their couple relationship. Therapists need to be appreciative and affirming of their clients' preferred identities and life goals, and they also need to value and honor their clients' strengths instead of directly or indirectly advancing their own standards for well-functioning individuals and relationships.

Given that the therapist–client relationship and alliance is a two-way street, sometimes therapists with minoritized social identities work with couples with one or both members from a dominant group. In this book, we have not addressed ways in which therapists can address such therapist–client differences, including options the therapist has when a client has exhibited a microaggression toward the therapist.

In addition to enhancing one's knowledge about diverse client couples, therapists need to consider ways in which generic CBCT principles and methods should be tailored to client needs. To date, a limited number of research and clinical publications have addressed strategies for making such adjustments to assessment and treatment within CBCT or other major couple therapy theoretical models (Epstein et al., 2012; Epstein, Falconier, & Dattilio, 2020). For example, the CBCT focus on enhancing clear and direct expression of one's thoughts and emotions may have some universal benefits for couples from diverse cultural backgrounds, but varying cultural norms about consequences of such open communication must be taken into account. In addition, identifying partners' standards for a good relationship is a component of CBCT that likely is relevant across cultures, but identifying what constitutes an unrealistic standard in a particular culture requires knowledge of relevant beliefs and traditions. Similarly, therapists need to modify interventions for sexual incompatibility between partners that are based on heteronormative and binary gender models. Much more work is needed if couple therapies such as CBCT are to meet the needs of diverse clients around the world. Nevertheless, we believe that CBCT provides a theoretical foundation and flexible framework for assessment and treatment planning that prepares therapists to be helpful to couples with diverse characteristics and challenges in their intimate relationships.

In Chapter 2, we noted the growth in the delivery of mental health services, including couple therapy, via telehealth methods. Given the advantages online therapy offers for clients, especially easy access to treatment for clients who live far from providers, and removal of logistical barriers such as the need for child care during visits to a therapist's office, telehealth couple therapy likely will continue to be a popular option. Because conducting CBCT requires that the therapist pay close attention to probing for partners' moment-to-moment thought processes and emotional responses, and to observing their behavioral interactions closely, the immediacy of observing a couple on high-quality video equipment has the potential to work well. However, clinicians must adjust to some constraints of observing and interacting with couples online. For example, on the one hand, having a couple share one screen allows the therapist to observe live behavioral interactions, which cannot occur in a comparable manner if they participate on separate screens from different locations. On the other hand, sharing a screen forces the couple to sit very close to each other, which may trigger negative cognitions and emotional responses in high-conflict couples. Thus, therapists need to tailor the way they have members of a couple participate based on each couple's level of distress and conflict. In addition, the therapist's ability to observe partners' nonverbal behavior is limited by the extent to which the clients' camera shows more than their heads and torsos. Although research has indicated that therapy via telehealth can be as effective as in-person therapy (Doss, Knopp, Wrape, & Morland, 2023), more research is needed on the effectiveness of particular telehealth CBCT assessment and intervention methods, including risks that exist in treating couples with partner aggression online (see Chapter 5).

Finally, throughout this book we have noted the major influences that contextual conditions (e.g., extended family, structural racism, community resources, job stresses, local and national economic and social factors) have on couple relationships. Epstein and Baucom (2002) presented an enhanced CBCT approach that increased attention to assessment and interventions for such contextual factors. At the same time, it still is easy for practitioners of CBCT and other therapy models to focus mostly on cognitive, emotional, and behavioral processes occurring within the dyad, particularly as the therapist observes them occurring during sessions. We hope our expanded attention to contextual factors in this book will contribute to clinicians routinely applying a broad contextual framework in their efforts to help couples overcome difficulties and achieve greater happiness in their relationships.

References

Abramowitz, J. S., Baucom, D. H., Wheaton, M. G., Boeding, S., Fabricant, L. E., Paprocki, C., & Fischer, M. S. (2013). Enhancing exposure and response prevention for OCD: A couple-based approach. *Behavior Modification, 37,* 189–210.

Achenbach, T. M., Ivanova, M. Y., Rescorla, L. A., & Dumas, J. A. (2017). Transdiagnostic dimensional assessment of psychopathology in later life. *Current Behavioral Neuroscience Reports, 4,* 167–175.

Achenbach, T. M., & Rescorla, L. A. (2021). *Manual for the ASEBA school-age forms & profiles.* Burlington: University of Vermont, Research Center for Children, Youth, and Families.

Afifi, T. O., MacMillan, H., Cox, B. J., Asmundson, G. J., Stein, M. B., & Sareen, J. (2009). Mental health correlates of intimate partner violence in marital relationships in a nationally representative sample of males and females. *Journal of Interpersonal Violence, 24,* 1398–1417.

Ahmadabadi, Z., Najman, J. M., Williams, G. M., Clavarino, A. M., d'Abbs, P., & Tran, N. (2020). Intimate partner violence and subsequent depression and anxiety disorders. *Social Psychiatry and Psychiatric Epidemiology, 55,* 611–620.

Allen, E. S., Atkins, D. C., Baucom, D. H., Snyder, D. K., Gordon, K. C., & Glass, S. P. (2005). Intrapersonal, interpersonal, and contextual factors in engaging in and responding to extramarital involvement. *Clinical Psychology, 12,* 101–143.

Allen, M. L., Garcia-Huidobro, D., Hurtado, G. A., Allen, R., Davey, C. S., Forster, J. L., . . . Svetaz, M. V. (2012). Immigrant family skills-building to prevent tobacco use in Latino youth: Study protocol for a community-based participatory randomized controlled trial. *Trials, 13,* 242–251.

Ambrosi, C. C., Kavanagh, S., & Havighurst, S. S. (2022). The development of an adapted coparenting program: Tuning in to Kids Together. *International Journal of Systemic Therapy, 33,* 1–22.

American Association of Marriage and Family Therapy. (2017). Best practices in the online practice of couple and family therapy. Retrieved from *www.aamft.org/online_education/online_therapy_guidelines_2.aspx.*

American Psychiatric Association. (2022). *Diagnostic and statistical manual of mental disorders* (5th ed., text rev.). Washington, DC: Author.

American Psychological Association. (2017, November 1). Stress in America: The state of our nation. Retrieved from *www.apa.org/news/press/releases/stress/2017/state-nation.pdf.*

An, S., Ji, L.–J., Marks, M., & Zhang, Z. (2017). Two sides of emotion: Exploring positivity and negativity in six basic emotions across cultures. *Frontiers in Psychology, 8.* Retrieved from *www.ncbi.nlm.nih.gov/pmc/articles/PMC5397534.*

Anderson, H. (2007). The heart and spirit of collaborative therapy: The philosophical stance "A way of being" in relationship and conversation. In H. Anderson & D. Gehart (Eds.), *Collaborative therapy: Relationships and conversations that make a difference* (pp. 43–61). New York: Routledge.

Anderson, R. E., McKenny, M., Mitchell, A., Koku, L., & Stevenson, H. C. (2018). EMBRacing racial stress and trauma: Preliminary feasibility and coping responses of a racial socialization intervention. *Journal of Black Psychology, 44,* 25–46.

Anderson, R. E., Metzger, I., Applewhite, K., Sawyer, B., Jackson, W., Flores, S., . . . Carter, R. (2020). Hands up, now what? Black families' reactions to racial socialization interventions. *Journal of Youth Development, 15,* 93–109.

Anzani, A., Lindley, L., Prunas, A., & Galupo, P. (2021). "I use all the parts I'm given": A qualitative investigation of trans masculine and nonbinary individuals' use of body during sex. *International Journal of Sexual Health, 33,* 58–75.

Aponte, H. J., & Carlsen, C. J. (2009). An instrument for person-of-the-therapist supervision. *Journal of Marital and Family Therapy, 35,* 395–405.

Archer, J. (2000). Sex differences in aggression between heterosexual partners: A meta-analytic review. *Psychological Bulletin, 126,* 651–680.

Archuleta, K. L. (2013). Couples, money, and expectations: Negotiating financial management roles to increase relationship satisfaction. *Marriage and Family Review, 49*, 391–411.

Atkins, D. C., Marin, R. A., Lo, T. T., Klann, N., & Hahlweg, K. (2010). Outcomes of couples with infidelity in a community-based sample of couple therapy. *Journal of Family Psychology, 24*, 212–216.

Ayon, C., Williams, L. R., Marsiglia, F. F., Ayers, S., & Kiehne, E. (2015). A latent profile analysis of Latino parenting: The infusion of cultural values on family conflict. *Families in Society: The Journal of Contemporary Social Services, 96*, 203–210.

Aytac, I. A., & Rankin, B. H. (2009). Economic crisis and marital problems in Turkey: Testing the family stress model. *Journal of Marriage and Family, 71*, 756–767.

Babcock, J. C., & LaTaillade, J. J. (2000). Evaluating interventions for men who batter. In J. Vincent & E. N. Jouriles (Eds.), *Domestic violence: Guidelines for research-informed practice* (pp. 37–77). London: Jessica Kingsley.

Bandura, A. (1977). *Social learning theory*. Englewood Cliffs, NJ: Prentice Hall.

Bandura, A., & Walters, R. H. (1963). *Social learning and personality development*. New York: Holt, Rinehart & Winston.

Barbach, L. (2000). *For yourself: The fulfillment of female sexuality*. New York: Signet.

Barker, M.-J., & Iantaffi, A. (2019). *Life isn't binary: On being both, beyond, and in-between*. London: Jessica Kingsley.

Barkley, R. A. (2020). *Taking change of ADHD* (4th ed.). New York: Guilford Press.

Barkley, R. A., & Benton, C. M. (2013). *Your defiant child: 8 steps to better behavior* (2nd ed.). New York: Guilford Press.

Barkley, R. A., Robin, A. L., & Benton, C. M. (2014). *Your defiant teen: 10 steps to resolve conflict and rebuild your relationship* (2nd ed.). New York: Guilford Press.

Barlow, D. H., Farchione, T. J., Fairholme, C. P., Ellard, K. K., Boisseau, C. L., Allen, L. B., & May, J. T. E. (2018). *Unified protocol for transdiagnostic treatment of emotional disorders: Therapist guide* (2nd ed.). New York: Oxford University Press.

Barlow, D. H., Sauer-Zavala, S., Carl, J. R., Bullis, J. R., & Ellard, K. K. (2014). The nature, diagnosis, and treatment of neuroticism: Back to the future. *Clinical Psychological Science, 2*, 344–365.

Basson, R. (2001). Using a different model for female sexual response to address women's problematic low sexual desire. *Journal of Sex and Marital Therapy, 27*, 395–403.

Bastian., B., Kuppens, P., De Roover, K., & Diener, E. (2014). Is valuing positive emotion associated with life satisfaction? *Emotion, 14*, 639–645.

Bates, E. A., Archer, J., & Graham-Kevan, N. (2017). Do the same risk and protective factors influence aggression toward partners and same-sex others? *Aggressive Behavior, 43*, 163–175.

Baucom, D. H., & Epstein N. (1990). *Cognitive-behavioral marital therapy*. New York: Brunner/Mazel.

Baucom, D. H., Epstein, N. B., Fischer, M. S., Kirby, J. S., & LaTaillade, J. J. (2023). Cognitive behavioral couple therapy. In J. L. Lebow & D. K. Snyder (Eds.), *Clinical handbook of couple therapy* (6th ed., pp. 53–78). New York: Guilford Press.

Baucom, D. H., Epstein, N., Rankin, L. A., & Burnett, C. K. (1996). Assessing relationship standards: The Inventory of Specific Relationship Standards. *Journal of Family Psychology, 10*, 72–88.

Baucom, D. H., Epstein, N., Sayers, S., & Sher, T. G. (1989). The role of cognitions in marital relationships: Definitional, methodological, and conceptual issues. *Journal of Consulting and Clinical Psychology, 57*, 31–38.

Baucom, D. H., Fischer, M. S., Corrie, S., Worrell, M., & Boeding, S. E. (2020). *Treating relationship distress and psychopathology in couples: A cognitive-behavioural approach*. London: Routledge.

Baucom, D. H., & Lester, G. W. (1986). The usefulness of cognitive restructuring as an adjunct to behavioral marital therapy. *Behavior Therapy, 17*, 385–403.

Baucom, D. H., Porter, L. S., Kirby, J. S., Gremore, T. M., Wiesenthal, N., Aldridge, W., . . . Keefe, F. J. (2009). A couple-based intervention for female breast cancer. *Psycho-Oncology, 8*, 276–283.

Baucom, D. H., Porter, L. S., Kirby, J. S., & Hudepohl, J. (2012). Couple-based interventions for medical problems. *Behavior Therapy, 43*, 61–76.

Baucom, D. H., Sayers, S. L., & Sher, T. G. (1990). Supplementing behavioral marital therapy with cognitive restructuring and emotional expressiveness training: An outcome investigation. *Journal of Consulting and Clinical Psychology, 58*, 636–645.

Baucom, D. H., Shoham, V., Mueser, K. T., Daiuto, A. D., & Stickle, T. R. (1998). Empirically supported couples and family therapies for adult problems. *Journal of Consulting and Clinical Psychology, 66*, 53–88.

Baucom, D. H., Snyder, D. K., & Gordon, K. (2009). *Helping couples get past the affair: A clinician's guide*. New York: Guilford Press.

Baucom, D. H., Whisman, M. A., & Paprocki, C. (2012). Couple-based interventions for psychopathology. *Journal of Family Therapy, 34*, 250–270.

Baumeister, R. F., & Leary, M. R. (1995). The need to belong: Desire for interpersonal attachments as a fundamental human motivation. *Psychological Bulletin, 117*, 497–529.

Beach, S. R. H., Dreifuss, J. A., Franklin, K. J., Kamen, C., & Gabriel, B. (2008). Couple therapy and the treatment of depression. In A. S. Gurman (Ed.), *Clinical handbook of couple therapy* (4th ed., pp. 545–566). New York: Guilford Press.

Beach, S. R. H., Sandeen, E. E., & O'Leary, K. D. (1990). *Depression in marriage: A model for etiology and treatment*. New York: Guilford Press.

Beck, A. T. (1976). *Cognitive therapy and the emotional disorders*. New York: International Universities Press.

Beck, A. T. (1988). *Love is never enough*. New York: Harper & Row.

Beck, A. T., Emery, G., & Greenberg, R. L. (1985). *Anxiety disorders and phobias: A cognitive perspective*. New York: Basic Books.

Beck, A. T., Epstein, N., Brown, G., & Steer, R. A. (1988). An inventory for measuring clinical anxiety: Psychometric properties. *Journal of Consulting and Clinical Psychology, 56*, 893–897.

Beck, A. T., Rush, A. J., Shaw, B. F., & Emery, G. (1979). *Cognitive therapy of depression*. New York: Guilford Press.

Beck, A. T., Steer, R. A., & Brown, G. K. (1996). *Manual for the Beck Depression Inventory–II*. San Antonio, TX: Psychological Corporation.

Beck, J. S. (2021). *Cognitive behavior therapy: Basics and beyond* (3rd ed.). New York: Guilford Press.

Belsky, J., & Hsieh, K. H. (1998). Patterns of marital change during the early childhood years: Parenting personality, coparenting, and division-of-labor correlates. *Journal of Family Psychology, 12*, 511–528.

Benson, L. A., McGinn, M. M., & Christensen, A. (2012). Common principles of couple therapy. *Behavior Therapy, 43*, 25–35.

Bergeron, S., Rosen, N. O., Pukall, C. F., & Corsini-Munt, S. (2020). Genital pain in women and men. In K. S. K. Hall & Y. M. Binik (Eds.), *Principles and practice of sex therapy* (6th ed., pp. 180–201). New York: Guilford Press.

Bettinger, M. (2004). A systems approach to sex therapy with gay male couples. *Journal of Couple and Relationship Therapy, 3*, 65–74.

Biever, J. L., Bobele, M., & North, M. W. (1998). Therapy with intercultural couples: A postmodern approach. *Counselling Psychology Quarterly, 11*, 181–188.

Bilal, A., & Abbasi, N. (2020). Cognitive-behavioral sex therapy: An emerging treatment option for nonorganic erectile dysfunction in young men: A feasibility pilot study. *Journal of Sexual Medicine, 8*, 396–407.

Binik, Y. M., & Meana, M. (2009). The future of sex therapy: Specialization or marginalization? *Archives of Sexual Behavior, 38*, 1016–1027.

Birchler, G. R., Fals-Stewart, W. & O'Farrell, T. J. (2008). Couple therapy for alcoholism and drug abuse. In A. S. Gurman (Ed.), *Clinical handbook of couple therapy* (4th ed., pp. 523–544). New York: Guilford Press.

Bo, A., Durand, B., & Wang, Y. (2022). A scoping review of parent-involved ethnic and racial socialization programs. *Children and Youth Services Review, 144*, January. Retrieved from *https://doi.org/10.1016/j.childyouth.2022.106750*.

Bodenmann, G. (1995). A systemic-transactional conceptualization of stress and coping in couples. *Swiss Journal of Psychology/Schweizerische Zeitschrift für Psychologie/Revue Suisse de Psychologie, 54*(1), 34–49.

Bodenmann, G. (1997). Dyadic coping: A systemic-transactional view of stress and coping among couples: Theory and empirical findings. *European Review of Applied Psychology, 47*, 137–140.

Bodenmann, G. (2000). *Stress und coping bei paaren* [*Stress and coping in couples*]. Göttingen, Germany: Hogrefe.

Bodenmann, G. (2005). Dyadic coping and its significance for marital functioning. In T. Revenson, K. Kayser, & G. Bodenmann (Eds.), *Couples coping with stress: Emerging perspectives on dyadic coping* (pp. 33–50). Washington, DC: American Psychological Association.

Bodenmann, G. (2008). *DCI—Dyadisches Coping Inventar, Manual* [*The Dyadic Coping Inventory Manual*]. Bern, Goettingen: Huber & Hogrefe.

Bodenmann, G., Randall, A. K., & Falconier, M. K. (2016). Coping in couples: The systemic transactional model (STM). In M. K. Falconier, A. K. Randall, & G. Bodenmann (Eds.), *Couples coping with stress: A cross-cultural perspective* (pp. 5–22). New York: Routledge.

Bowlby, J. (1969). *Attachment and loss: Vol. 1. Attachment*. New York: Basic Books.

Bowlby, J. (1988). *A secure base*. New York: Basic Books.

Bronfenbrenner, U. (1979). *The ecology of human development: Experiments by nature and design*. Cambridge, MA: Harvard University Press.

Brossio, J. A., Basson, R., Driscoll, M. Correia, S., & Brotto, L. A. (2018). Mindfulness-based group therapy for men with situational erectile dysfunction: A mixed-methods feasibility analysis and pilot study. *Journal of Sexual Medicine, 15*, 1478–1490.

Brotto, L. A., Chivers, M. L., Millman, R. D., & Albert, A. (2016). Mindfulness-based sex therapy improves genital-subjective arousal concordance in women with sexual desire/arousal difficulties. *Archives of Sexual Behavior, 45*, 1907–1921.

Bulik, C. M., Baucom, D. H., & Kirby, J. S. (2012). Treating anorexia nervosa in the couple context. *Journal of Cognitive Psychotherapy, 26*, 19–33.

Bulik, C. M., Baucom, D. H., Kirby, J. S., & Pisetsky, E. (2011). Uniting couples (in the treatment of) anorexia nervosa (UCAN). *International Journal of Eating Disorders, 44*, 19–28.

Burgoyne, C., Clarke, V., & Burns, M. (2011). Money management and view of civil partnership in same-sex couples: Results from a UK survey of non-heterosexuals. *The Sociological Review, 59*, 685–706.

Bustamante, R. M., Nelson, J. A., Henriksen Jr., R. C., & Monakes, S. (2011). Intercultural couples: Coping with culture-related stressors. *The Family Journal: Counseling and Therapy for Couples and Families, 19*, 154–164.

Butler, E. A., Lee, T. L., & Gross, J. J. (2007). Emotion regulation and culture: Are the social consequences of emotion suppression culture-specific? *Emotion, 7,* 30–48.

Buunk, A. P., Dijkstra, P., & Massar, K. (2018). The universal threat and temptation of extradyadic affairs. In A. L. Vangelisti & D. Perlman (Eds.), *The Cambridge handbook of personal relationships* (2nd ed., pp. 353–364). New York: Cambridge University Press.

Calzada, E. J., Huang, K. Y., Anicama, C., Fernandez, Y., & Brotman, L. M. (2012). Test of a cultural framework of parenting with Latino families. *Cultural Diversity and Ethnic Minority Psychology, 18,* 285–296.

Campbell, L., & Fletcher, G. J. O. (2015). Romantic relationships, ideal standards, and mate selection. *Current Opinion in Psychology, 1,* 97–100.

Cano, A., & O'Leary, K. D. (1997). Romantic jealousy and affairs: Research and implications for couple therapy. *Journal of Sex and Marital Therapy, 23,* 249–275.

Carlson, R. G., Rhoades, G. K., Johnson, S., Stanley, S. M., & Markman, H. J. (2023). Relationship enhancement and distress prevention. In J. L. Lebow & D. K. Snyder (Eds.), *Clinical handbook of couple therapy* (6th ed., pp. 639–655). New York: Guilford Press.

Carney, M. M., & Barner, J. R. (2012). Prevalence of partner abuse: Rates of emotional abuse and control. *Partner Abuse, 3,* 286–335.

Cartwright, C. (2011). Transference, countertransference, and reflective practice in cognitive therapy. *Clinical Psychologist, 15,* 112–120.

Carver, C. S. (1997). You want to measure coping but your protocol's too long: Consider the Brief COPE. *International Journal of Behavioral Medicine, 4,* 92–100.

Chambless, D. L. (2012). Adjunctive couple and family intervention for patients with anxiety disorders. *Journal of Clinical Psychology: In Session, 68,* 548–560.

Chambless, D. L., Allred, K. M., Chen, F. F., McCarthy, K. S., Milrod, B., & Barber, J. P. (2017). Perceived criticism predicts outcome of psychotherapy for panic disorder: Replication and extension. *Journal of Consulting and Clinical Psychology, 85,* 37–44.

Christensen, A. (1987). Detection of conflict patterns in couples. In K. Hahlweg & M. J. Goldstein (Eds.), *Understanding major mental disorder: The contribution of family interaction research* (pp. 250–265). New York: Family Process Press.

Christensen, A., Atkins, D. C., Baucom, B., & Yi, J. (2010). Marital status and satisfaction five years following a randomized clinical trial comparing traditional versus integrative behavioral couple therapy. *Journal of Consulting and Clinical Psychology, 78,* 225–235.

Christensen, A., Atkins, D. C., Berns, S., Wheeler, J., Baucom, D. H., & Simpson, L. E. (2004). Traditional versus integrative behavioral couple therapy for significant and chronically distressed married couples. *Journal of Consulting and Clinical Psychology, 72,* 176–191.

Christensen, A., Dimidjian, S., Martell, C. R., & Doss, B. D. (2023). Integrative behavioral couple therapy. In J. L. Lebow & D. K. Snyder (Eds.), *Clinical handbook of couple therapy* (6th ed., pp. 79–103). New York: Guilford Press.

Christopher, C., Umemura, T., Mann, T., Jacobvitz, D. B., & Hazen, N. L. (2015). Marital quality over the transition to parenthood as a predictor of coparenting. *Journal of Child and Family Studies, 24,* 3636–3651.

Clark., R., Coleman, A. P., & Novak, J. D. (2004). Brief report: Initial psychometric properties of the everyday discrimination scale in black adolescents. *Journal of Adolescence, 27,* 363–368.

Coard, S. I., Wallace, S. A., Stevenson, H. C., & Brotman, L. M. (2004). Towards culturally relevant preventive interventions: The consideration of racial socialization in parent training with African American families. *Journal of Child and Family Studies, 13,* 277–293.

Coker, A. L., Davis, K. E., Arias, I., Desai, S., Sanderson, M., Brandt, H. M., & Smith, P. H. (2002). Physical and mental health effects of intimate partner violence for men and women. *American Journal of Preventive Medicine, 24,* 260–268.

Commission on Accreditation for Marriage and Family Education. (2004). *Marriage and family therapy core competencies.* Retrieved from *https://www.coamfte.org/Documents/COAMFTE/Accreditation/Resources/MFTCoreCompetencies(December202004).pdf.*

Conte, H. R., Ratto, R., & Karusa, T. (1996). The Psychological Mindedness Scale: Factor structure and relationship to outcome of psychotherapy. *Journal of Psychotherapy Practice and Research, 5,* 250–259.

Costa, D., Hatzidimitriadou, E., Ionnidi-Kapolou, E., Lindert, J., Soares, J. J. F., Sundin, O., . . . Barros, H. (2016). Male and female physical intimate partner violence and socio-economic position: A cross-sectional international multicentre study in Europe. *Public Health, 139,* 44–52.

Crenshaw, A. O., Christensen, A., Baucom, D. H., Epstein, N. B., & Baucom, B. R. W. (2017). Revised scoring and improved reliability for the Communication Patterns Questionnaire. *Psychological Assessment, 29,* 913–925.

Crippen, C. L. (2011). Working with intercultural couples and families: Exploring cultural dissonance to identify transformative opportunities. Retrieved from *http://counselingoutfitters.com/vistas/vistas11/Article_21.pdf.*

Cutrona, C. (1996). *Social support in couples.* Thousand Oaks, CA: Sage.

Daneshpour, M. (2003). Lives together, worlds apart? The lives of multicultural Muslim couples. *Journal of Couple and Relationship Therapy, 2,* 57–71.

Darwiche, J., Carneiro, C., Imesch, C., Nunes, C. E., & de Roten, Y. (2022). Parents in couple therapy: An intervention targeting marital and coparenting relationships. *Family Process, 61,* 490–506.

Dattilio, F. M. (2010). *Cognitive-behavioral therapy with couples and families: A comprehensive guide for clinicians.* New York: Guilford Press.

Dattilio, F. M., & Epstein, N. B. (2016). Cognitive-behavioral couple and family therapy. In T. L. Sexton & J. Lebow (Eds.), *Handbook of family therapy: The science and practice of working with families and couples* (4th ed., pp. 89–119). New York: Routledge.

Dattilio, F. M., Kazantzis, N., Shinkfield, G., & Carr, A. G. (2011). A survey of homework use, experience of barriers to homework, and attitudes about the barriers to homework among couples and family therapists. *Journal of Marital and Family Therapy, 37,* 121–136.

Dattilio, F. M., & Padesky, C. A. (1990). *Cognitive therapy with couples.* Sarasota, FL: Professional Resource Exchange.

Davies, P. T., Martin, M. J., & Cicchetti, D. (2012). Delineating the sequelae of destructive and constructive interparental conflict for children within an evolutionary framework. *Developmental Psychology, 48,* 939–955.

Dearing, R. L., & Tangney, J. P. (2011). Introduction: Putting shame in context. In R. L. Dearing & J. P. Tangney (Eds.), *Shame in the therapy hour* (pp. 3–19). Washington, DC: American Psychological Association.

Deater-Deckard, K. (2004). *Parenting stress.* New Haven, CT: Yale University Press.

Deries, K. M., Mak, J. Y., Garcia-Moreno, C., Petzold, M., Child, J. C., Falder, B., . . . Pallitto, C. (2013). The global prevalence of intimate partner violence against women. *Science, 340,* 1527–1528.

Dew, J., Britt, S., & Huston, S. (2012). Examining the relationship between financial issues and divorce. *Family Relations, 61,* 615–628.

Diamond, A. (2013). Executive functions. *Annual Review of Psychology, 64,* 135–168.

Dobson, K. S., & Dozois, D. J. A. (Eds.). (2019). *Handbook of cognitive-behavioral therapies* (4th ed.). New York: Guilford Press.

Dobson, K. S., & Kendall, P. C. (Eds.). (1993). *Psychopathology and cognition.* San Diego, CA: Academic Press.

Dobson, K. S., Poole, J. C., & Beck, J. S. (2018). The fundamental cognitive model. In R. L. Leahy (Ed.), *Science and practice in cognitive therapy: Foundations, mechanisms, and applications* (pp. 29–47). New York: Guilford Press.

Doherty, W. J., Harris, S. M., & Wilde, J. L. (2015). Discernment counseling for "mixed-agenda" couples. *Journal of Marital and Family Therapy, 42,* 246–255.

Domenech Rodríguez, M. M., Donovick, M. R., & Crowley, S. L. (2009). Parenting styles in a cultural context: Observations of "protective parenting" in first-generation Latinos. *Family Process, 48,* 195–210.

Doss, B. D., Cicila, L. N., Hsueh, A. C., Morrison, K. R., & Cahart, K. (2014). A randomized controlled trial of brief coparenting and relationship interventions during the transition to parenthood. *Journal of Family Psychology, 28,* 483–494.

Doss, B. D., Knopp, K. C., Wrape, E. R., & Morland, L. A. (2023). Telehealth and digital couple interventions. In J. L. Lebow & D. K. Snyder (Eds.), *Clinical handbook of couple therapy* (6th ed., pp. 656–676). New York: Guilford Press.

Doss, B. D., Simpson, L. E., & Christensen, A. (2004). Why do couples seek marital therapy? *Professional Psychology, 35,* 608–614.

Duarte, C. S., Klotz, J., Elkington, K., Shrout, P. E., Canino, G., Eisenberg, R., . . . Bird, H. (2020). Severity and frequency of antisocial behaviors: Late adolescence/young adulthood Antisocial Behavior Index. *Journal of Child and Family Studies, 29,* 1200–1211.

Durtschi, J., Soloski, K. L., & Kimmes, J. (2017). The dyadic effects of supportive coparenting and parental stress on relationship quality across the transition to parenthood. *Journal of Marital & Family Therapy, 43,* 308–321.

Dylman, A. S., & Bjärtå, A. (2019). When your heart is in your mouth: The effect of second language use on negative emotions, *Cognition and Emotion, 33,* 1284–1290.

Eaton, N. R., Rodriguez-Seijas, C., Carragher, N., & Krueger, R. F. (2015). Transdiagnostic factors of psychopathology and substance use disorders: A review. *Social Psychiatry and Psychiatric Epidemiology, 50,* 171–182.

Eckhardt, C. I., Murphy, C. M., Whitaker, D. J., Sprunger, J., Dykstra, R., & Woodard, K. (2013). The effectiveness of intervention programs for perpetrators and victims of intimate partner violence. *Partner Abuse, 4,* 196–231.

Ehrensaft, M. K. (2009). Family and relationship predictors of psychological and physical aggression. In K. D. O'Leary & E. M. Woodin (Eds.), *Psychological and physical aggression in couples: Causes and interventions* (pp. 99–118). Washington, DC: American Psychological Association.

Eidelson, R. J., & Epstein, N. (1982). Cognition and relationship maladjustment: Development of a measure of dysfunctional relationship beliefs. *Journal of Consulting and Clinical Psychology, 50,* 715–720.

Ellis, A. (1962). *Reason and emotion in psychotherapy.* New York: Lyle Stuart.

Ellis, A., Sichel, J. L., Yeager, R. J., DiMattia, D. J., & DiGiuseppe, R. (1989). *Rational-emotive couples therapy.* New York: Pergamon.

Ellsberg, M., Jansen, H. A., Heise, L., Watts, C. H., & Garcia-Moreno, C. (2008). Intimate partner violence and women's physical and mental health in the

WHO Multi-Country Study on Women's Health and Domestic Violence: An observational study. *The Lancet, 371,* 1165–1172.

Epstein, N. (1982). Cognitive therapy with couples. *American Journal of Family Therapy, 10*(1), 5–16.

Epstein, N. B., & Baucom, D. H. (2002). *Enhanced cognitive-behavioral therapy for couples: A contextual approach.* Washington, DC: American Psychological Association.

Epstein, N. B., Baucom, D. H., Burnett, C. K., & Rankin, L. A. (1990). *The Inventory of General Relationship Standards.* Unpublished scale, Department of Family Science, University of Maryland, College Park.

Epstein, N. B., Baucom, D. H., Kirby, J. S., & LaTaillade, J. J. (2019). Cognitive-behavioral couple therapy. In K. S. Dobson & D. J. A. Dozois (Eds.), *Handbook of cognitive-behavioral therapies* (4th ed., pp. 433–463). New York: Guilford Press.

Epstein, N. B., Berger, A. T., Fang, J. J., Messina, L., Smith, J. R., Lloyd, T. D., . . . Liu, Q. X. (2012). Applying Western-developed family therapy models in China. *Journal of Family Psychotherapy, 23,* 217–237.

Epstein, N. B., Chen, F., & Beyder-Kamjou, I. (2005). Relationship standards and marital satisfaction in Chinese and American couples. *Journal of Marital and Family Therapy, 31,* 59–74.

Epstein, N. B., Dattilio, F. M., & Baucom, D. H. (2016). Cognitive-behavior couple therapy. In T. L. Sexton & J. Lebow (Eds.), *Handbook of family therapy* (4th ed., pp. 361–386). New York: Routledge.

Epstein, N. B., & Falconier, M. K. (2011). Shame in couple therapy. In R. Dearing & J. P. Tangney (Eds.), *Shame in the therapy hour.* Washington, DC: American Psychological Association.

Epstein, N. B., & Falconier, M. K. (2014). Cognitive-behavioral therapies for couples and families. In J. L. Wetchler & L. L. Hecker (Eds.), *An introduction to marriage and family therapy* (2nd ed., pp. 259–318). New York: Brunner-Routledge.

Epstein, N. B., & Falconier, M. K. (2017). Shame in couple relationships. In J. Fitzgerald (Ed.), *Foundations for couples' therapy: Research for the real world* (pp. 374–383). New York: Routledge.

Epstein, N. B., Falconier, M. K., & Dattilio, F. M. (2020). Cultural factors in the practice of couple and family therapy. In W. K. Halford & F. J. R. van de Vijver (Eds.), *Cross-cultural family research and practice* (pp. 479–521). New York: Elsevier.

Epstein, N. B., LaTaillade, J. J., & Werlinich, C. A. (2023). Couple therapy for partner aggression. In J. L. Lebow & D. K. Snyder (Eds.), *Clinical handbook of couple therapy* (6th ed., pp. 391–412). New York: Guilford Press.

Epstein, N., Schlesinger, S. E., & Dryden, W. (Eds.). (1988). *Cognitive-behavioral therapy with families.* New York: Brunner/Mazel.

Epstein, N. B., & Werlinich, C. A. (1999). *The Relationship Issues Survey: A measure of areas of couple conflict.* Unpublished measure, Department of Family Science, University of Maryland, College Park.

Eyberg, S. M., & Members of the Child Study Laboratory. (1999). Integrity checklists and session materials. In *Parent–Child Interaction Therapy manual.* Gainesville: University of Florida. Available from *www.PCIT.org.*

Falconier, M. K. (2010). Female anxiety and male depression: Links between economic strain and psychological aggression in Argentinean couples. *Family Relations, 59,* 424–238.

Falconier, M. K., & Epstein, N. B. (2010). Relationship satisfaction in Argentinian couples under economic strain: Gender differences in a dyadic stress model. *Journal of Social and Personal Relationships, 27,* 781–799.

Falconier, M. K., & Epstein, N. B. (2011). Couples undergoing financial strain: What we know and we can do. *Family Relations, 60,* 303–317.

Falconier, M. K., & Jackson, J. (2020). Economic strain and couple relationship functioning: A meta-analysis. *International Journal of Stress Management, 27,* 311–325.

Falconier, M. K., & Kim, J. (2015). *TOGETHER: A Program for Couples to Improve Stress Management, Communication, and Financial Management Skills—Revised Manual for Trainers.* Unpublished manual, available from Mariana K. Falconier, PhD, Department of Family Science, University of Maryland, College Park, MD 20742.

Falconier, M., Kim, J., & Lachowicz, M. J. (2023). Together—A couples' program integrating relationship and financial education: A randomized controlled trial. *Journal of Social and Personal Relationships, 40,* 333–359.

Falconier, M. K., & Kuhn, R. (2019). Dyadic coping in couples: A conceptual integration and a review of the empirical literature. *Frontiers in Psychology, 10,* Article 571. Retrieved from *https://doi.org/10.3389/fpsyg.2019.00571.*

Falconier, M. K., Randall, A. K., & Bodenmann, G. (2016). Cultural considerations in understanding dyadic coping across cultures. In M. K. Falconier, A. K. Randall, & G. Bodenmann (Eds.), *Couples coping with stress: A cross-cultural perspective* (pp. 23–35). New York: Routledge.

Falconier, M. K., Rusu, P., & Bodenmann, G. (2019). Initial validation of the Dyadic Coping Inventory for Financial Stress. *Stress and Health, 35,* 367–381.

Falicov, C. J. (1995). Cross-cultural marriages. In N. Jacobson & A. Gurman (Eds.), *Clinical handbook of couple therapy* (2nd ed., pp. 231–246). New York: Guilford Press.

Feinberg, M. E. (2003). The internal structure and

ecological context of coparenting: A framework for research and intervention. *Parent: Science and Practice, 3*, 95–131.

Feinberg, M. E., Brown, L. D., & Kan, M. L. (2012). A multi-domain self-report measure of coparenting. *Parenting: Science and Practice, 12*, 1–21.

Feinberg, M. E., Jones, D. E., Hostetler, M. L., Roettger, M. E., Paul, I. M., & Ehrenthal, D. B. (2016). Couple-focused prevention at the transition to parenthood a randomized trial: Effects on coparenting, parenting, family violence and parent and child adjustment. *Prevention Science, 17*, 751–764.

Feldman, P. J., Cohen, S., Hamrick, N., & Lepore, S. J. (2004). Psychological stress, appraisal, emotion and cardiovascular response in a public speaking task. *Psychology and Health, 19*, 353–368.

Fischer, M. S., Baucom, D. H., & Cohen, M. J. (2016). Cognitive-behavioral couple therapies: Review of the evidence for the treatment of relationship distress, psychopathology, and chronic health conditions. *Family Process, 55*, 423–442.

Fishman, H. C. (2012). *Intensive structural therapy: Treating families in their social context.* New York: Basic Books.

Fiske, S. T., & Taylor, S. E. (1991). *Social cognition* (2nd ed.). New York: McGraw-Hill.

Fletcher, G. J. O., Overall, N. C., Friesen, M. D., & Nicolls, C. L. (2018). Social cognition in romantic relationships. In A. L. Vangelisti & D. Perlman (Eds.), *The Cambridge handbook of personal relationships* (2nd ed., pp. 230–242). Cambridge, UK: Cambridge University Press.

Fletcher, G. J. O., Simpson, J. A., Campbell, L., & Overall, N. C. (2013). *The science of intimate relationships.* New York: Wiley-Blackwell.

Florin, I., Nostadt, A., Reck, C., Franzen, U., & Jenkins, M. (1992). Expressed emotion in depressed patients and their partners. *Family Process, 31*, 163–172.

Foeman, A., & Nance, T. (2002). Building new cultures, reframing old images: Success strategies of interracial couples. *Howard Journal of Communication, 13*, 237–249.

Folkman, S., & Lazarus, R. S. (1988). *Ways of Coping Questionnaire: Research Edition.* Palo Alto, CA: Consulting Psychologists Press.

Forbush, K. T., South, S. C., Krueger, R. F., Iacono, W. G., Clark, L. A., Keel, P. K., . . . Watson, D. (2010). Locating eating pathology within an empirical diagnostic taxonomy: Evidence from a community-based sample. *Journal of Abnormal Psychology, 119*, 282–292.

Forgatch, M. S. (1994). *Parenting through change: A training manual.* Eugene: Oregon Social Learning Center.

Forgatch, M. S., & DeGarmo, D. S. (1999). Parenting through change: An effective prevention program for single mothers. *Journal of Consulting and Clinical Psychology, 67*, 711–724.

Forman, T. A., Williams, D. R., & Jackson, J. S. (1997). Race, place, and discrimination. *Perspectives on Social Problems, 9*, 231–261.

Frederick, D. A., & Fales, M. R. (2016). Upset over sexual versus emotional infidelity among gay, lesbian, bisexual, and heterosexual adults. *Archives of Sexual Behavior, 45*, 175–191.

Freedman, J., & Combs, G. (2023). Narrative couple therapy. In J. L. Lebow & D. K. Snyder (Eds.), *Clinical handbook of couple therapy* (6th ed., pp. 227–249). New York: Guilford Press.

Freeman, A., & McCloskey, R. D. (2003). Impediments to effective psychotherapy. In R. L. Leahy (Ed.), *Roadblocks in cognitive behavioral therapy* (pp. 24–48). New York: Guilford Press.

Freud, S. (1910). *The future prospects of psycho-analytic therapy.* In J. Strachey (Ed. and Trans.), *The standard edition of the complete psychological works of Sigmund Freud* (Vol. XI, pp. 139–151). London: Hogarth Press.

Frieze, I. H. (2005). Female violence against intimate partners: An introduction. *Psychology of Women Quarterly, 29*, 229–237.

Frühauf, S., Gerger, H., Schmidt, H. M., Munder, T., & Barth, J. (2013). Efficacy of psychological interventions for sexual dysfunction: A systematic review and meta-analysis. *Archives of Sexual Behavior, 42*, 915–933.

Fruzzetti, A. E., McLean, C., & Erikson, K. M. (2019). Mindfulness and acceptance interventions in cognitive-behavioral therapy. In K. S. Dobson and D. J. A. Dozois (Eds.), *Handbook of cognitive-behavioral therapies* (4th ed., pp. 271–296). New York: Guilford Press.

Fruzzetti, A. E., & Payne, L. (2015). Couple therapy and borderline personality disorder. In A. S. Gurman, J. L. Lebow, & D. K. Snyder (Eds.), *Clinical handbook of couple therapy* (5th ed., pp. 606–634). New York: Guilford Press.

Funk, J. L., & Rogge, R. D. (2007). Testing the rule with item response theory: Increasing precision of measurement for relationship satisfaction with the Couples Satisfaction Index. *Journal of Family Psychology, 21*, 572–583.

Fusco, R. A. (2010). Intimate partner violence in interracial couples: A comparison to white and ethnic minority monoracial couples. *Journal of Interpersonal Violence, 25*, 1785–1800.

Gambescia, N., Weeks, G. R., & Hertlein, K. M. (2021). *A clinician's guide to systemic sex therapy* (3rd ed.). New York: Routledge.

Gao, M., Du, H., Davies, P. T., & Cummings, E. M. (2019). Marital conflict behaviors and parenting: Dyadic links over time. *Family Relations, 68*, 135–149.

Garcia, D. R. (2006). Mixed marriages and transnational families in the intercultural context: A case study of African Spanish couples in Catalonia. *Journal of Ethnic and Migration Studies, 32*, 403–433.

Garner, C., Person, M., Goddard, C., Patridge, A., & Bixby, T. (2019). Satisfaction in consensual nonmonogamy. *The Family Journal: Counseling and Therapy for Couples and Families, 27,* 115–121.

Gattis, K. S., Simpson, L. E., & Christensen, A. (2008). What about the kids? Parenting and child adjustment in the context of couple therapy. *Journal of Family Psychology, 22,* 833–842.

Girard, A., & Wooley, S. R. (2017). Using Emotionally Focused Therapy to treat sexual desire discrepancy in couples. *Journal of Sex and Marital Therapy, 43,* 720–735.

Girard, J. M., Wright, A. G. C., Beeney, J. E., Lazarus, S. A., Scott, L. N., Stepp, S. D., & Pilkonis, P. A. (2017). Interpersonal problems across levels of the psychopathology hierarchy. *Comprehensive Psychiatry, 79,* 53–69.

Glass, S. P. (2003). *Not 'just friends': Protect your relationship from infidelity and heal the trauma of betrayal.* New York: Free Press.

Goetz, J. L., Spencer-Rodgers, J., & Peng, K. (2008). Dialectical emotions: How cultural epistemologies influence the experience and regulation of emotional complexity. In *Handbook of Motivation and Cognition across Cultures* (pp. 517–539). San Diego, CA: Academic Press.

Goldman, R. N., & Greenberg, L. S. (2006). Promoting emotional expression and emotion regulation in couples. In D. K. Snyder, J. A. Simpson, & J. N. Hughes (Eds.), *Emotion regulation in couples and families* (pp. 231–248). Washington, DC: American Psychological Association.

Gonzales, K. L., Noonan, C., Goins, R. T., Henderson, W. G., Beals, J., Manson, S. M., . . . Roubideaux, Y. (2016). Assessing the Everyday Discrimination Scale among American Indians and Alaska Natives. *Psychological Assessment, 28,* 51–58.

Gonzales, N. A., Deardorff, J., Formoso, D., Barr, A., Jr., & Barrera, M. (2006). Family mediators of the relation between acculturation and adolescent mental health. *Family Relations, 55,* 318–330.

Gonzales, N. A., Dumka, L. E., Millsap, R. E., Gottschall, A., McClain, D. B., Wong, J. J., . . . Kim, S. Y. (2012). Randomized trial of a broad preventive intervention for Mexican American adolescents. *Journal of Consulting and Clinical Psychology, 80,* 1–16.

Goodman, R. (2001). Psychometric properties of the Strengths and Difficulties Questionnaire. *Journal of the American Academy of Child and Adolescent Psychiatry, 40,* 1337–1345.

Gordon, K. C., Mitchell, E. A., Baucom, D. H., & Snyder, D. K. (2023). Couple therapy for infidelity. In J. L. Lebow & D. K. Snyder (Eds.), *Clinical handbook of couple therapy* (6th ed., pp. 413–433). New York: Guilford Press.

Gottman, J. M. (1979). *Marital interaction: Experimental investigations.* New York: Academic Press.

Gottman, J. M. (1994). *What predicts divorce? The relationship between marital processes and marital outcomes.* Hillsdale, NJ: Erlbaum.

Gottman, J. M. (1999). *The marriage clinic: A scientifically based marital therapy.* New York: Norton.

Gratz, K. L., & Roemer, L. (2004). Multidimensional assessment of emotion regulation and dysregulation: Development, factor structure, and initial validation of the difficulties in emotion regulation scale. *Journal of Psychopathology and Behavioral Assessment, 26,* 41–54.

Green, R-J., & Mitchell, V. (2015). Gay, lesbian, and bisexual issues in couple therapy. In A. S. Gurman, J. L. Lebow, & D. K. Snyder (Eds.), *Clinical handbook of couple therapy* (5th ed., pp. 489–511). New York: Guilford Press.

Greenberg, L. S., & Goldman, R. N. (2008). *Emotion-focused couples therapy: The dynamics of emotion, love, and power.* Washington, DC: American Psychological Association.

Gross, J. J. (Ed.). (2014). *Handbook of emotion regulation* (2nd ed.). New York: Guilford Press.

Gross, J. J., & John, O. P. (2003). Individual differences in two emotion regulation processes: Implications for affect, relationships, and well-being. *Journal of Personality and Social Psychology, 85,* 348–362.

Gudykunst, W. B., Matsumoto, Y., Ting-Toomey, S., Nishida, T., Kim, K., & Heyman, S. (1996). The influence of cultural individualism-collectivism, self construals, and individual values on communication styles across cultures. *Human Communication Research, 22,* 510–543.

Gurman, A. S., & Kniskern, D. P. (1978). Research on marital and family therapy: Progress, perspective and prospect. In S. Garfield & A. Bergin (Eds.), *Handbook of psychotherapy and behavior change* (2nd ed., pp. 817–901). New York: Wiley.

Guttman, G. (2020). Sex and couples therapy: Biopsychosocial and relationship therapy. In T. Nelson (Ed.). *Integrative sex and couples therapy: A therapist's guide to new and innovative approaches* (pp. 1–16). Eau Claire, WI: PESI Publishing and Media.

Hahlweg, K. (2004). Kategoriensystem für Partnerschaftliche Interaktion (KPI): Interactional Coding System (ICS). In P. K. Kerig & D. H. Baucom (Eds.), *Couple observational coding systems* (pp. 127–142). Mahwah, NJ: Erlbaum.

Hahlweg, K., Reisner, L., Kohli, G., Vollmer, M., Schindler, L., & Revenstorf, D. (1984). Development and validity of a new system to analyze interpersonal communication. KPI: Kategoriensystem für Partnerschaftliche Interaktion. In K. Hahlweg & N. S. Jacobson (Eds.), *Marital interaction: Analysis and modification* (pp. 182–198). New York: Guilford Press.

Halford, W. K. (2011). *Marriage and relationship education: What works and how to provide it.* New York: Guilford Press.

Halford, W. K., & Moore, E. N. (2002). Relationship education and the prevention of couple relationship problems. In A. S. Gurman & N. S. Jacobson (Eds.), *Clinical handbook of couple therapy* (3rd ed., pp. 400–419). New York: Guilford Press.

Halgunseth, L. C., Ispa, J. M., & Rudy, D. (2006). Parental control in Latino families: An integrated review of the literature. *Child Development, 77*, 1282–1297.

Hall, K. S. K., & Binik, Y. M. (Eds.). (2020). *Principles and practice of sex therapy* (6th ed.). New York: Guilford Press.

Hall, K. S. K., & Graham, C. A. (2020). The privileging of pleasure: Sex therapy in global cultural context. In K. S. K. Hall & Y. M. Binik (Eds.), *Principles and practice of sex therapy* (6th ed., pp. 243–268). New York: Guilford Press.

Hangen, F., Crasta, D., & Rogge, R. D. (2020). Delineating the boundaries between nonmonogamy and infidelity: Bringing consent back into definitions of consensual nonmonogamy with latent profile analysis. *Journal of Sex Research, 57*, 438–457.

Hankerson, S. H., Moise, N., Wilson, D., Waller, B. Y., Arnold, K. T., Duarte, C., . . . Shim, R. (2022). The intergenerational impact of structural racism and cumulative trauma on depression. *American Journal of Psychiatry, 179*, 434–440.

Hardy, K. V., & Laszloffy, T. A. (1995). The cultural genogram: Key to training culturally competent family therapists. *Journal of Marital and Family Therapy, 21*, 227–237.

Haseli, A., Shariati, M., Nazari, A. M., Keramat, A., & Emamian, M. H. (2019). Infidelity and its associated factors: A systematic review. *Journal of Sexual Medicine, 16*, 1155–1169.

Helms, H. M., Supple, A. J., Su, J., Rodriguez, Y., Cavanaugh, A. M., & Hengstebeck, N. D. (2014). Economic pressure, cultural adaptation stress, and marital quality among Mexican-origin couples. *Journal of Family Psychology, 28*, 77–87.

Hertlein, K. M., & Weeks, G. R. (2007). Two roads diverging in a wood: The current state of infidelity research and treatment. *Journal of Couple and Relationship Therapy, 6*, 95–107.

Hertlein, K. M., Wetchler, J. L., & Piercy, F. P. (2005). Infidelity: An overview. *Journal of Couple and Relationship Therapy, 4*, 5–16.

Heyman, R. E. (2004). Rapid Marital Interaction Coding System (RMICS). In P. K. Kerig & D. H. Baucom (Eds.), *Couple observational coding systems* (pp. 67–93). Mahwah, NJ: Erlbaum.

Heyman, R. E., & Neidig, P. H. (1997). Physical aggression couples treatment. In W. K. Halford & H. J. Markman (Eds.), *Clinical handbook of marriage and couples intervention* (pp. 589–617). Chichester, UK: Wiley.

Hiew, D. N., Halford, W. K., van de Vijver, F. J. R., & Liu, S. (2015). The Chinese-Western Intercultural Couple Standards Scale. *Psychological Assessment, 27*, 816–826.

Hilton, J. M., & Devall, E. L. (1997). The Family Economic Strain Scale: Development and evaluation of the instrument with single- and two-parent families. *Journal of Family and Economic Issues 18*, 247–271.

Hodge, D. R. (2005). Spiritual ecograms: A new assessment instrument for identifying clients' strengths in space and across time. *Families in Society, 86*, 287–296.

Hofmann, S. G., & Asmundson, G. J. G (2017). *The science of cognitive behavioral therapy*. San Diego, CA: Academic Press.

Holland, A. S., & McElwain, N. L. (2013). Maternal and paternal perceptions of coparenting as a link between marital quality and the parent–toddler relationship. *Journal of Family Psychology, 27*, 117–126.

Holmberg, M., Arver, S., & Dhejne, C. (2020). Improving sexual function and pleasure in transgender persons. In K. S. K. Hall & Y. M. Binik (Eds.), *Principles and practice of sex therapy* (6th ed., pp. 423–452). New York: Guilford Press.

Holzapfel, J., Randall, A., Tao, C., & Iida, M. (2018). Intercultural couples' internal stress, relationship satisfaction, and dyadic coping. *Interpersona: An International Journal on Personal Relationships, 12*, 145–163.

Hooley, J. M. (2007). Expressed emotion and relapse of psychopathology. *Annual Review of Clinical Psychology, 3*, 329–352.

Hooley, J. M., & Miklowitz, D. J. (2018). Families and mental disorders. In J. N. Butcher & J. M. Hooley (Eds.), *APA handbook of psychopathology: Psychopathology: Understanding, assessing, and treating adult mental disorders* (pp. 687–703). Washington, DC: American Psychological Association.

Hrapczynski, K. M., Epstein, N. B., Werlinich, C. A., & LaTaillade, J. J. (2011). Changes in negative attributions during couple therapy for abusive behavior: Relations to changes in satisfaction and behavior. *Journal of Marital and Family Therapy, 38*, 117–132.

Ivanova, M. Y., Achenbach, T. M., Rescorla, L. A., Turner, L. V., Ahmeti-Pronaj, A., Au, A., . . . Zasepa, E. (2015). Syndromes of self-reported psychopathology for ages 18–59 in 29 societies. *Journal of Psychopathology and Behavioral Assessment, 37*, 171–183.

Jacobson, N. S., & Christensen, A. (1996). *Integrative couple therapy: Promoting acceptance and change*. New York: Norton.

Jacobson, N. S., & Margolin, G. (1979). *Marital therapy: Strategies based on social learning and behavior exchange principles*. New York: Brunner/Mazel.

Jacobson, N. S., & Truax, P. (1991). Clinical significance: A statistical approach to defining meaningful change in psychotherapy research. *Journal of Consulting and Clinical Psychology, 59*, 12–19.

Janoff-Bulman, R. (1992). *Shattered assumptions: Towards a new psychology of trauma*. New York: The Free Press.

Jeanfreau, M. M., Jurich, A. P., & Mong, M. D. (2014).

Risk factors associated with women's marital infidelity. *Contemporary Family Therapy, 36,* 327–332.

Johnson, M. P. (1995). Patriarchal terrorism and common couple violence: Two forms of violence against women. *Journal of Marriage and the Family, 57,* 283–294.

Johnson, M. P. (2006). Conflict and control: Gender symmetry and asymmetry in domestic violence. *Violence against Women, 12,* 1003–1018.

Johnson, S. M. (1996). *The practice of emotionally focused marital therapy.* New York: Brunner/Mazel.

Johnson, S. M., Simakhodskaya, Z., & Moran, M. (2018). Addressing issues of sexuality in couples therapy: Emotionally Focused Therapy meets sex therapy. *Current Sexual Health Reports, 10*(2), 65–71.

Johnson, S. M., Wiebe, S. A., & Allan, R. (2023). Emotionally focused couple therapy. In J. L. Lebow & D. K. Snyder (Eds.), *Clinical handbook of couple therapy* (6th ed., pp. 127–150). New York: Guilford Press.

Jose, A., & O'Leary, K. D. (2009). Prevalence of partner aggression in representative and clinic samples. In K. D. O'Leary & E. M. Woodin (Eds.), *Psychological and physical aggression in couples: Causes and interventions* (pp. 15–35). Washington, DC: American Psychological Association.

Kahn, S. Y., Epstein, N. B., & Kivlighan, D. M. (2015). Couple therapy for partner aggression: Effects on individual and relational well-being. *Journal of Couple and Relationship Therapy. 14,* 95–115.

Kaplan, H. S. (1974). *The new sex therapy.* New York: Brunner/Mazel.

Kar, H. L., & Garcia-Moreno, C. (2009). Partner aggression across cultures. In K. D. O'Leary & E. M. Woodin (Eds.), *Psychological and physical aggression in couples: Causes and interventions* (pp. 59–75). Washington, DC: American Psychological Association.

Karam, E., & Sprenkle, D. (2010). The research-informed clinician: A guide to training the next generation MFT. *Journal of Marital and Family Therapy, 36,* 307–319.

Kaufman, E. A., Xia, M., Fosco, G., Yaptangco, M., Skidmore, C. R., & Crowell, S. E. (2016). The Difficulties in Emotion Regulation Scale Short Form (DERS-SF): Validation and replication in adolescent and adult samples. *Journal of Psychopathology and Behavioral Assessment, 38,* 443–455.

Kazdin, A. E. (2009). *The Kazdin method for parenting the defiant child.* Boston: Houghton Mifflin Harcourt.

Kennedy, B. (2022). *Good inside: A guide to becoming the parent you want to be.* New York: HarperCollins.

Kerig, P. K., & Baucom, D. H. (Eds.) (2004). *Couple observational coding systems.* New York: Routledge.

Kerr, M. E., & Bowen, M. (1988). *Family evaluation: An approach based on Bowen theory.* New York: Norton.

Kessler, R. C., Berglund, P., Demler, O., Jin, R., Merikangas, K. R., & Walters, E. E. (2005). Lifetime prevalence and age-of-onset distributions of DSM-IV disorders in the National Comorbidity Survey Replication. *Archives of General Psychiatry, 62,* 593–602.

Khan, T., Österman, K., & Björkqvist, K. (2019). Victimization from three types of intimate partner aggression and mental health concomitants among women in Pakistan. *Journal of Educational, Health and Community Psychology, 8,* 355–374.

Killian, K. D. (2015). Couple therapy and intercultural relationships. In A. S. Gurman, J. L. Lebow, & D. K. Snyder (Eds.), *Clinical handbook of couple therapy* (5th ed., pp. 512–528). New York: Guilford Press.

Kim, H., Epstein, N. B., Hancock, G. R., Hurtado, G. A., Svetaz, M. V., & Allen, M. (2022). Latent change modeling of Latino parent–child conflict and pathways to mental health. *Journal of Marriage and Family, 85,* 518–538.

Kinnunen, U., & Feldt, T. (2004). Economic stress and marital adjustment among couples: Analyses at the dyadic level. *European Journal of Social Psychology, 34,* 519–532.

Kissil, K., Carneiro, R., & Aponte, H. (2018). Beyond duality: The relationship between the personal and the professional selves of the therapist in the Person of the Therapist Training. *Journal of Family Psychotherapy, 29 ,*71–86.

Kleinplatz, P. J., Charest, M., Paradis, N., Rosen, L., & Ramsay, T. O. (2022). The effectiveness of in-person versus remote group couples therapy for the treatment of low sexual desire or frequency. *Journal of Sexual Medicine, 19,* S156–S157.

Knobloch-Fedders, L. M., Pinsoff, W. M., & Mann, B. J. (2004). The formation of the therapeutic alliance in couple therapy. *Family Process, 43,* 425–442.

Knudson-Martin, C., & Kim, L. (2023). Socioculturally attuned couple therapy. In J. L. Lebow & D. K. Snyder (Eds.), *Clinical handbook of couple therapy* (6th ed., pp. 267–291). New York: Guilford Press.

Knudson-Martin, C., McDowell, T., & Bermudez, J. M. (2020). Sociocultural attunement in systemic family therapy. In K. S. Wampler (Ed.), *The handbook of systemic family therapy* (Vol. 1, pp. 619–637). New York: Wiley Blackwell.

Kotov, R., Chang, S-W., Fochtmann, L. J., Mojtabai, R., Carlson, G. A., Sedler, M. J., & Bromet, E. J. (2011). Schizophrenia in the internalizing-externalizing framework: A third dimension? *Schizophrenia Bulletin, 37,* 1168–1178.

Krahé, B., & Abbey, A. (2013). Guest editorial: Intimate partner violence as a global problem: International and interdisciplinary perspectives. *International Journal of Conflict and Violence, 7,* 198–202.

Krahé, B., Bieneck, S., & Möller, I. (2005). Partner violence from an international perspective. *Sex Roles, 52,* 807–827.

Kröger, C., Reißner, T., Vasterling, I., Schütz, K., & Kliem, S. (2012). Therapy for couples after an affair:

A randomized-controlled trial. *Behaviour Research and Therapy, 50,* 786–796.

Kwok, S., & Wong, D. (2000). Mental health of parents with young children in Hong Kong: The roles of parenting stress and parenting self-efficacy. *Child and Family Social Work, 5,* 57–65.

Labrecque, L. T., & Whisman, M. A. (2017). Attitudes toward and prevalence of extramarital sex and descriptions of extramarital partners in the 21st century. *Journal of Family Psychology, 31,* 952–957.

LaTaillade, J. J., Epstein, N. B., & Werlinich, C. A. (2006). Conjoint treatment of intimate partner violence: A cognitive behavioral approach. *Journal of Cognitive Psychotherapy, 20,* 393–410.

Laumann, E., Gagnon, J., Michael, R., & Michaels, S. (1994). *The social organization of sexuality: Sexual practices in the United States.* Chicago: University of Chicago.

Laumann, E., Paik, A., & Rosen, R. (1999). Sexual dysfunction in the United States: Prevalence and perspectives. *Journal of the American Medical Association, 261,* 537–544.

Lazarus, R. S., & Folkman, S. (1984). *Stress, appraisal, and coping.* New York: Springer.

Le, Y., Treter, M. O., Roddy, M. K., & Doss, B. D. (2021). Coparenting and parenting outcomes of online relationship interventions for low-income couples. *Journal of Family Psychology, 35,* 1033–1039.

Leahy, R. L. (1996). *Cognitive therapy: Basic principles and applications.* Northvale, NJ: Jason Aronson.

Leahy, R. L. (2007). Schematic mismatch in the therapeutic relationship: A social cognitive model. In P. Gilbert & R. L. Leahy (Eds.), *The therapeutic relationship in the cognitive behavioral psychotherapies* (pp. 229–254). New York: Routledge.

Leahy, R. L. (2015). *Emotional schema therapy.* New York: Guilford Press.

Leahy, R. L. (2017). *Cognitive therapy techniques: A practitioner's guide* (2nd ed.). New York: Guilford Press.

Leahy, R. L. (2019). *Emotional schema therapy: Distinctive features.* New York: Routledge.

Leahy, R. L., Holland, S. J. F., & McGinn, L. K. (2012). *Treatment plans and interventions for depression and anxiety disorders* (2nd ed.). New York: Guilford Press.

Lebow, J., & Snyder, D. K. (2022). Couple therapy in the 2020s: Current status and emerging developments. *Family Process, 61,* 1359–1385.

Lebow, J. L., & Snyder, D. K. (Eds.). (2023). *Clinical handbook of couple therapy* (6th ed.). New York: Guilford Press.

Leeker, O., & Carlozzi, A. (2014). Effects of sex, sexual orientation, infidelity expectations, and love on distress related to emotional and sexual infidelity. *Journal of Marital and Family Therapy, 40,* 68–91.

Lev, A. I. (2004). *The complete lesbian and gay parenting guide.* New York: Berkley Books.

Leventhal, A. M. & Zvolensky, M. J. (2015). Anxiety, depression, and cigarette smoking: A transdiagnostic vulnerability framework to understanding emotion–smoking comorbidity. *Psychological Bulletin, 141,* 176–212.

Levine, S. B. (2014). Infidelity. In Y. M. Binik & K. S. K. Hall (Eds.), *Principles and practice of sex therapy* (5th ed., pp. 399–415). New York: Guilford Press.

Levine, S., Risen, C., & Althof, S. (2016). *Handbook of clinical sexuality for mental health professionals* (3rd ed.). New York: Routledge.

Linehan, M. M. (1993). *Cognitive-behavioral treatment of borderline personality disorder.* New York: Guilford Press.

Linehan, M. M. (2015). *DBT skills training handouts and worksheets* (2nd ed.). New York: Guilford Press.

Long, L. L., Burnett, J. A., & Valorie Thomas, R. (2006). *Sexuality counseling: An integrative approach.* London: Pearson.

Lusterman, D. D. (2005). Marital infidelity: The effects of delayed traumatic reaction. *Journal of Couple and Relationship Therapy, 4,* 71–81.

Macintosh, H. B., Hall, J., & Johnson, S. M. (2007). Forgive and forget: A comparison of emotionally focused and cognitive behavioral models of forgiveness and intervention in the context of couple infidelity. In P. R. Peluso (Ed.), *Infidelity: A practitioner's guide to working with couples in crisis* (pp. 127–148). New York: Routledge.

Mackay, J., Bowen, E., Walker, K., & O'Doherty, L. (2018). Risk factors for female perpetrators of intimate partner violence within criminal justice settings: A systematic review. *Aggression and Violent Behavior, 41,* 128–146.

Marcu, I., Oppenheim, D., & Koren-Karie, N. (2016). Parental insightfulness is associated with cooperative interactions in families with toddlers. *Journal of Family Psychology, 30,* 927–934.

Marcus, D. K., Hughes, K. T., & Arnau, R. C. (2008). Health anxiety, rumination, and negative affect: A mediational analysis. *Journal of Psychosomatic Research, 64,* 495–501.

Margolin, G., Gordis, E. B., & John, R. S. (2001). Coparenting: A link between marital conflict and parenting in two-parent families. *Journal of Family Psychology, 15,* 3–21.

Mark, K. P., & Schuman, D. L. (2020). A scoping review of the practice recommendations of secrets in couple's therapy. *Journal of Family Psychotherapy, 31,* 56–71.

Markman, H. J., & Rhoades, G. K. (2012). Relationship education research: Current status and future directions. *Journal of Marital and Family Therapy, 38,* 169–200.

Markman, H. J., Stanley, S. M., & Blumberg, S. L. (2010). *Fighting for your marriage: Positive steps for preventing divorce and preserving a lasting love* (3rd ed.). San Francisco: Jossey-Bass.

Markus, H. R. (2004). Culture and personality: Brief for

an arranged marriage. *Journal of Research in Personality, 38*, 75–83.

Martell, C. R., & Prince, S. E. (2005). Treating infidelity in same-sex couples. *Journal of Clinical Psychology, 61*, 1429–1438.

Martin, D. J., Garske, J. P., & Davis, M. K. (2000). Relation of the therapeutic alliance with outcome and other variables: A meta-analytic review. *Journal of Consulting and Clinical Psychology, 68*, 438–450.

Masters, W., & Johnson, V. (1966). *Human sexual response*. Boston: Little, Brown.

Masters, W. M., & Johnson, V. (1970). *Human sexual inadequacy*. Boston: Little, Brown.

Mastromanno, B. K., Kehoe, C. E., Wood, C. E., & Havighurst, S. E. (2021). A randomized-controlled pilot study of the one-to-one delivery of Tuning in to Kids: Impact on emotion socialization, reflective functioning, and childhood behaviour problems. *Emotional and Behavioural Difficulties, 26*, 359–374.

Mauss, I. B., & Butler, E. A. (2010). Cultural context moderates the relationship between emotion control values and cardiovascular challenge versus threat responses. *Biological Psychology, 84*, 521–530.

McCabe K., & Yeh M. (2009). Parent-Child Interaction Therapy for Mexican Americans: A randomized clinical trial. *Journal of Clinical Child and Adolescent Psychology, 38*, 753– 759.

McClelland, D. C. (1987). *Human motivation*. Cambridge, UK: Cambridge University Press.

McCool-Myers, M., Theurich, M., Zuelke, A., Knuettel, H., & Apfelbacher, C. (2018). Predictors of female sexual dysfunction: A systematic review and qualitative analysis through gender inequality paradigms. *BMC Women's Health, 18*(1), 108.

McCrady, B. S., Epstein, E. E., & Holzhauer, C. G. (2023). Couple therapy for alcohol problems. In J. L. Lebow & D. K. Snyder (Eds.), *Clinical handbook of couple therapy* (6th ed., pp. 554–575). New York: Guilford Press.

McDowell, T., Knudson-Martin, C., & Bermudez, M. J. (2022). *Socioculturally attuned therapy* (2nd ed.). New York: Routledge.

McEvoy, P. M., Nathan, P., & Norton, P. J. (2009). Efficacy of transdiagnostic treatments: A review of published outcome studies and future research directions. *Journal of Cognitive Psychotherapy, 23*, 20–33.

McGoldrick, M., Gerson, R., & Petry, S. (2020). *Genograms: Assessment and treatment* (4th ed.). New York: Norton.

McHale, J. P. (2011). Assessing coparenting. In J. P. McHale & K. M. Lindahl (Eds.), *Coparenting: A conceptual and clinical examination of family systems* (pp. 147–170). Washington, DC: American Psychological Association.

McHale, J. P., & Irace, K. (2011). Coparenting in diverse family systems. In J. P. McHale & K. M. Lindahl (Eds.). *Coparenting: A conceptual and clinical examina-*

tion of family systems (pp. 15–37). Washington, DC: American Psychological Association.

McHale, J. P., & Lindahl, K. M. (Eds.). (2011). *Coparenting: A conceptual and clinical examination of family systems*. Washington, DC: American Psychological Association.

McNally, R. J. (2002). Anxiety sensitivity and panic disorder. *Biological Psychiatry, 52*, 938–946.

Meichenbaum, D. (1977). *Cognitive-behavior modification*. New York: Plenum.

Meichenbaum, D. (1985). *Stress inoculation training*. New York: Pergamon Press.

Messinger, A. M. (2011). Invisible victims: Same-sex IPV in the national violence against women survey. *Journal of Interpersonal Violence, 26*, 2228–2243.

Metz, M. E., & Epstein, N. B. (2002). Assessing the role of relationship conflict in sexual dysfunction. *Journal of Sex and Marital Therapy, 28*, 139–164.

Metz, M. E., Epstein, N. B., & McCarthy, B. (2018). *Cognitive-behavioral therapy for sexual dysfunction*. New York: Routledge.

Metz, M. E., & McCarthy, B. W. (2011). *Enduring desire: Your guide to lifelong intimacy*. New York: Routledge.

Meyer, I. H. (2003). Prejudice, social stress, and mental health in lesbian, gay, and bisexual populations: Conceptual issues and research evidence. *Psychological Bulletin, 129*, 674–697.

Meyers, R. J., Smith, J. E., Serna, B., & Belon, K. E. (2013). Community reinforcement approaches: CRA and CRAFT. In P. M. Miller (Ed.), *Interventions for addiction: Comprehensive addictive behaviors and disorders* (Vol. 3, pp. 47–55). San Diego, CA: Academic Press.

Midy, T. (2018). The examination of discrimination and social bias toward interracial relationships. *Graduate Dissertations and Theses, 84*. Available at *https://orb.binghamton.edu/cgi/viewcontent.cgi?article=1089&context=dissertation_and_theses*.

Mikulincer, M., & Shaver, P. R. (2016). *Attachment in adulthood: Structure, dynamics, and change* (2nd ed.). New York: Guilford Press.

Miller, R. B., Yorgason, J. B., Sandberg, J., & White, M. B., 2003). Problems that couples bring to therapy: A view across the family life cycle. *The American Journal of Family Therapy, 31*, 395–407.

Mistry, R. S., Vandewater, E. A., Huston, A. C., & McLoyd, V. C. (2002). Economic well-being and children's social adjustment: The role of family process in an ethnically diverse low-income sample. *Child Development, 73*, 935–951.

Miyamoto, Y., Ma, X., & Petermann, A. G. (2014). Cultural differences in hedonic emotion regulation after a negative event. *Emotion, 14*, 804–815.

Moller, N. P., & Vossler, A. (2015). Defining infidelity in research and couple counseling: A qualitative study. *Journal of Sex and Marital Therapy, 41*, 487–497.

Monson, C. M., & Fredman, S. J. (2012). *Cognitive-*

behavioral conjoint therapy for posttraumatic stress disorder: Harnessing the healing power of relationships. New York: Guilford Press.

Monson, C. M., & Fredman, S. J. (2023). Couple therapy for posttraumatic stress disorder. In J. L. Lebow & D. K. Snyder (Eds.), *Clinical handbook of couple therapy* (6th ed., pp. 533–553). New York: Guilford Press.

Moors, A. C., Matsick, J. L., Ziegler, A., Rubin, J. D., & Conley, T. D. (2013). Stigma toward individuals engaged in consensual nonmonogamy: Robust and worthy of additional research. *Analyses of Social Issues and Public Policy, 13,* 52–69.

Mueser, K. T., & Gingerich, S. (2006). *The complete family guide to schizophrenia.* New York: Guilford Press.

Mumford, D. J., & Weeks, G. R. (2003). The money genogram. *Journal of Family Psychotherapy, 14*(3), 33–44.

Murphy, C. M., & Eckhardt, C. I. (2005). *Treating the abusive partner: An individualized cognitive-behavioral approach.* New York: Guilford Press.

Murphy, C. M., & Hoover, S. A. (1999). Measuring emotional abuse in dating relationships as a multifactorial construct. *Violence and Victims, 14,* 39–53.

Murphy, S. E., Jacobvitz, D. B., & Hazen, N. L. (2016). What's so bad about competitive coparenting? Family-level predictors of children's externalizing symptoms. *Journal of Child and Family Studies, 25,* 1684–1690.

Murray, D. W., Rosanbalm, K., & Christopoulos, C. (2016). *Self-regulation and toxic stress: Implications for programs and practice.* Report #2015–97 to the Office of Planning, Research and Evaluation, Administration for Children and Families, U.S. Department of Health and Human Services.

Naragon-Gainey, K. (2010). Meta-analysis of the relations of anxiety sensitivity to the depressive and anxiety disorders. *Psychological Bulletin, 136,* 128–150.

Negy, C., & Snyder, D. K. (2000). Relationship satisfaction of Mexican American and nonHispanic White American interethnic couples: Issues of acculturation and clinical intervention. *Journal of Marital and Family Therapy, 26,* 293–304.

Nelson, T. (Ed.). (2020). *Integrative sex and couples therapy: A therapist's guide to new and innovative approaches.* Eau Claire, WI: PESI Publishing and Media.

Neppl, T. K., Senia, J. M., & Donnellan, M. B. (2016). Effects of economic hardship: Testing the family stress model over time. *Journal of Family Psychology, 30,* 12–21.

Newman, C. F. (2018). Cognitive-behavioral therapy for the reduction of suicide risk. In R. L. Leahy (Ed.), *Science and practice in cognitive therapy: Foundations, mechanisms, and applications* (pp. 233–252). New York: Guilford Press.

Nezu, A. M., Nezu, C. M., & Hays, A. M. (2019). Emotion-centered problem-solving therapy. In K. S. Dobson & D. J. A. Dozois (Eds.), *Handbook of cognitive-behavioral therapies* (4th ed., pp. 171–190). New York: Guilford Press.

Ng, Y. K. (2002). East-Asian happiness gap. *Pacific Economic Review, 7,* 51–63.

Nichols, M. (2014). *Therapy with LGBTQ clients.* In Y. M. Binik & K. S. K. Hall (Eds.), *Principles and practice of sex therapy* (5th ed., pp. 309–333). New York: Guilford Press.

Nichols, M. P., & Davis, S. (2016). *Family therapy: Concepts and methods* (11th ed.). Hoboken, NJ: Pearson.

Niec, L. N. (Ed.) (2018). *Handbook of Parent-Child Interaction Therapy: Innovations and applications for research and practice.* Cham, Switzerland: Springer Nature.

Nolen-Hoeksema, S., Stice, E., Wade, E., & Bohon, C. (2007). Reciprocal relations between rumination and bulimic, substance abuse, and depressive symptoms in female adolescents. *Journal of Abnormal Psychology, 116,* 198–207.

Nolen-Hoeksema, S., & Watkins, E. R. (2011). A heuristic for developing transdiagnostic models of psychopathology: Explaining multifinality and divergent trajectories. *Perspectives on Psychological Science, 6,* 589–609.

Northey, W. F. (2002). Characteristics and clinical practices of marriage and family therapists: A national survey. *Journal of Marital and Family Therapy, 28,* 487–494.

Norton, P. J. (2012). *Group cognitive-behavioral therapy of anxiety: A transdiagnostic treatment manual.* New York: Guilford Press.

Norton, P. J., & Philipp, L. M. (2008). Transdiagnostic approaches to the treatment of anxiety disorders: A quantitative review. *Psychotherapy: Theory, Research, Practice, Training, 45,* 214–226.

Nunes, C. E., Pascual-Leone, A., de Roten, Y., Favez, N., & Darwiche, J. (2020). Resolving coparenting dissatisfaction in couples: A preliminary task analysis study. *Journal of Marital and Family Therapy, 47,* 21–35.

Nussbeck, F. W., & Jackson, J. B. (2016). Measuring dyadic coping across cultures. In M. K. Falconier, A. K. Randall, & G. Bodenmann (Eds.), *Couples coping with stress: A cross-cultural perspective* (pp. 36–53). New York: Routledge.

O'Farrell, T. J., & Fals-Stewart, W. (2006). *Behavioral couples therapy for alcoholism and drug abuse.* New York: Guilford Press.

O'Farrell, T. J., Murphy, C. M., Stephan, S. H., Fals-Stewart, W., & Murphy, M. (2004). Partner violence before and after couples-based alcoholism treatment for male alcoholic patients: The role of treatment involvement and abstinence. *Journal of Consulting and Clinical Psychology, 72,* 202–217.

Olayide, O., & Clisdell, E. (2017). Intimate partner violence prevention and reduction: A review of literature. *Health Care for Women International, 38,* 439–462.

O'Leary, K. D. (2008). Couple therapy and physical aggression. In A. S. Gurman (Ed.), *Clinical handbook of couple therapy* (4th ed., pp. 478–498). New York: Guilford Press.

O'Leary, K. D. (2015). Time for dyadic treatments for low-level partner aggression. *Journal of Clinical Psychiatry, 76,* e824–825.

O'Leary, K. D., & Maiuro, R. D. (2001). *Psychological abuse in violent domestic relations.* New York: Springer.

O'Leary, K. D., Smith Slep, A. M., & O'Leary, S. G. (2007). Multivariate models of men's and women's partner aggression. *Journal of Consulting and Clinical Psychology, 75,* 752–764.

Papernow, P. L. (2023). Therapy with stepfamily couples. In J. L. Lebow & D. K. Snyder (Eds.)., *Clinical handbook of couple therapy* (6th ed., pp. 492–511). New York: Guilford Press.

Papp, L. M., Cummings, E. M., & Goeke-Morey, M. C. (2009). For richer, for poorer: Money as a topic of marital conflict in the home. *Family Relations, 58,* 91–103.

Parra Cardona, J., Holtrop, K., Cordóva, D., Escobar-Chew, A. R., Horsford, S., Tams, L., . . . Fitzgerald, H. E. (2009). "Queremos aprender": Latino immigrants' call to integrate cultural adaptation with best practice knowledge in a parenting intervention. *Family Process, 48,* 211–231.

Parra Cardona, J. R., Domenech-Rodriguez, M., Forgatch, M., Sullivan, C., Bybee, D., Holtrop, K., . . . Bernal, G. (2012). Culturally adapting an evidence-based parenting intervention for Latino immigrants: The need to integrate fidelity and cultural relevance. *Family Process, 51,* 56–72.

Pascoe, E. A., & Richman, S. L. (2009). Perceived discrimination and health: A meta-analytic review. *Psychological Bulletin, 135,* 531–554.

Patterson, G. R. (1982). *Coercive family process.* Eugene, OR: Castalia.

Patterson, L. Q. P., Handy, A. B., & Brotto, L. A. (2017). A pilot study of eight-session mindfulness-based cognitive therapy adapted for women's sexual interest/arousal disorder. *Journal of Sex Research, 54,* 850–861.

Peacock, E. J., & Wong, P. T. P. (1990). Stress appraisal measures (SAM): A multidimensional approach to cognitive appraisals. *Stress Medicine, 6,* 227–236.

Pepping, C. A., Halford, W. K., Cronin, T. J., & Lyons, A. (2020). Couple relationship education for same-sex couples: A preliminary evaluation of Rainbow Couple CARE. *Journal of Couple and Relationship Therapy, 19,* 230–249.

Perez, J. E., Riggio, R. E., & Kopelowicz, A. (2007). Social skill imbalances in mood disorders and schizophrenia. *Personality and Individual Differences, 42,* 27–36.

Pew Research Center. (2015, June 2). Interfaith marriage is common in U.S., particularly among the recently wed. Available at *www.pewresearch.org/fact-tank/2015/06/02/interfaith-marriage.*

Pew Research Center. (2017a, May 18). Intermarriage in the U.S. 50 years after *Loving v. Virginia.* Available at *www.pewresearch.org/social-trends/2017/05/18/intermarriage-in-the-u-s-50-years-after-loving-v-virginia.*

Pew Research Center. (2017b, November 15). Assaults against Muslims in U.S. surpass 2001 level. Available at *www.pewresearch.org/fact-tank/2017/11/15/assaults-against-muslims-in-u-s-surpass-2001-level.*

Pew Research Center. (2019). Marriage and cohabitation in the U.S. Available at *www.pewresearch.org/social-trends/2019/11/06/marriage-and-cohabitation-in-the-u-s.*

Pew Research Center. (2020, July 22). Before COVID-19, Many Latinos worried about their place in America and had experienced discrimination. Available at *www.pewresearch.org/fact-tank/2020/07/22/before-covid-19-many-latinos-worried-about-their-place-in-america-and-had-experienced-discrimination.*

Pew Research Center. (2021a, March 18). Majority of Americans see at least some discrimination against Black, Hispanic, and Asian people in the U.S. Available at *www.pewresearch.org/fact-tank/2021/03/18/majorities-of-americans-see-at-least-some-discrimination-against-black-hispanic-and-asian-people-in-the-u-s.*

Pew Research Center. (2021b, April 11). One-third of Asian Americans fear threats, physical attacks and most say violence against them is rising. Available at *www.pewresearch.org/fact-tank/2021/04/21/one-third-of-asian-americans-fear-threats-physical-attacks-and-most-say-violence-against-them-is-rising.*

Pew Research Center. (2021c, May 11). Jewish Americans in 2020. Available at *www.pewforum.org/2021/05/11/marriage-families-and-children.*

Pew Research Center. (2021d, July 7). On some demographic measures, people in same-sex marriages differ from those in opposite-sex marriages. Available at *www.pewresearch.org/fact-tank/2021/07/07/on-some-demographic-measures-people-in-same-sex-marriages-differ-from-those-in-opposite-sex-marriages.*

Pico-Alfonso, M. A., Garcia-Linares, M. I., Celda-Navarro, N., Blasco-Ros, C., Echeburúa, E., & Martinez, M. (2006). The impact of physical, psychological, and sexual intimate male partner violence on women's mental health: Depressive symptoms, posttraumatic stress disorder, state anxiety, and suicide. *Journal of Women's Health, 15,* 599–611.

Pittman, P. S., Kamp Dush, C., Pratt, K. J., & Wong, J. D. (2023). Interracial couples at risk: Discrimination, well-being, and health. *Journal of Family Issues.* Available at *https://doi.org/10.1177/0192513X221150994.*

Planalp, S., Fitness, J., & Fehr, B. A. (2018). The roles of emotion in relationships. In A. L. Vangelisti & D. Perlman (Eds.), *The Cambridge handbook of personal relationships* (2nd ed., pp. 256–267). Cambridge, UK: Cambridge University Press.

Poulsen, S. S. (2003). Therapists' perspectives on working with interracial couples. In V. Thomas, T. A. Karis, & J. L. Wetchler (Eds.), *Clinical issues with interracial couples: Theories and research* (pp. 163–177). New York: Haworth.

Prado, G., & Pantin, H. (2011). Reducing substance use and HIV health disparities among Hispanic youth in the U.S.A.: The Familias Unidas program of research. *Intervención Psicosocial, 20*, 63–73.

Prawitz, A. D., Garman, E. T., Sorhaindo, B., O'Neill, B., Kim, J., & Drentea, P. (2006). The Incharge Financial Distress/Financial Well-being Scale: Development, administration, and score interpretation. *Financial Counseling and Planning, 17*, 34–50.

Pretzer, J., Epstein, N., & Fleming, B. (1991). The Marital Attitude Survey: A measure of dysfunctional attributions and expectancies. *Journal of Cognitive Psychotherapy: An International Quarterly, 5*, 131–148.

Price, S. J., Price, C. A., & McKenry, P. C. (2010). Families coping with change: A conceptual overview. In S. J. Price, C. A. Price, & P. C. McKenry (Eds.), *Families and change: Coping with stressful events and transitions* (4th ed., pp. 1–23). Thousand Oaks, CA: Sage.

Pronk, T. M., Finkenauer, C., & Kuijer, R. G. (2017). Self-regulation in close relationships. In J. Fitzgerald (Ed.), *Foundations for couples' therapy: Research for the real world* (pp. 345–354). New York: Routledge.

Proulx, C., Helms, H., & Buehler, C. (2007). Marital quality and personal well-being: A meta-analysis. *Journal of Marriage and Family, 69*, 576–593.

Pruett, M. K., & Donsky, T. (2011). Coparenting after divorce: Paving pathways for parental cooperation, conflict resolution, and redefined family roles. In J. P. McHale & K. M. Lindahl (Eds.), *Coparenting: A conceptual and clinical examination of family systems* (pp. 231–250). Washington, DC: American Psychological Association.

Quinn, W. H., Dotson, D., & Jordan, K. (1997). Dimensions of therapeutic alliance and their associations with outcome in family therapy. *Psychotherapy Research, 7*, 429–438.

Rathus, J. H., & Sanderson, W. C. (1999). *Marital distress: Cognitive behavioral interventions for couples.* Northvale, NJ: Jason Aronson.

Raytek, H. S., McCrady, B. S., Epstein, E. E., & Hirsch, L. S. (1999). Therapeutic alliance and the retention of couples in conjoint alcoholism treatment. *Addictive Behaviors, 24*, 317–330.

Rehman, U. S., Gollan, J., & Mortimer, A. R. (2008). The marital context of depression: Research, limitations, and new directions. *Clinical Psychology Review, 28*, 179–198.

Reinholt, N., Aharoni, R., Winding, C., Rosenberg, N., Rosenbaum, B., & Arnfred, S. (2017). Transdiagnostic group CBT for anxiety disorders: The unified protocol in mental health services. *Cognitive Behaviour Therapy, 46*, 29–43.

Repond, G., Darwiche, J., El Ghaziri, N., & Antonietti,

J. (2019). Coparenting in stepfamilies: A cluster analysis. *Journal of Divorce and Remarriage, 60*, 211–233.

Resick, P. A. (2018). Cognitive therapy for posttraumatic stress disorder. In R. L. Leahy (Ed.), *Science and practice in cognitive therapy: Foundations, mechanisms, and applications* (pp. 358–375). New York: Guilford Press.

Revenstorf, D., Hahlweg, K., Schindler, L., & Vogel, B. (1984). Interaction analysis of marital conflict. In K. Hahlweg & N. S. Jacobson (Eds.), *Marital interaction: Analysis and modification* (pp. 159–181). New York: Guilford Press.

Rietmeijer, C. A., Bull, S. S., & McFarlane, M. (2001). Sex and the Internet. *AIDS, 15*, 1433–1434.

Riley, K. E., & Park, C. L. (2014). Problem-focused vs. meaning-focused coping as mediators of the appraisal-adjustment relationship in chronic stressors. *Journal of Social and Clinical Psychology, 33*, 587–611.

Risen, C. B. (2010). Listening to sexual stories. In S. B. Levine, C. B. Risen, & S. E. Althof (Eds.). *Handbook of clinical sexuality for mental health professionals* (2nd ed., pp. 3–20). New York: Routledge.

Rizvi, S. L., & King, A. M. (2019). Dialectical behavior therapy. In K. S. Dobson & D. J. A. Dozois (Eds.), *Handbook of cognitive-behavioral therapies* (4th ed., pp. 297–317). New York: Guilford Press.

Robert Wood Johnson Foundation. (2017a, October). *Discrimination in America: Experiences and views of African Americans.* Available at *file:///Users/mariana-falconier/Downloads/rwjf441128%20(2).pdf*.

Robert Wood Johnson Foundation. (2017b, November). *Discrimination in America: Experiences and views of Native Americans.* Available at: *file:///Users/mariana-falconier/Downloads/rwjf441678.pdf*.

Robila, M., & Krishnakumar, A. (2005). Effects of economic pressure on marital conflict in Romania. *Journal of Family Psychology, 19*, 246–251.

Rodriguez, J., McKay, M. M., & Bannon Jr., W. M., (2008). Role of racial socialization in relation to parenting practices and youth behavior: An exploratory analysis. *Social Work in Mental Health, 6*, 30–54.

Rollè, L., Giardina, G., Caldarera, A. M., Gerino, E., & Brustia, P. (2018). When intimate partner violence meets same sex couples: A review of same sex intimate partner violence. *Frontiers in Psychology, 9*, Article 1506. *https:/doi:10.3389/fpsyg.2018.01506*

Romano, D. (2001). *Intercultural marriage: Promises and pitfalls* (3rd ed.). Yarmouth, ME: Intercultural Press.

Roos, L. G., O'Connor, V., Canevello, A., & Bennett, J. M. (2018). Post-traumatic stress and psychological health following infidelity in unmarried young adults. *Stress and Health, 35*, 468–479.

Rosenbaum, A., & Kunkel, T. S. (2009). Group interventions for intimate partner violence. In K. D. O'Leary & E. M. Woodin (Eds.), *Psychological and physical aggression in couples: Causes and interventions* (pp. 191–210). Washington, DC: American Psychological Association.

Rosenblatt, P., & Stewart, C. C. (2004). Challenges in cross-cultural marriage: When she is Chinese and he Euro-American. *Sociology Focus, 37,* 43–58.

Roth, R. M., Isquith, P. K., & Gioia, G. A. (2005). *Behavior Rating Inventory of Executive Function—Adult Version.* Lutz, FL: Assessment Resources.

Rubel, A. N., & Bogaert, A. F. (2015). Consensual nonmonogamy: Psychological well-being and relationship quality correlates. *Journal of Sex Research, 52,* 961–982.

Rubinsky, V. (2019). Identity gaps and jealousy as predictors of satisfaction in polyamorous relationships. *Southern Communication Journal, 84,* 17–29.

Rutter, P. A. (2012). Sex therapy with gay male couples using affirmative therapy. *Sex and Relationship Therapy, 27,* 35–45.

Rutter, P. A., Leech, N. N., Anderson, M., & Saunders, D. (2010). Couples counseling for a transgender-lesbian couple: Student counselors' comfort and discomfort with sexuality counseling topics. *Journal of GLBT Family Studies, 6,* 68–79.

Rychlowska, M., Miyamoto, Y., Matsumoto, D., Hess, U., Gilboa-Schechtman, E., Kamble, S., . . . Niedenthal, P. M. (2015). Heterogeneity of long-history migration explains cultural differences in reports of emotional expressivity and the functions of smiles. *Proceedings of the National Academy of Sciences, 112,* E2429–E2436.

Safran, J. D., & Segal, Z. V. (1990). *Interpersonal process in cognitive therapy.* New York: Basic Books.

Sainii, M., Pruett, M. K., Alschech, J., & Suchchyk, A. R. (2019). A pilot study to assess coparenting across family structures (CoPAFS). *Journal of Child and Family Studies, 28,* 1392–1401.

Schachner, D. A., Shaver, P. R., & Mikulincer, M. (2003). Adult attachment theory, psychodynamics, and couple relationships: An overview. In S. M. Johnson & V. E. Whiffen (Eds.), *Attachment processes in couple and family therapy* (pp. 18–42). New York: Guilford Press.

Scheitle, C. P., & Ecklund, E. H. (2020). Individuals' experience with religious hostility, discrimination, and violence: Findings from a national survey. *Socius: Sociological Research for a Dynamic World.* https://doi.org/10.1177/2378023120967815

Schlesinger, S. E., & Epstein, N. B. (2007). Couple problems. In F. M. Dattilio & A. Freeman (Eds.), *Cognitive-behavioral strategies in crisis intervention* (3rd ed., pp. 300–326). New York: Guilford Press.

Schoppe-Sullivan, S. J., Mangelsdorf, S. C., Frosch, C. A., & McHale, J. L. (2004). Associations between coparenting and marital behavior from infancy to the preschool years. *Journal of Family Psychology, 18,* 194–207.

Schumacher, J. A., Feldbau-Kohn, S., Smith Slep, A. M., & Heyman, R. E. (2001). Risk factors for male-to-female partner physical abuse. *Aggression and Violent Behavior, 6,* 281–352.

Schumm, J. A., O'Farrell, T. J., Murphy, C. M., & Fals-Stewart, W. (2009). Partner violence before and after couples-based alcoholism treatment for female alcoholic patients. *Journal of Consulting and Clinical Psychology, 77,* 1136–1146.

Segrin, C. (2000). Social skills deficits associated with depression. *Clinical Psychology Review, 20,* 379–403.

Serban, I., Salvati, M., & Enea, V. (2022). Sexual orientation and infidelity-related behaviors on social media sites. *International Journal of Environmental Research in Public Health, 19,* 15659. Available at https://doi.org/10.3390/ijerph192315659.

Seshadri, G., & Knudson-Martin, C. (2013). How couples manage interracial and intercultural differences. Implications for clinical practice. *Journal of Marital and Family Therapy, 39,* 43–58.

Shadish, W. R., & Baldwin, S. A. (2003). Meta-analysis of MFT interventions. *Journal of Marital and Family Therapy, 29,* 547–570.

Shadish, W. R., & Baldwin, S. A. (2005). Effects of behavioral marital therapy: A meta-analysis of randomized controlled trials. *Journal of Consulting and Clinical Psychology, 73,* 6–14.

Sharara, F., GBD 2019 Police Violence US Subnational Collaborators, & Wool, E. E. (2021). Fatal police violence by race and state in the USA, 1980–2019: A network meta-regression. *The Lancet, 398,* 1239–1255.

Shelton, M. (2013). *Family pride: What LGBT families should know about navigating home, school, and safety in their neighborhoods.* Boston: Beacon Press.

Simons, J. S., & Carey, M. P. (2001). Prevalence of sexual dysfunctions: Results from a decade of research. *Archives of Sexual Behavior, 30,* 177–219.

Sims, T., Tsai, J. L., Jiang, D., Wang, Y., Fung, H. H., & Zhang, X. (2015). Wanting to maximize the positive and minimize the negative: Implications for mixed affective experience in American and Chinese contexts. *Journal of Personality and Social Psychology, 109,* 292–315.

Singh, R., Killian, K. D., Bhugun, D., & Tseng, S-T. (2020). Clinical work with intercultural couples. In K. S. Wampler & A. J. Blow (Eds.), *The handbook of systemic family therapy* (Vol. 3, pp. 155–183). New York: Wiley.

Singla, R. (2015). *Intermarriage and mixed parenting, promoting mental health and wellbeing: Crossover love.* New York: Palgrave Macmillan.

Skinner, A. L., & Hudac, C. M. (2017). "Yuck, you disgust me!" Affective bias against interracial couples. *Journal of Experimental Social Psychology, 68,* 68–77.

Skinner, B. F. (1953). *Science and human behavior.* New York: Macmillan.

Skinner, B. F. (1971). *Beyond freedom and dignity.* New York: Knopf.

Slep, A. M., Foran, H. M., Heyman, R. E., & Snarr, J. D.

(2010). Unique risk and protective factors for partner aggression in a large scale Air Force survey. *Journal of Community Health, 35,* 375–383.

Snyder, D. K. (1997). *Marital Satisfaction Inventory—Revised (MSI-R).* Torrance, CA: Western Psychological Services.

Snyder, D. K., Baucom, D. H., & Gordon, K. C. (2007). *Getting past the affair: A program to help you cope, heal, and move on—together or apart.* New York: Guilford Press.

Snyder, D. K., & Mitchell, A. E. (2008). Affective-reconstructive couple therapy. In A. S. Gurman (Ed.), *Clinical handbook of couple therapy* (4th ed., pp. 353–382). New York: Guilford Press.

Solomon, S. (n.d.). Money habitudes. Available at *www.moneyhabitudes.com.*

Solomon, S. E., Rothblum, E. D., & Balsam, K. F. (2005). Money, housework, sex, and conflict: Same-sex couples in civil unions, those not in civil unions, and heterosexual married siblings. *Sex Roles, 52* (9/10), 561–575.

Soloski, K. L., & Deitz, S. L. (2016). Managing emotional responses in therapy: An adapted EFT supervision approach. *Contemporary Family Therapy, 38,* 361–372.

Spanier, G. B. (1976). Measuring dyadic adjustment: New scales for assessing the quality of marriage and similar dyads. *Journal of Marriage and the Family, 38,* 15–28.

Spector, I. P., Carey, M. P., & Steinberg, L. (1996). The Sexual Desire Inventory: Development, factor structure, and evidence of reliability. *Journal of Sex and Marital Therapy, 22,* 175–190.

Spencer, K. G., Iantaffi, A., & Bockting, W. (2017). Treating sexual problems in transgender clients. In Z. D. Peterson (Ed.), *The Wiley handbook of sex therapy* (pp. 291–305). Chichester, UK: Wiley.

Spitzer, R. L., Kroenke, K., Williams, J. B. W., & Lowe, B. (2006). A brief measure for assessing generalized anxiety disorder. *Archives of Internal Medicine, 166,* 1092–1097.

Spivak, H. R., Jenkins, E. L., VanAudenhove, K., Lee, D., Kelly, M., & Iskander, J. (2014). CDC grand rounds: A public health approach to prevention of intimate partner violence. *Morbidity and Mortality Weekly Report, 63*(2), 38–41.

Sprenkle, D. H., Davis, S. D., & Lebow, J. L. (2009). *Common factors in couple and family therapy.* New York: Guilford Press.

Spring, J. A. (2020). *After the affair: Healing the pain and rebuilding trust when a partner has been unfaithful* (3rd ed.). New York: HarperCollins.

St. Vil, N. M., Leblanc, N. M., & Giles, K. N. (2021). The who and why of consensual nonmonogamy among African Americans. *Archives of Sexual Behavior, 50,* 1143–1150.

Stanley, S. M., Rhoades, G. K., & Markman, H. J. (2006)

Sliding versus deciding: Inertia and the premarital cohabitation effect. *Family Relations, 55,* 499–509.

Stefano, J. D., & Oala, M. (2008). Extramarital affairs: Basic considerations and essential tasks in clinical work. *The Family Journal: Counseling and Therapy for Couples and Families, 16,* 13–19.

Stein, G. L., Coard, S. I., Gonzalez, L. M., Kiang, L., & Sircar, J. K. (2021). One talk at a time: Developing an ethnic-racial socialization intervention for Black, Latinx, and Asian American families. *Journal of Social Issues, 77,* 1014–1036.

Stith, S. M., & McCollum, E. E. (2009). Couples treatment for psychological and physical aggression. In K. D. O'Leary & E. M. Woodin (Eds.), *Psychological and physical aggression in couples: Causes and interventions* (pp. 233–250). Washington, DC: American Psychological Association.

Stith, S. M., McCollum, E. E., & Rosen, K. H. (2011). *Couples therapy for domestic violence: Finding safe solutions.* Washington, DC: American Psychological Association.

Stith, S. M., Smith, D. B., Penn, C. E., Ward, D. B., & Tritt, D. (2004). Intimate partner physical abuse perpetration and victimization risk factors: A meta-analytic review. *Aggression and Violent Behavior, 10,* 65–98.

Straus, M. A. (2009). Why the overwhelming evidence on partner physical violence by women has not been perceived and is often denied. *Journal of Aggression, Maltreatment and Trauma, 18,* 552–571.

Straus, M. A., Hamby, S. L., Boney-McCoy, S., & Sugarman, D. B. (1996). The revised Conflict Tactics Scales (CTS2): Development and preliminary psychometric data. *Journal of Family Issues, 17,* 283–316.

Stuart, R. B. (1980). *Helping couples change: A social learning approach to marital therapy.* New York: Guilford Press.

Sue, D. W., Capodilupo, C. M., Torino, G. C., Bucceri, J. M., Holder, A., Nadal, K. L., & Esquilin, M. (2007). Racial microaggressions in everyday life: Implications for clinical practice. *American Psychologist, 62,* 271–285.

Sue, D. W., & Sue, D. (2003). *Counseling the culturally diverse: Theory and practice* (4th ed.). Hoboken, NJ: Wiley.

Sugg, N. (2015). Intimate partner violence: Prevalence, health consequences, and intervention. *Medical Clinics of North America, 99,* 629–649.

Taylor, S. (2014). *Anxiety sensitivity: Theory, research, and treatment of the fear of anxiety.* New York: Routledge.

Teubert, D., & Pinquart, M. (2010). The association between coparenting and child adjustment: A meta-analysis. *Parenting: Science and Practice, 10,* 286–307.

Thibaut, J. W., & Kelley, H. H. (1959). *The social psychology of groups.* New York: Wiley.

Timm, T. M., & Blow, A. J. (1999). Self-of-the-therapist work: A balance between removing restraints and identifying resources, *Contemporary Family Therapy, 21*, 331–351.

Ting-Toomey, S., & Oetzel, J. (2001). *Managing intercultural conflict effectively*. Thousand Oaks, CA: Sage.

Tobin, D. L., Holroyd, K. A., Reynolds, R. V., & Wigal, J. K. (1989) The hierarchical factor structure of Coping Strategies Inventory. *Cognitive Therapy and Research, 13*, 343–361.

Troy, A. B., Lewis-Smith, J., & Laurenceau, J.-P. (2006). Interracial and intraracial romantic relationships: The search for differences in satisfaction, conflict, and attachment style. *Journal of Social and Personal Relationships, 23*, 65–80.

Tsai, J. L., Knutson, B., & Fung, H. H. (2006). Cultural variation in affect valuation. *Journal of Personality and Social Psychology, 90*, 288–307.

Tubbs, C. Y., & Rosenblatt, P. C. (2003). Assessment and intervention with Black-White multiracial couples. *Journal of Couple and Relationship Therapy, 2*, 115–129.

United Nations Department of Economic and Social Affairs. (2015). World population prospects. Available at *https://population.un.org*.

Van Egeren, L. A., & Hawkins, D. P. (2004). Coming to terms with coparenting: Implications of definition and measurement. *Journal of Adult Development, 11*, 165–178.

Varnum, M. E. W., & Grossmann, I. (2017). Cultural change: The how and the why. *Perspectives on Psychological Science, 12*, 956–972.

Varnum, M. E. W., & Grossmann, I. (2021). The psychology of cultural change: Introduction to the special issue. *American Psychologist, 76*, 833–837.

Vaudan, C., Darwiche, J., & de Roten, Y. (2016). L'Intervention Systemique Breve [The Brief Systemic Intervention]. In N. Favez, & J. Darwiche (Eds.), *Les interventions de couple et de famille. Modèles empiriquement validés et applications thérapeutiques* [Couple and family interventions. Empirically validated models and therapeutic applications] (pp. 251–268). Brussels: Mardaga.

Vishkin, A., Bloom, P. B.-N., Schwartz, S. H., Solak, N., & Tamir, M. (2019). Religiosity and emotion regulation. *Journal of Cross-Cultural Psychology, 50*, 1050–1074.

Vishkin, A., Bloom, P. B.-N., & Tamir, M. (2019). Always look on the bright side of life: Religiosity, emotion regulation and well-being in a Jewish and Christian sample. *Journal of Happiness Studies, 20*, 427–447.

Voisin D., Berringer, K., Takahashi, L., Burr, S., & Kuhnen, J. (2016). No safe havens: Protective parenting strategies for African American youth living in violent communities. *Violence and Victims, 31*, 523–536.

Vowels, L. M., Vowels, M. J., & Mark, K. P. (2022). Is infidelity predictable? Using explainable machine learning to identify the most important predictors of infidelity. *Journal of Sex Research, 59*, 224–237.

Voydanoff, P., & Donnelly, B. W. (1988). Economic distress, family coping, and quality of family life. In P. Voydanoff & L. C. Majka (Eds.), *Families and economic distress: Coping strategies and social policy* (pp. 97–116). Beverly Hills, CA: Sage.

Waldman, K., & Rubalcava, L. (2005). Psychotherapy with intercultural couples: A contemporary psychodynamic approach. *American Journal of Psychotherapy, 59*, 227–245.

Weeks, G. R., & Gambescia, N. (2015). Couple therapy and sexual problems. In A. S. Gurman, J. Lebow, & D. K. Snyder, (Eds.), *Clinical handbook of couple therapy* (5th ed., pp. 635–656). New York: Guilford Press.

Weeks, G. R., Gambescia, N., & Hertlein, K. M. (2020). The intersystem approach to sex therapy. In K. M. Hertlein, N. Gambescia, & Weeks, G. R. (Eds.), *Systemic sex therapy* (3rd ed., pp 1–12). New York: Routledge.

Weeks, G. R., Gambescia, N., & Jenkins, R. E. (2003). *Treating infidelity: Therapeutic dilemmas and effective strategies*. New York: Norton.

Wei, M., Russell, D. W., Mallinckrodt, B., & Vogel, D. L. (2007). The Experiences in Close Relationships Scale (ECR)—short form: Reliability, validity, and factor structure. *Journal of Personality Assessment, 88*, 187–204.

Weiss, R. L. (1978). The conceptualization of marriage from a behavioral perspective. In T. J. Paolino & B. S. McCrady (Eds.). *Marriage and marital therapy: Psychoanalytic, behavioral, and systems theory perspectives* (pp. 165–239). New York: Brunner/Mazel.

Weiss, R. L. (1980). Strategic behavioral martial therapy: Toward a model for assessment and intervention. In J. P. Vincent (Ed.), *Advances in family intervention, assessment and theory* (Vol. 1, pp. 229–271). Greenwich, CT: JAI.

Weiss, R. L., Hops, H., & Patterson, G. R. (1973). A framework for conceptualizing marital conflict, a technology for altering it, some data for evaluating it. In L. A. Hamerlynck, L. C. Handy, & E. J. Mash (Eds.), *Behavior change: Methodology, concepts and practice* (pp. 309–342). Champaign, IL: Research Press.

Whisman, M. A. (2001). The association between depression and marital dissatisfaction. In S. R. Beach (Ed.), *Marital and family processes in depression: A scientific foundation for clinical practice* (pp. 3–24). Washington, DC: American Psychological Association.

Whisman, M. A., & Baucom, D. H. (2012). Intimate relationships and psychopathology. *Clinical Child and Family Psychology Review, 15*, 4–13.

Whisman, M. A., Beach, S. R. H., & Davila, J. (2023). Couple therapy for depression or anxiety. In J. L. Lebow, & D. K. Snyder (Eds.), *Clinical handbook of couple therapy* (6th ed., pp. 576–594). New York: Guilford Press.

Whisman, M. A., Dixon, A. E., & Johnson, B. (1997).

Therapists' perspectives of couple problems and treatment issues in couple therapy. *Journal of Family Psychology, 11,* 361–366.

Whisman, M. A., & Uebelacker, L. A. (2003), Comorbidity of relationship distress and mental and physical health problems. In D. K. Snyder & M. A. Whisman (Eds.) *Treating difficult couples* (pp. 3–26). New York: Guilford Press.

White, M., & Epston, D. (1990). *Narrative means to therapeutic ends.* New York: Norton.

Wincze, J., & Weisberg, R. (2015). *Sexual dysfunction* (3rd ed.). New York: Guilford Press.

Wolska, M. (2011). Marital therapy/couples therapy: Indications and contraindications. *Archives of Psychiatry and Psychotherapy, 13,* 57–64.

World Health Organization. (1993). *The ICD-10 classification of mental and behavioural disorders.* Geneva: Author.

World Health Organization. (2017). *Depression and other common mental disorders: Global health estimates.* Geneva: Author.

Yancey, G. (2007). Experiencing racism: Differences in the experiences of whites married to blacks and non-black racial minorities. *Journal of Comparative Family Studies, 38,* 197–213.

Yoo, J., & Miyamoto, Y. (2018). Cultural fit of emotions and health implications: A psychosocial resources model. *Social Personality Psychology Compass, 1,* 1–19.

Yoon, J. E., & Lawrence, E. (2013). Psychological victimization as a risk factor for the developmental course of marriage. *Journal of Family Psychology, 27,* 53–64.

Zemp, M., & Bodenmann, G. (2018). Family structure and the nature of couple relationships: Relationship distress, separation, divorce, and repartnering. In M. R. Sanders & A. Morawska (Eds.), *Handbook of parenting and child development across the lifespan* (pp. 415–440). Heidelberg, Germany: Springer.

Zilbergeld, B. (1999). *The new male sexuality* (revised ed.). New York: Bantam.

Zvolensky, M. J., Garey, L., Fergus, T. A., Gallagher, M. W., Viana, A. G., Shepherd, J. M., . . . Schmidt, N. B. (2018). Refinement of anxiety sensitivity measurement: The Short Scale Anxiety Sensitivity Index (SSASI). *Psychiatry Research, 269,* 549–557.

Index

Note. *f* following a page number indicates a figure.